Progressive Mothers, Better Babies

JOE R. AND TERESA LOZANO LONG SERIES IN
LATIN AMERICAN AND LATINO ART AND CULTURE

Progressive Mothers, Better Babies

RACE, PUBLIC HEALTH, AND THE STATE
IN BRAZIL, 1850–1945

By Okezi T. Otovo

University of Texas Press Austin

Requests for permission to reproduce material from this work should be
sent to:
    Permissions
    University of Texas Press
    P.O. Box 7819
    Austin, TX 78713-7819
    www.utexas.edu/utpress/about/bpermission.html

♾ The paper used in this book meets the minimum requirements of
ANSI/NISO Z39.48-1992 (R1997) (Permanence of Paper).

LIBRARY OF CONGRESS CATALOGING-IN-PUBLICATION DATA
Otovo, Okezi T., author.
    Progressive mothers, better babies : race, public health, and the state in
Brazil, 1850–1945 / by Okezi T. Otovo. — First edition.
        pages   cm. — (Joe R. and Teresa Lozano Long series in Latin
American and Latino art and culture)
    Includes bibliographical references and index.
    ISBN 978-1-4773-0883-7 (cloth : alk. paper)
    ISBN 978-1-4773-0905-6 (pbk. : alk. paper)
    ISBN 978-1-4773-0884-4 (library e-book)
    ISBN 978-1-4773-0885-1 (non-library e-book)
    1. Motherhood—Brazil—History—19th century. 2. Motherhood—
Brazil—History—20th century. 3. Public health—Brazil—History—
19th century. 4. Public health—Brazil—History—20th century.
5. Women, Black—Race identity—Brazil. 6. Women's health services—
Brazil. 7. Public health—Social aspects—Brazil. 8. Health care
reform—Brazil—History. I. Title. II. Series: Joe R. and Teresa
Lozano Long series in Latin American and Latino art and culture.
    HQ759.O886 2016
    306.874′3—dc23   2015033636

10.7560/308837

For my parents

Contents

Acknowledgments

ONE OF THE MOST CHALLENGING BUT REWARDING aspects of doing historical research is that the sources, the questions, and the conclusions seem to have their own volition. The endeavor then becomes a quest to harness and respond to the directions that the work itself has insisted its author take. The best one can hope for in this pursuit is to have a community of like-minded allies who offer support and expertise as you find ways to meet the work on its own terms and then push it to rich, rigorous, and unexpected places.

This book, therefore, is the product of my participation in a number of vibrant intellectual communities beginning at Georgetown University, where I was fortunate to work with Bryan McCann, John Tutino, and Meredith McKittrick and to be a member of a raucous and stimulating graduate community. I give special thanks to Bryan, whose wise counsel helped this research to develop. Most recently, I have benefited from the collegiality and encouragement of my many colleagues in the Department of History and the Program in African and African Diaspora Studies at Florida International University. I am grateful that during the gestation years of this book I have found myself in such good company.

In Brazil, as I researched and composed this work, I had more allies than I could reasonably thank. I gratefully acknowledge the staff at the Liga Álvaro Bahia contra a Mortalidade Infantil at the Hospital Martagão Gesteira, who opened their doors and documents to me and embraced my crusade to excavate this rich history right from the beginning. I thank my colleagues in the research group História da Assistência à Saúde, and particularly Renilda Barreto, Gisele Sanglard, Ana Paula Vosne Martins, and Martha de Luna Freire, who share my obsession with the history of public health and social welfare. Fellow travelers on this scholarly mission to claim, investigate, and disseminate Afro-Brazilian history Luciana da Cruz Brito, Edvan Brito, and

Sales Augusto do Santos have inspired and educated me even when they did not know they were doing so. I thank Yuko Miki, Jessica Graham, Camillia Cowling, and Manuella Meyer for years of friendly and productive conversations during various archival, congressional, and digital scholarly encounters.

I would also like to acknowledge the Ford Foundation, whose support made much of my archival research in Brazil possible. Smaller summer grants from the University of Vermont and Florida International University supported this research as well. I further note that a section of chapter 5 appeared as "The Gender of Social Welfare: Maternalism and Paternalism in Bahia's Estado Novo," in the Brazilian journal *Revista da Associação Brasileira de Pesquisadores(as) Negros(as)* 6, no. 14 (2014): 110–128. Prior to that, I explored some of the themes that appear in this book in "From *Mãe Preta* to *Mãe Desamparada*: Maternity and Public Health in Post-Abolition Bahia," *Luso-Brazilian Review* 48, no. 2 (2011): 164–191.

I extend my appreciation to many colleagues near and far who carefully read and provided insightful feedback on parts of this larger work along the way: Tamara Walker, Christen Smith, Abigail McGowan, Paul Deslandes, Elizabeth Heath, Keisha-Khan Perry, Rebecca Friedman, Bianca Premo, Alexandra Cornelius, Kirsten Wood, Caroline Faria, and Anadelia Romo. I am especially indebted to April Merleaux and Martine Jean, who were generous enough to read and respond to the entire manuscript. I thank James Green and Barbara Weinstein, who have been long-term supporters of my work and valuable guides to the universe of Brazilian history as well as the profession of academia.

Strong groups are a vital part of the long processes that bring books to life, so I take advantage of this opportunity to show my work. I thank the Junior Faculty Working Group at the University of Vermont and the African and African Diaspora Studies Works-In-Progress Series at Florida International University. At the University of Texas Press, I thank Kerry Webb, Angelica Lopez, and the entire production and marketing team. Two anonymous reviewers also provided thoughtful critiques that helped strengthen the final version of this book.

To my parents, Benson Otovo and Earnestine Otovo; my sister, Amelia Otovo; my brother, Eric Otovo; and my close friends Renee Littleton, Jean-Jacques Ahouansou, Mavis Gragg, Simone Manigo-Truell dos Santos, and Raimundo dos Santos, I give my heartfelt gratitude for supporting me in all the ways that are most meaningful.

Finally, the men, women, and children who populate this book and I have been on quite a journey together. In various modes and at different junctures, they have managed to perplex, humor, sadden, inspire, and infuriate me. In return, I hope I have done the complexities of their lives proper justice.

Abbreviations

APEB	Arquivo Público do Estado da Bahia (Public Archive of the State of Bahia)
CPDOC	Centro de Pesquisa e Documentação de História Contemporânea do Brasil (Center for Research and Documentation of Contemporary Brazilian History)
DNC	Departamento Nacional da Criança (National Children's Department)
FAMEB	Faculdade de Medicina da Bahia (Bahia School of Medicine)
IBGE	Instituto Brasileiro de Geografia e Estatística (Brazilian Institute of Geography and Statistics)
IPAI	Instituto de Protecção e Assistencia á Infancia (Childhood Protection and Assistance Institute)
LBA	Legião Brasileira de Assistência (Brazilian Assistance Legion)
Liga	Liga Bahiana contra a Mortalidade Infantil (Bahian League against Infant Mortality)
SCMB	Santa Casa de Misericórdia da Bahia
SUS	Sistema Único de Saúde (Unified Health Care System)

Note on Orthography and Currency

F OR PROPER NAMES AND INSTITUTIONAL NAMES, I
have retained the spelling used in the historical documentation: for example, Liga Bahiana contra a Mortalidade Infantil and Instituto
de Protecção e Assistencia á Infancia (IPAI), rather than their present-day
spellings. This is also the case in the notes and the bibliography. All other
Portuguese words in the text appear with their present-day spellings.

Brazil adopted the milreis currency in 1846. One thousand reis was written as one milreis (1$000). One thousand milreis equaled one *conto*, written
as 1:000$000. Within the text, I have simplified the format for ease of read-
ing. In 1942, Brazil adopted the cruzeiro. At the time of its introduction, the
cruzeiro equaled one thousand reis. The cruzeiro remained Brazil's currency
until 1967, beyond the periodization of this book.

Introduction

I T WAS NO ACCIDENT THAT WHEN THE PROVINCIAL government of Bahia sought to appoint an abolitionist society to disburse manumission funds in 1870, they selected the Sociedade Libertadora Sete de Setembro, named for Brazil's independence day, and stipulated that the society privilege enslaved girls who were "at the age of puberty."[1] Many slave societies recognized that black women's reproductive labor held particular significance for the perpetuation of the institution and its ultimate dismantling. And naming the abolition society after the Seventh Day of September, the symbolic birth of the nation, reified this complex set of associations. The provincial government established this relationship with Sete de Setembro just a year before the General Assembly of the Empire passed the Law of Free Womb on September 28, 1871. With it, the Assembly created a new category in the relationship between mother and child, the mother a slave and the child an untainted "innocent." This choice of language was also intentional—a compromise that elided the multiple fictions of the ownership of human beings and the disembodiment of the productive womb from the bonded black female body.[2] Abundantly clear in the nineteenth century was that upon the childbirth and child-rearing activities of women of color rested the very nature of Brazil's economic, political, and social structure, of the order of things. Then, as in the century that followed, mothering, women's labor, and racialized servitude were (often brutal) realities as much as they were metaphorical fictions for a changing nation. In a certain sense, Brazil itself followed the womb.[3]

By the opening decades of the twentieth century, mothers, babies, and family health occupied the minds of many Brazilians who pondered the state of their young republic. As the nation reimagined and reconstructed itself following the end of slavery (1888) and empire (1889), successful mothering and healthy child rearing emerged as essential components of those processes—at least according to dominant voices in medicine and policy making. Concern over maternal and child health and welfare united diverse interests in favor of what many considered an imperative and urgent national issue whose relevance far superseded familial well-being. This era witnessed an explosion of private organizations, state institutions, and new legislation, and their maternal and pronatal missions quickly combined with the charitable impulses of wealthy citizens. Despite differing approaches, advocates, politicians, and intellectuals agreed that healthy mothers and children were fundamental to propelling Brazil forward in a difficult age, an indispensable step in the quest for a successful and prosperous century.

This book's central argument is that all of these complex ideas, experiences, and versions of motherhood, public health, and national identity were intimately, inseparably related and pivotal to the political, cultural, and social climate of Brazil between 1850 and 1945. The new opportunities and differentiations that emerged with the institutionalization of maternal and child health and welfare hold great significance for understanding the transitions of this critical period. In the northeastern province, later state, of Bahia, maternalism was institutionalized into policies in specific ways designed to "modernize" the masses and to link Bahia to the larger reformist fervor of the era. At the center of this were poor Bahian women of color, who were finding much-needed medical assistance and social aid while constructing and negotiating a new but conservative connection to the modernizing efforts of reformists and the state. Thereby, they laid claim to inclusion in the modern state, but one predicated on many older notions of their social "place." My study explores the significance and impact of Brazilian maternalism from Bahia, a state that helped set the national tone through medical scholarship and clinical work in favor of women's and children's health and welfare while it was declining in political clout and economic relevance. Within the larger framework, I tackle maternalism from various directions: the academic production of Brazil's medical community; the clinical practice and assistance projects of private agencies; the experiences of mothers of color and their families; and the networks created between practitioners, reformist physicians and advocates, and their state and federal governments.

Though maternalism was a worldwide movement, which proposed that women possess a unique, naturalized orientation toward the care of children, this book situates the study in Brazil and from Bahia.[4] With "maternalism," I refer to intersecting medical and cultural discourses, health policies and institutions, and the construction of a welfare state—all with mothers and women's child-rearing activities at their core. Brazilian maternalism reflected and advanced various liberal projects, including the secularization and medicalization of family dynamics. On the household level, reformists hoped health and hygiene would replace piety as the gauge of family morality and would distinguish privileged and progressive families from those that were less so. On the professional front, an emerging sector of physicians, deeply engaged in the local community and committed to social reform, sought and often gained national prominence by interweaving medical concerns with issues of societal change and governance. These arguments found many adherents beyond medical circles; physicians helped establish a widely shared consensus that Brazilian development absolutely depended on social reform guided by scientific interventions.

Brazilian maternalism emerged during a period when many feared the foundations of society were in flux. As it did for many of their counterparts around the world, the anxiety of Brazilian intellectuals, politicians, and economic elites over the "social question," a euphemism for the capacity or politicization of the working class, coalesced into vehement calls for reform. The Brazilian social question seemed even more dire, given the abolition of slavery in 1888, culminating a long process that began in 1850 with the end of the slave trade, and the proclamation of the republic shortly thereafter. Brazil's slave society endured longer than anywhere else in the Americas, and the nation's turn to republicanism came nearly a century later than it did for its South American neighbors. The context of the deconstruction of slavery differentiates Brazil from similar contemporary movements in other places and helps explain the wresting of family welfare from the private to the public sphere. Assuming that science and medicine could tame perceived chaos, induce progress, and even promote racial "improvement," physicians at the medical schools of Bahia and Rio de Janeiro carried the reform mission forward and, as a professional class, had unprecedented influence on the First Republican state. Several reformist theories and projects crafted in those academic environments placed family dynamics, and particularly the scientific rearing of healthy children, as the linchpin in escaping nineteenth-century "backwardness" and achieving twentieth-century "modernity."

At the inauguration of the Liga Bahiana contra a Mortalidade Infantil (Bahian League against Infant Mortality) in 1923, headquartered in the capital city of Salvador, for example, the founder Dr. Joaquim Martagão Gesteira referred to the new organization as a "humanitarian and patriotic crusade."[5] Infant mortality was a serious and tragic issue in Brazil, with as many as three hundred children per thousand dying before their second birthdays in major cities like Salvador and Rio de Janeiro. This had been the case for decades but had garnered little organized attention. The creation of a League against Infant Mortality resulted from debates and advocacy work at the Bahia School of Medicine that began back in the mid-nineteenth century.

On that inaugural day, Dr. Gesteira urged the fortunate mothers in his audience (potential benefactors) not to forget the "others," those "less happy but no less diligent mothers in the city's humble homes who suffer the heartbreak" of childhood illness and mortality.[6] Several years later, *senhorinha* Leticia Trigueiros heeded the doctor's call by pursuing specialized training in scientific child rearing and community advocacy through a pioneering program offered by the League. In her words, "Today, more than ever, we see evidence of the problems concerning Maternity and Childhood and the evolution of human society," which Trigueiros attributed to "incessant social transformation."[7]

By the 1930s, "incessant transformation," maternity, and child rearing were pressing issues for the government as well, even at the highest levels. On Christmas Eve of 1932, President Getúlio Vargas pronounced in evocative eugenic language that "no other patriotic cause [was] as intimately linked to the perfection of the race and the progress of the nation as the protection and health of children."[8] The president, the symbolic father of the nation, hoped state protection of women and children would help transform husbands and fathers into cooperative and productive workers. For Vargas, mothers and children were a means to a developmentalist end. Appointed Governor Juracy Magalhães, the president's representative in Bahia, listed maternal and child welfare among the key accomplishments of his own term in office, "envisioning the future of the race" by providing for those women making "the sublime sacrifice of maternity."[9] The Magalhães administration funded several well-baby clinics in Salvador, a Maternal Shelter for women who lacked "paternal assistance," a specialized residence for foundling children, and a Maternity Hospital.

Ten years later, in June of 1942, a twenty-four-year-old cook, Domingas de Jesus, gave birth to her twin sons, Antonio and Carlos, in that Maternity Hospital, opting for biomedical birthing rather than the expertise of a traditional midwife. Partnerless and lacking resources to care for her four children, Domingas de Jesus received monthly stipends from the Bahian League against Infant Mortality and the state government on the condition that she breast-feed her newborns. For the League and the state, providing maternal stipends of this kind helped prevent infant mortality and child abandonment. Similarly, when her partner was interned in a local hospital, a thirty-nine-year-old domestic servant named Maria Felina de Oliveira faced serious need and enrolled with her two-month-old son Duval in the same assistance program. Antonio, Carlos, and Duval were all registered in the well-baby clinic at Salvador's Fifth Health Post, also a requirement for those receiving benefits.[10] At times, mothers in need found social assistance through the advocacy and intervention of partner organizations like the Legião Brasileira de Assistência (LBA; Brazilian Assistance Legion), a national network of prominent, philanthropic women who pledged their efforts on behalf of "social works that support the health, education, and well-being of children."[11] Thus, the family lives and domestic work of Domingas de Jesus and Maria Felina de Oliveira; the clinical practice and advocacy of physicians, staffers, midwives, and women's organizations; the sponsorship and influence of philanthropists; and local and national politics and social policies all wound together. And from the reformists' perspective, the advances made in mothers' and children's health gave Bahia a claim to coauthorship of Brazilian modernity. This book both teases these multiple elements of maternalism apart and analyzes their interconnectedness in aggregate.

Mothering and child rearing in sickness and in health were integral everyday activities for families as well as part of community knowledge and culture, individual and shared expertise, and gendered and racialized labor practices. Families of the popular classes had their own maternalist politics, which were among multiple interpretations of mothering and child rearing that were in conversation over the decades examined in this book even if not always in agreement. Domingas de Jesus and Maria Felina de Oliveira certainly understood motherhood differently than did Leticia Trigueiros, whose family would have employed women like Jesus and Oliveira to perform child-rearing labor in her household. While families always responded to internal dynamics and those closest to home, Brazilians of all backgrounds also navigated shifting political and economic ground between 1850 and 1945. Most important, and clearly connected to family and the labor of birthing, rearing, and caring for children, were the abolition of slavery, the fall of Brazil's empire, and the accompanying creation of a liberal republic. And abolition was a multistep process that began in 1850 when Brazil definitively ended the slave trade and forced the reproduction of the institution exclusively upon black women's bodies.

While conservative, these transitions were deeply consequential to family life and to servitude relations within households, especially in Bahia—one of the most important slave societies in the Atlantic network where bondage had long been the reference point for a complexity of relationships of labor and hierarchy. Brazilians experienced the transformations between 1850 and 1945 with greater and lesser intensity, depending on myriad factors. However, it is clear that republicanism and abolition marked continuities as well as change and did not signal a radical break between the early nineteenth century and that century's close.

These transitions, therefore, give rise to a number of questions that are the primary purpose of this book. Why did maternalism emerge in the late nineteenth century, and how, specifically, were the resultant ideas, policies, and institutions reflective or constitutive of their larger social and political context, a context marked by the enduring importance of race through changing state structures and regimes? Why was there a particular emphasis on poor families and poor women's child-rearing activities with their own children and those in their care? Moreover, what were the consequences of these developments for those women and families and their "place," particularly as Brazilians of color, within the transforming nation and nationality? Finally, in what ways did maternalism and its institutionalization simultaneously evidence reformism and conservatism in the construction of the medicalized welfare state? The answers to these questions establish that maternalism as ideology and history was jointly constructed by rhetoric and institution, by medicine and culture, by practitioners (biomedical and traditional) and clients, and by public and private resources. Despite political change, the fallout from centuries of racialized and gendered inequality, institutionalized through slavery until 1888, remained visible in Bahian maternalism well into the twentieth century.

BAHIA: MOTHERS REAL AND IMAGINED

The state of Bahia figures prominently in this book—home to Brazil's first colonial capital and jewel of the Portuguese Empire due to the wealth of sugar produced on the backs of hundreds of thousands of enslaved Africans and Afro-Brazilians. Bahia experienced a rather sharp fall from eminence when the sugar industry faltered in the eighteenth century, and its relegation was sealed by the late nineteenth century when the coffee-producing and then industrial South rose to dominate national politics and the economy. Modern Bahia, however, is almost completely absent from Brazilian historiography—written by scholars based in US or Brazilian universities. The unfortunate imbalance between colonial and imperial histories and scholarship investigating post-1889 reinforces the erroneous assumption that Bahia (and the Northeast generally) has little to offer to the study of "modern" Brazil in all its complexity and contradiction. Yet Bahia proves a distinctive and fertile site to analyze modern public health policy, maternalism, and race. On the one hand, this choice is for practical reasons, a reflection of the preeminence of the Bahia School of Medicine's leadership in theorizing and institutionalizing maternalism even on the national level. On the other hand, the chapters that follow play with cultural symbolism as well as the lived and institutional realities of maternal and children's health and welfare. For maternalism's cultural politics, situating this study in Bahia is exceptionally rich due to the long-standing association between motherhood and the conception of Bahia as a place.

Contemporary scholars and observers repeated certain stock scripts from the nineteenth century about Bahia's place within the national imaginary, scripts loaded with racialized maternal metaphors. Bahia, nicknamed the "Mulata Velha," was the site of tradition—the genesis, birthplace, or font of something essential that nurtured the whole of Brazil.[12] Far more than a generic conservatism, Bahia supposedly embodied a generative and nourishing quality that conjured both race and gender. "A Mulata Velha," or "the Old Black Mammy," was a generous, loyal, and submissive woman of color. Her body either birthed or sustained culture, transmitting continuity with generations past for her own children and for those whom she suckled. She was either a literal mother or a figurative one and, by extension, one critical element in the social reproduction of Brazil, for better or worse.

The renowned sociologist Gilberto Freyre played with these ideas in a 1926 poem, reflecting on the sights, sins, and smells of Bahia—a place that smelled "of food, of incense, of *mulatas.*"[13] Freyre painted an evocative picture of the streets of Salvador, "Old black women from Brazil / selling *mingau, angu, acarajé* / Old black women with bright red shawls / sagging breasts / mothers of the most beautiful *mulatas* of Brazil / *mulatas* with plump breasts, nipples erect / as if ready to breastfeed all of Brazil."[14] Reflecting the racially democratic spirit of the times, the 1942 version of this same poem declared that the breasts of Bahia's *mulatas* were "erect as if ready to breastfeed a multitude of whites."[15] For Freyre, Bahia and its emblematic women of color were a comforting reminder of simpler, less ambiguous times. Clearly the author cast these *baianas* in a servile role, as Patricia Pinho has argued, "conditioning their existence [and their bodies] to the pleasure of others."[16] Beyond the promise of culinary and erotic delights, Freyre imbued his archetypal Bahian *negras* and *mulatas* with maternal affection even as he conflated that filial attachment with sexual desire.

While Freyre reveled in the symbolic merger of brown female bodies and Bahia as a place, critics who evoked the "Old Black Mammy" not so subtly intimated that the state was antiquated and peripheral. From this perspective, casting Bahia as a "Mulata Velha" was derogatory—not necessarily a negation of the black maternal and sexual role Freyre cherished, but this reference to race, femininity, and domestic relations was decidedly negative. This contrast illustrates the ways Bahia has been "alternately romanticized and denigrated, [and] has served both as a cradle of Brazilian national identity and as an embarrassing symbol of Brazil's backwardness."[17] To a turn-of-the-century progress-obsessed elite, Old Black Mammies were on the wrong side of history.

To observers, women of color culturally typified Bahia in its urbanity, not just on the plantations of the Recôncavo. For his part, Freyre praised Salvador's fecundity in a celebratory elegy, calling the capital Brazil's "mother-city" and "the wet nurse of all of her cities."[18] In her investigation of the Candomblé religion and its faithful, the American anthropologist Ruth Landes famously christened Salvador the "City of Women," owing to the authority of the mother-priestesses (*mães de santo*) that she witnessed in the *terreiros* (houses of worship) during a 1938 research trip.[19] Landes's assessment of female urban space in the "city of women" contributes two crucial points about Bahia's maternal metaphors. First, like many who preceded her, when Landes characterized the city of Bahia as a woman, she did not mean just any woman. To the author, Afro-Brazilian womanhood was essential to the local culture, and in the private spaces of worship, she observed rituals of kinship and hierarchy based on spiritual metaphors of motherhood, family, and African ethnicity. Her "city of women" was not a wet nurse, not a servant, but a place that evidenced gendered sources of power. Second, Landes's interpretation drew a relationship between the private gendered dynamics inside the *terreiros* and *soteropolitano* (Salvadoran) society at large. Thus, the symbolism was neither exclusive to Candomblé nor a meaningless abstraction; it was explicitly grounded in her observations and in the lived experiences of Bahian women and men.

Whatever bias one may read into Freyre's and Landes's interpretations, these scholars witnessed and extrapolated from a very real aspect of life in Salvador da Bahia. Anyone passing through the center of town in the 1920s or 1930s would have noticed the buzz of working women going about their business in the streets, often with their children trailing behind. Like Rio de Janeiro, this city was home to thousands of women whose labors took them into public spaces with regularity.[20] Many of the women of color out and about on Salvador's bustling streets would have been domestic servants, in addition to the food vendors. They were nannies, wet nurses, cooks, and laundresses. Their labor reflected the racialized and gendered dynamic of household servitude, a deeply embedded social and economic attribute inherited from centuries of slavery. The point is that household servants, women of color, and mothers were highly visible and integral to public life. Moreover, for thousands of women, the experiences of motherhood, servitude, and race relations were intimately intertwined.

It was also the case that private family dynamics helped construct, reproduce, and reinforce various characteristics of Brazilian society in general, both locally and beyond Bahia. Olívia Gomes da Cunha has aptly termed this relationship the "intimate articulation" between the end of slavery and the dynamics of turn-of-the century household hierarchies.[21] Da Cunha argues that "rather than standing in simple and supposedly natural contrast to the public domain, domestic space contain[ed] social relations prevailing in other spheres of social life—signally, those symbolic hierarchies that mark distinctions of gender, class, and ethnicity."[22] The significance of the home and its link to broader social relations was not lost on turn-of-the-century Bahian health reformers either. The Brazilian home and its inhabitants emerged as a key target for medical interventions that sought not just to improve the sanitation of the home as a space but also to effect the proper ordering through science of relations between household members, including parents (especially mothers) and their children, female domestics and their patrons, female domestics and their charges, and family units and their health-care practitioners. For Bahian reformers, what happened inside the home undoubtedly manifested and generated larger social patterns—or problems—and those household experiences were the starting point for transforming both.

For many families, axioms of servitude, patronage, and dependence also mitigated domestic space. This kind of ranking between families and within them was a central part of the inequalities that anchored social relations and must be taken seriously in any investigation of Brazilian social history. Another natural contrast between house and street exemplified the gender, class, and racial distinctions characterizing the larger society beyond the walls of the private sphere: household domestics also maintained intimate relationships *beyond* the realm of the homes in which they labored. Often the closest ties these women had were with persons who literally lived several streets away. Domestic servants and their children feature prominently in this book because the great majority of women accessing Bahian public health resources worked in household service. In cultural or folkloric accounts, female domestics appeared foremost as appendages to the patriarchal home, even if cherished and integral members of it. Just as the position of domestics in their patrons' homes established and refracted social relations at large, the spatial separation of domestics from their own partners, spouses, relatives, children, and friends was a consequence of historical and contemporary inequalities.[23] Gender, class, and race relations marked those who served in the home and those who were served.

On the intellectual side, physicians at Bahia's School of Medicine were deeply engaged in academic dialogues about family medicine in which maternity, race, and gender also played a dominant role. Whether or not local physicians concurred that Bahia was on the wrong side of history, they staunchly believed that their home state was not destined to remain there. Bahia may not have had an influx of European immigrants or rapid industrialization as signifiers of progress, as did São Paulo and Rio de Janeiro, but the state could invest in its "human capital" through maternal and child health and welfare programs. Ideologically, medical theories about motherhood and cultural ideas overlapped and informed one another. By definition and due to the Brazilian context, Bahian maternalist medicine had a great deal to say about black mammies, breast-feeding, folk midwives, and the practice of motherhood; medical discourse and practice, therefore, could not escape being loaded with symbolic and cultural meanings.

Shifting notions of race and its relation to society provided the greatest impetus for the development of Brazilian maternalism and root a worldwide phenomenon in uniquely Brazilian terms. Science and medicine seemed to hold the most potential for addressing the "social question" because many physicians and other intellectuals believed that, in Brazil, the problem was a historical and hereditary one. The inconvenient history of Brazil's long devotion to race-based slavery had supposedly created conditions that needed to be overcome in the quest to "modernize"; these racialized social conditions could be either biological or cultural depending on the proponent.[24] Of relevance here is not simply the existence of racist doctrine, though there was plenty of that, but also the fact that critics in Bahia and elsewhere decried what they understood to be societal distortions engendered by centuries of reliance on slavery for domestic labor and all manner of services, trades, and commercial and agricultural production. One of those distortions, according to these arguments, was a long-standing inattention to the education and health of the popular classes, whose labor Brazil desperately needed for a productive twentieth century. Patriarchalism and the dependence on household servitude meant that families made their own decisions about health and welfare without seeking the expertise of medical professionals. Similarly, families relied on women's knowledge passed among relatives as well as between and among midwives, wet nurses, and nursemaids, leading to "superstitious" birthing and child-rearing habits that endangered the lives of children. These women—"inept wet nurses," "sinister midwives," and "apathetic mothers"—symbolically embodied Brazil's inadequacies at the turn of the century.

Beyond domestics and their children, Brazilian health reformists paid special attention to working-class families in general. Over the course of the period I examine in this book, health and welfare became the primary means through which poor families as a unit maintained a connection to the state, bringing both opportunities and problematic assumptions. Reformists and bureaucrats conceptualized the need to improve the health of poor families in distinct ways from the assumptions they held about privileged families' health. When considering poor families, they prepared for a battle against ignorance and resistance to change—all for the greater good of rearing healthy future laborers for Brazilian development. In Bahia, reformists envisioned the poor family unit as one with mother and child at its center, different from the patriarchal model typical of privileged families. Regardless of social class, reformists certainly saw mothers as potential agents of social change and their child-rearing activities as the cornerstone for transforming Brazil into a modern twentieth-century nation.

While I highlight local specificities and context in this book, I staunchly reject the notion that Bahia is somehow inherently so distinct from other areas of Brazil as to render any conclusions based on its history peculiar or provincial. To make that argument would mean to fall into the same historical trap of essentialism that already plagues cultural understandings of Bahia and the Northeast generally. Bahian society did reflect certain local dynamics—as would any state in Brazil—that are significant to understanding maternalism in history, particularly since there is an important emphasis here on local bureaucracy, public health infrastructure, and welfare policies. The existence and importance of the School of Medicine also distinguished Bahia, and Rio de Janeiro, from the rest of Brazil. Lilia Moritz Schwarcz has analyzed the competing but complementary schools of thought emanating from Bahia and Rio de Janeiro, elucidating the vital role that both faculties played in articulating the medical interest in bodies as a means of perfecting the nation.[25] Pushing that argument even further, Stanley Blake has argued that many of Brazil's *national* racial discourses were born in the northeastern academy and disseminated to points south from there.[26] Bahian medicine was absolutely fundamental to that process, and I explore the intersections of racial discourses with both the theory and practice of maternal and child health and welfare throughout this book. Thus, Bahia is the protagonist of this story, coloring it in meaningful ways, but it is likewise part of the larger history of Brazilian schemes to "modernize" through health reform and to create a twentieth-century welfare state.

THE POLITICS OF BRAZILIAN HEALTH REFORM

A final analytical note relates to the fact that maternalism was one expression of a greater trend within Brazilian public health reform. Scholars of the First Republic (1889–1930) have confirmed that new public health initiatives helped significantly advance the expansion of the federal state, pushing the reach of government into loosely integrated interior areas and neglected urban ones.[27] The parallel history of Brazil's institutionalization of women's and children's health and welfare is an underexplored story even though the maternalism movement is foundational to any full understanding of public health in the growing state.

Brazil's great sanitation and disease-eradication efforts of the era and the maternalist movement all hinged on the same set of assumptions. According to sanitation experts, Brazil could overcome perceived racial limitations and a lack of cohesion or integration through health reform, thereby bolstering human capacity (for labor) and the nation's economic development and international prominence in turn. Therefore, a shared conception of the functionality of health reform and its implications beyond the individual, family, or even community level characterized a diversity of medical projects across Brazil in the early twentieth century. Moreover, though persistent, ideas about race were not static. If anything, twentieth-century science modernized racial discourse and adapted it to fit the aspirations of a nation recently emerging from slavery and monarchy. Thus, these health movements were historical in the proper sense; reform projects like the sanitation and maternalist movements responded not simply to the fact of health deficiencies but to changing perceptions of their repercussions.

On the maternal and child health side, the state and federal governments initially took a backseat to the reformist zeal of urban doctors and benevolent organizations. This was true in Bahia and in Rio de Janeiro, which also had a flourishing maternalist movement. Though maternal health and welfare did not attract the type of federal interest during the First Republic as it would in the subsequent Vargas years (1930–1945), both maternalist and sanitation advocates evoked the same language of national regeneration. The difference was that private organizations, founded and directed by groups of physicians, led the effort to add neighborhood family clinics to Brazil's rather inadequate health infrastructure. The medical community in Brazil's major cities, so adamantly convinced of the necessity and potential of social reform and so disappointed with the perceived failures of republican government, pulled together private resources and founded health and welfare clinics serving local poor communities free of charge. In Bahia, two such organizations offered a litany of services to families in need: the Childhood Protection and Assistance Institute, or Instituto de Protecção e Assistencia á Infancia (IPAI, founded in 1903), and the Bahian League against Infant Mortality (Liga, founded in 1923). Along with the Santa Casa de Misericórdia, an old colonial confraternity, they were the most important nongovernmental health organizations in Bahia, and their histories are treated in detail in chapters 2–4 of this book. These types of organizations and their leaders maintained complicated fiscal and administrative relationships with state and federal bureaucracies. Private agencies, in turn, enjoyed the sponsorship of prosperous and charitable families whose donations augmented or even exceeded the agencies' public grants. New health services, therefore, also provided an opportunity for wealthy Brazilians to exercise an updated version of patronage and philanthropy, solidifying the link between private benefactors and public social welfare.[28]

Physicians and their champions launched unprecedented campaigns to medicalize both state and society, whether through maternalism and pronatalism or disease eradication and sanitation. Meanwhile, millions of Brazilian families went about their everyday lives, impacted in certain ways by some of the changes in medical ideas and public health and welfare projects and unaware of or uninterested in others. I highlight the significance and consequence of the medicalization of women's and children's health and welfare, that is, where and in what ways it mattered for families as well as its limitations. Brazil's health landscape was varied and highly localized in the nineteenth century, as was the case in many other areas of the world. As that century progressed, biomedical practitioners increased their competition with midwives, healers, and other empiricists by undermining their rivals to the public at large and asserting a stark differentiation between scientific and "traditional" methods.[29] Many of these local practitioners were lower-class women—and many were women of color. Brazilian medicine simultaneously experienced a professionalization process as physicians jockeyed for public space and influence against other rising liberal professionals.[30] Conquering the ideological legitimacy and infrastructure necessary to occupy a significant societal and political role was a gradual, contested, and partial process. But over the decades analyzed in this book, more and more families gave credence to biomedical approaches to treating the body and sought the expertise of biomedical specialists over more established practitioners.

Tracing maternalism demonstrates that Bahian society was still wrestling with the cultural baggage of differentiated experiences of motherhood, femininity, and family left over from Brazil's slavocracy well into the 1940s. Because medical theories and practices intertwined with assumptions about race, gender, and class, the encounter between families and physicians was in some ways conditioned by cultural expectations on both sides. Yet the sheer access that urban Brazilians had to family medical care by the 1930s represented a watershed change from the prior century and a rather rapid one. Families may have sought out health and welfare programs for reasons other than reforming a problematic working-class majority—their architects' intention—yet maintaining maternal and child health was an arena where family and medical interests largely converged.

Between the years of 1930 and 1945, when this investigation concludes, this convergence of family, medical, and state interests was firmly consolidated. During this period, the nationalizing projects of President Getúlio Vargas and his Estado Novo administration (1937–1945), in particular, rhetorically and corporately integrated the multiethnic working classes into a greater patriotic and developmentalist logic. Part labor pacification and part mobilization, laborers and working-class families were a fundamental cog in the national machine for President Vargas, part of a seamless whole of a race-less Brazilian identity. For Vargas, the "Father of the Poor," greater access to social services and a larger investment in health and education were critical steps to increasing the productive capacity and well-being of the working class—a type of "eugenic nationalism."[31] The Estado Novo take on working-class families had an interesting gendered dimension as well because new policies aimed to secure greater economic security for male heads of household, working-class patriarchy, while restricting women to the home, barring the (very common) circumstance of financial necessity.

Domestic servants did not have a clear place within the Estado Novo policies on "women's and children's protection," either as mothers or as workers. But within the specific realm of the Bahian maternal and child health movement, they most certainly did. In Bahia, female household servants were the majority of mothers *and* the majority of female workers. Due to the political climate inspired by Vargas-era programs and legislation, Bahian maternalist advocates articulated their local efforts as vital contributions to a larger national project. In fact, maternalism became Bahia's best link to Estado Novo nation-building-through-popular-incorporation, since the state lacked a significant industrial working class. On the practical side, poor families of the 1930s and 1940s found more preventative and treatment options for mothers and children than ever before. These families did not always access services for the reason or in the manner that organizers intended, and certainly the availability of services was never sufficient in the Bahian case to meet the degree of need, but over the long term, many families and reformists came to expect social assistance to be a function of the state, in conjunction with private agencies.

SOURCES, APPROACHES, AND TERMINOLOGIES

Naturally, racial analysis in Brazilian health care is more complicated than simply determining the appropriate translations and definitions based on institutional context. Rooting out any understanding of race as it influenced ideologies and experiences of public health can be difficult and risky. It is difficult because the turn of the twentieth century witnessed quite a bit of change in Brazilian thinking on race, and therein lies the risk as well, because applying anachronous conceptions of race or failing to accurately depict context would certainly not aid in understanding this book's themes. Even within that period of transformation, I argue, as have many others, that race continued to hold deep significance. Rather than a bifurcated dichotomy of black and white, in this book I use terminology that suggests colors of skin tone, as this better approximates the language within the source documents. For example, I translate *"preto"* as "black" and *"pardo," "moreno,"* and *"mulato"* as "brown." The chapters that follow also utilize the phrase "of color" to refer to Brazilians of African descent.

For sources and documents, this book draws upon a diversity of print and archival materials. Medical journals, such as the *Gazeta Médica da Bahia* and *Pediatria e Puericultura*, were the most important theoretical organs of the Bahian medical community. Dissertations written by graduating students at the School of Medicine also unveil the development of maternalist medicine. Maternalist ideals and accomplishments consistently appeared on the pages of local newspapers as well. On the institutional side, this research follows several decades of the experiences of clients and practitioners at the Bahian League against Infant Mortality (Liga) and the Santa Casa de Misericórdia, already mentioned, as well as a few less prominent associations. In terms of public services, I draw upon the records of the various incarnations of clinical and administrative agencies sponsored by the state of Bahia between 1903 and 1945, including the Directorate for Infant and School-Age Hygiene, the Prenatal and Children's Hygiene Inspectorate, and the state Children's Department, as well as the federal Ministry of Education and Health on the national level.

Even in clinical records, racial designations fell out of fashion in the mid-twentieth century due to the widely shared conception of Brazilians as one united nationality that refused to fracture its presumed unity into categories based on skin tone. Generations of Brazilianist scholars have confirmed the enduring significance of race during that time period, and for the specific case of social policy, Jerry Dávila has cautioned against reading "hidden transcripts" of race as race-neutral.[32] For maternalism, a number of factors assist in making the dynamic of race quite visible. First, race was very often a major subject of consideration in medical journals due to both the cultural politics of Brazil described at the outset of this chapter and the lineage of medical discourses that Brazilian experts engaged, which were highly racialized by the mid-nineteenth century and continued to be so through the hegemony of eugenic thinking in the early twentieth. Second, demographic realities help simplify the racial issue because the overwhelming majority of women and children enrolled in Bahian maternal and child services were Brazilians of color. Given the racial demographics of the state in general and of the poor in particular, there is no reason to assume this customary pattern did not hold for sources related to patient populations for which racial data are missing. Finally, because of the demographic realities, physicians and health care practitioners were well aware of the racial composition of their patient population. Thus, even where explicit references to race were absent, I argue that when maternal and child advocates made reference to unfortunate, poor, single, "ignorant" mothers and their children, the image they conjured was that of a woman of color.

Unquestionably, physicians were not the only Brazilians whose concepts of mothering and family mattered. Average families' conceptions seem obscure to the historian. But where mothers do not speak in the sources, their actions elucidate an engagement with medical maternalism on their own terms and within the constraints and contingencies of the nascent welfare system. Furthermore, the point here is not that medical ideas were more meaningful than other philosophies about mothers, children, or health care. But given their relative discursive and political influence, it is important to recognize the power that the medical community wielded over the development of public health programs and institutions. This power was contested and progressed irregularly over time, but it was vital nonetheless for health projects and families' experiences with them. Thus, it is absolutely necessary to outline where the pertinent medical ideas came from; why these sets of ideas prevailed over other possibilities; and what the relationship was between medical knowledge, cultural knowledge, and the health programs that ultimately emerged.

Finally, I argue that symbol, rhetoric, and metaphor became entangled in medical discourse, and the medical view of maternalism created new meanings in turn. Methodologically, then, this book engages the reciprocal relation of theory to praxis. Ultimately, this approach illuminates the origins and consequences of Brazil's maternal and child health and welfare movement, opening new opportunities for poor women of color and their children within "acceptable" limits. Progressive motherhood posited the integration of women and, through women and children, poor families in general. Despite the incomplete notion of citizenship or incorporation implied within that movement, the birth of the public health system and its emphasis on family welfare redefined the relationship between the popular classes and their state—at least rhetorically. For thousands of Bahians, especially those under two years of age, the benefits of that new relationship were far more than rhetorical—they literally made the difference between life and death.

STRUCTURE OF THE BOOK

To examine the changing expectations and experiences of family health in relation to shifting medical, social, and political ideas and circumstances, the book begins in the mid-nineteenth century. It follows this history through the First Republic (1889–1930), during which Bahian maternal and child health and welfare became a major thrust of action for private medical and philanthropic organizations. The book concludes at the end of President Getúlio Vargas's Estado Novo administration in 1945, by which time public health and welfare had become significantly institutionalized and codified into the Brazilian state. This periodization expands the public/household articulation beyond the negotiations between masters and domestics postslavery to understand how the presence and activities of female domestic servants, especially those who worked with children, attracted the medical gaze. In addition to patron-servant relations, this book also prioritizes the experiences of domestics and their own families with the ever-expanding medicalized state.

The story begins with an exploration of Bahia, the "Mulata Velha"; Bahia itself is the main character of this first chapter, which focuses on health conditions, family dynamics, and ideological change. In it, I argue that maternalism emerged out of anxieties related to the end of slavery and empire in Brazil and blended both medical and cultural understandings of race, gender, and family. From chapter 1, the study tackles the experiences of mother-clients; popular practitioners, physicians, and advocates; and the institutional and bureaucratic infrastructure that organized and administered public health and welfare services. Each subsequent chapter is framed around a different "character" or actor in this history: the *Mãe Preta*, the *Curiosa*, the *Mãe Desnaturada*, and the *Pai dos Pobres*. The framing highlights the fact that all of these "characters" have both a cultural mythology and a real history that bring into relief the development and consequences of public health projects focused on mothers and children. The relationship between these idealized figures and actual families, reformists, and officials, along with the ways in which maternalism symbolized larger social and political dynamics, are discussed in detail at the end of chapter 1. In chapter 2, I argue that Bahian maternalist organizations emerged with an explicit focus on crafting better Brazilians for the new century while conceiving of black motherhood in ways that more resembled the old one.

The next three chapters overlap chronologically in their focus on the 1930s–1940s, years in which the maternalist movement turned its attention to aiding "motherless" children and developing welfare programs that would keep poor women and their children together (chapter 3), to discrediting and then ultimately negotiating with folk midwives and educating women in scientific child rearing (chapter 4), and to using the gains in Bahian mothers' and children's health and well-being for political leverage within the patriarchal working-class politics of the Vargas era (chapter 5). Across the chapters, I argue that maternal advocates certainly did not introduce changes in birthing, healing, and child rearing alone or uncontested. Brazilian families also made different choices from those that were the most typical approaches to health, to caregiving, and to need in an earlier period. The progression from the first chapter to the last exposes an increasingly interventionist medicalized project, consistently expanding its radius of action in new ways, and thereby linking families to the state government and to private agencies; the state to private organizations, their benefactors, and local practitioners; and finally, Bahian organizations to national ones. The intertwined cultural narratives and exchanges of maternalist health and welfare policy open up the interrelationship and inseparability between Bahian and Brazilian history.

CHAPTER ONE

Persistence and Change

THE *MULATA VELHA*

I N   T H E   N I N E T E E N T H   C E N T U R Y ,   W H E N   B R A Z I L I A N women needed expert advice on pregnancy, birthing, and children's health, they turned to their local midwife. When family members fell ill, they prepared home remedies and called upon healers and spiritual guides. When wealthy families needed child care, they entrusted the supervision and nourishment of their children to black and brown domestics. In extreme circumstances, families gave custody of their infants and small children to Catholic charity. By the mid-twentieth century, these traditions had significantly eroded—particularly in urban areas—as more and more families looked to biomedical advice to maintain their health and to "scientific" recommendations for household organization. The older traditions did not disappear, but something fundamental in the world of health and welfare shifted. These shifts were ideological and material, and they began in earnest in the second half of the nineteenth century, the decades under consideration in this chapter.

Brazil faced two significant "crises" during that period that played out in particular ways in Bahia: the long road to the abolition of slavery and the demise of the imperial government. Deconstructing slavery and empire required political and social changes that were closely tied to understandings of race and nationality, but many Brazilians also saw an opening to usher in societal transformations. The medical community in particular, in Bahia and elsewhere, argued that societal change began with the family—the fundamental unit in a patriarchal culture. Family dynamics and everyday familial decisions took on new significance. Furthermore, family, motherhood, and children were increasingly central topics in French medicine, adding more relevance and respectability to local discourses because international literature offered a conceptual framework for using medicine to harness and guide societal change. Thus, family health became highly politicized in the province of Bahia, in response to the medical gaze on social transformation and due to a deliberate effort to turn medical pretensions into reality.

Beyond medicine, ideas about race, family, and gender carried a great deal of cultural and historical significance, as is to be expected. Biomedical thought absorbed contemporaneous interpretations of Brazilian history and culture, especially as physicians and other intellectuals turned their attention toward change and intervention. Cultural symbols mattered vitally as medical theory attempted to create knowledge about mothers and the distinctions (by race, class, and family status) between them. Subsequently, medical influence branched outward as ideas that were invented in nineteenth-century medicine became essential to the foundation of "modern" public health programs and institutions in the early twentieth. Between 1850 and 1900, medical theories of motherhood took shape in the midst of Brazil's gradual abolition of slavery and rocky republicanism. As in the nation at large, these were dynamic decades in Bahia. Women's bodies and their child-rearing activities took center stage in the attempt to exploit the possibilities of the age and harness its inherent risks.

Customarily, Brazilian families tended to their own health matters with the help of largely independent healers, many of whom were women, but this was one of the social dynamics that modernizing reformists targeted for eradication. Biomedicine's spokesmen began a process of legitimizing the professional practice of scientific medical treatment; invalidating competing forms of thinking about the body, wellness, illness, and healing; and discrediting rival practitioners. In Bahia, medical reformists conceived of that ideological campaign as a battle against the long-standing domestic practices of families; the dire state of urban sanitation; the woefully inadequate public health facilities; and the effects of all of these shortfalls on the productivity, salubrity, and life span of the population at large. Reformists personified these problems into stock gendered characters: the incompetent black wet nurse; the superstitious and dangerous midwife; and the unnatural, failed mother. Such traditional women were products of Brazil's Mulata Velha and her retrograde tendencies. In truth, families' domestic practices *were* gendered and racialized, as were health and healing practices, due to Brazil's long history as a multiethnic yet unequal society. Thus, medical conceptions of family health and approaches designed to improve it were gendered and racialized as well. To combat presumed backwardness, Brazil needed to levy modern masculine knowledge (read as scientific, rational, and action oriented), enacted by men or women. Implementing health and welfare policy was only possible with the support of the final trope—the strong, active patriarch/patron. Finally, situating maternalism in Bahia must begin from a careful consideration of local health conditions and family patterns as well as the social, political, and intellectual currents of that complex period. While doing so, this chapter must afford precise attention to the women and men who populated this world, as this articulation between lived experience and discursive imaginary orients the chapters that follow.

A MULATA VELHA AND HER ENVIRONS (1850–1900)

In some ways, Bahia in the second half of the nineteenth century must have looked quite similar to the way it appeared in the colonial period. Bahia continued to be one of the largest provinces in the empire, with a capital city of nearly 100,000 residents overlooking the magnificent Bay of All Saints. São Salvador da Bahia de Todos os Santos was among the oldest and most populous cities in Brazil, a city with a diverse and multifaceted population where black and brown people constituted the majority of residents. Slavery was characteristic of the province, as it was of the empire as a whole, but Salvador also had a large free population of color. Free poor and enslaved men and women filled the streets of the city, selling food in the bustling marketplaces, carrying people and goods back and forth from the port, and tending to their own domestic needs and those of their masters and patrons. Impressive church structures dotted the urban landscape, including many that dated back to the earliest transfer of Catholic institutions from Portugal in the sixteenth century. And in less conspicuous spaces, followers of the Afro-Brazilian religion of Candomblé also congregated to celebrate and perpetuate their faith. In the countryside, Bahians cultivated and exported cacao, sugar, and tobacco just as their parents and grandparents had done for generations. *Coronelismo,* rule by powerful bosses, was characteristic of the vast interior of the state, where average people had limited rights and depended on relationships with local patrons. Political competition and violence were widespread in the interior and would only worsen by the close of the century as the advent of the republic brought increased power for state governments to exert over regional interests. Whether in Salvador or in the interior, Bahia continued to be an unequal society where a small, white elite owned most of the land and industry, and the majority of residents were marginalized into low-paying economic activities with little access to even basic education. This blanket statement only tells a portion of the story, however, because the many variations of color, ethnicity, birthplace, gender, class, legal status, and social connections ensured that social dynamics were not easily reduced to a simplistic formula of black versus white. To use Richard Graham's recent assertion, Salvador's being "a culture of rank and favor" did not preclude ample "room for negotiation."[1]

Despite continuities, Bahians wrestled with significant and controversial transformations post-1850. Far from static, Bahia's social, political, and intellectual landscapes were dynamic and contested. Still a *mulata* perhaps, but between 1850 and 1900, Bahia exemplified both old and new characteristics. The province experienced on a local level the general turbulence of national politics in the final decades of the century. This turmoil directly affected the lives of Bahians as it did for Brazilian communities across the empire. Slavery was a dying institution, and this was common knowledge even though the series of laws that abolished the institution emerged slowly over a span of nearly forty years. In Bahia, the end of the slave trade from Africa in 1850 preceded a period of violent uprisings, massive flight, and court cases over illegal bondage and abusive conditions. Resistance and revolt were not new to Bahia, but the end of the trade and the long, bloody war pitting Brazil, Argentina, and Uruguay against Paraguay (War of the Triple Alliance, 1864–1870) only exacerbated the demand to definitively bring Brazilian slavery to an end. The imperial army recruited thousands of Bahian men of free and enslaved status to join that effort, many against their will.

These conflicts had a number of significant results. While the enslaved demonstrated their antislavery sentiments through action, the climate of fear within the white population contributed to the rise of an antislavery discourse, especially within Bahia's medical community. Fear and antislavery views connected directly to a rampant anti-Africanism in Bahia that had worsened following the legendary Malê Revolt of 1835. Anti-African hostility concretized into new legislation, and free Africans found their rights to move around the city, to conduct economic activities, and to own property within it severely curtailed.[2] The law held Africans to a standard of "creolization" in determining their right to live without surveillance or even deportation. This bar of Brazilianness could even determine African women's rights to custody of their own children, as Jane-Marie Collins has found.[3] Bahians born in Africa certainly lived a "precarious freedom" following the revolt, and local anti-Africanism had reverberations across Brazil.[4]

Slavery declined rapidly as the century progressed. The enslaved population of 300,000 in 1864 fell just below 77,000 by 1887.[5] Slavery was no longer the main source of labor in the province, and holding slaves was no longer the primary marker of social status.[6] There was a significant rise in self-purchase as thousands bought their way out of bondage. Bahia's plantation agriculture was, in any case, only a shadow of the industry it had been in the seventeenth century when the wealth cultivated in northeastern sugar drove the Portuguese Empire. The booming coffee economy of southern Brazil provoked the sale and forced relocation of tens of thousands of enslaved Bahians, including many from Salvador. Many slave owners sold people to coffee plantations in order to take advantage of high prices, an economic reality once Brazil abolished the slave trade. São Paulo's enslaved population more than doubled between 1864 and 1884, for example. Brazil's southern region was rapidly changing due to urbanization, industrialization, and massive European immigration—all interconnected developments—which combined to push Bahia further to the periphery of national politics. A segment of wealthy Bahians diverted funds, which in a prior age could have found profit in the slave trade, into new sectors such as textiles and food production. Diversification had various results, including growth in state administration, helping to make local bureaucracy an avenue for social mobility. All of these transformations incited intense debates among *soteropolitanos* (residents of Salvador) about race and politics and Bahia's place in a nation contemplating its position on a larger stage.

Persistent and changing health conditions and family patterns help link these transformations with maternalism, establishing how race, maternity, and public health became interrelated. Like most urban port cities in the 1800s, Salvador's geography and commercial activities made residents vulnerable to contagious disease. Due to the circulation of people and poor sanitary conditions, recurring outbreaks plagued the City on the Bay, some of which were epidemic in scale, particularly at midcentury. Bahia was among the provinces most devastated by yellow fever, for example, which appeared periodically and most severely in 1850 and 1856. These outbreaks were highly destructive and difficult to combat. In 1850 alone, yellow fever claimed the lives of 3,000 city residents. During that same wave, more than 100,000 Rio de Janeiro residents (*cariocas*) suffered the illness. In 1855, Bahia experienced a catastrophic episode of cholera that resulted in food shortages, a terrified populace, and an estimated 25,000 fatalities across the province.[7] In all cases, the movement of people and goods, the precarious nature of city sanitation, and the scarcity of medical facilities meant that infectious diseases proliferated almost unchecked.

Interestingly, the severity of the midcentury epidemics contributed to an antislavery attitude in Bahia. Many Brazilians, including physicians at both medical schools, assumed that epidemic disease, such as yellow fever and "African fever," arrived on Brazil's shores via the slave ships. Some acknowledged the inhumane, degrading conditions of the trade that led to "smallpox, scurvy, chicken pox, scabies, measles, eye infections, and diphtheria" on the ships, not to mention the barbaric maimings and cripplings that occurred in transit.[8] Other critics, however, decried the slave ships as vessels that unloaded diseased African bodies directly into the city. Bahia's port, different from Rio de Janeiro's for example, did not have any official form of quarantine or treatment for the enslaved as they arrived. Connecting epidemic disease to slave ships served as further confirmation that the end of the transatlantic trade had been a step in the right direction. One scholar has argued that cholera "helped to seal the fate of the transatlantic slave trade to Brazil."[9] This reinforcement of antislavery in Bahia serves as a reminder that serious health conditions were never separate from the concerns of the society at large and its politics.

Unfortunately, the provincial government was not in a position to do much in the face of epidemic disease. The Public Hygiene Commission attempted, rather unsuccessfully, to respond to the cholera epidemic of 1855. Despite a rigorous mobilization, preventative measures largely failed; this was to be expected because the etiology of cholera was not defined at that time. Beyond that, Bahia simply lacked the necessary public health personnel, infrastructure, and sanitation procedures. This was a recurring theme throughout the century as Bahians faced grave public health problems without comprehensive, large-scale organization to address them. On the intellectual side, periods of epidemic disease were vitally important for the development of medical knowledge in Bahia. For the majority of the population, however, health and illness were matters to be addressed on a familial level.[10]

Given the conditions of periodic disease, poor public hygiene, and insufficient infrastructure, it is easy to imagine the difficulty of maintaining family health. Family was the center of social life for most Brazilians, although certainly some families, such as those of the enslaved, faced great constraints on their ability to remain cohesive and stable. In Bahia, family structure was quite varied, which should be unsurprising, given the diversity of legal status, class, color, religion, and ethnic origin—all features that influence the family as an institution. As expected, the wealthiest families are most visible in the historical record, providing a more concrete basis from which to describe typical patterns. In fact, the term "family" had specific class connotations. When locals spoke of "*famílias baianas*," or "Bahian families," they referred to respectable elite families whose unions were legitimized by the Catholic Church and whose male heads of household protected and exerted control over wives, children, servants, and other dependents.[11] Among the *famílias baianas*, well-to-do ladies lived in seclusion (at least stereotypically) in their homes or in retirement homes such as the Recolhimento do Santo Nome de Jesus maintained by the esteemed confraternity, the Santa Casa de Misericórdia. In 1847, 123 women and girls lived at the Recolhimento, which also housed a school of primary letters for recluses and small numbers of poor girls from the community who were invited to study free of charge.[12] Two smaller retirement homes existed in Salvador as well, Perdões and São Raymundo, both founded in the early eighteenth century.[13]

As was typical of Brazil, families with wealth to protect married strategically; thus, the members of Bahia's elite formed a small, interconnected community. Managing slaves, servants, and dependents was also characteristic of wealthy and even middle-class families, who formed a small but important segment of society. Being served in a private, autonomous space was a sign of status and position, an important means by which the privileged distinguished themselves from the poor. Many poor families did not meet these criteria of legitimacy, patriarchy, and servitude, making their unions less respectable in the minds of the wealthier classes. Despite these generalizations, rigid codes of honor and strict distinctions between the familial and behavioral patterns of the haves and have-nots were always more of an ideal than a reality.

Contemporary accounts and histories of poor families are more difficult to find. Some recurring observations allow for a general characterization of the majority of Bahian families. Among the poor, consensual unions were more common than marriages formalized through the Church. Patriarchal authority was also typical in poorer families, though female-headed households with children were commonplace. As compared to wealthier families, the poor seemed to experience a greater sense of mobility. The necessities of making a living brought men and women into publicly shared space more frequently, in the marketplaces, on street corners, in the plazas, at the ports, and at the public water fountains. Working people's mobility provided opportunities for association with neighbors, vendors, and shopkeepers, and thus alternative community formation and a degree of autonomy.[14] During the waning years of slavery, kinship ties were fundamental in helping many Bahians secure their freedom from captivity. Extended families of color often included free, freed, and enslaved members. Bahians defined familial bonds broadly, including informally adopted children and godparents. Additionally, kinship applied to spiritual and ethnic ties of maternity, fraternity, and hierarchy within Afro-Brazilian religious culture.[15]

Concubinage and single motherhood were common facets of Brazilian family dynamics in the 1800s. Perhaps the greatest illustration of this in colonial Bahia comes from the *devassa* (judicial inquiry) of 1813 in which an Ecclesiastical Visitor toured twelve southern villages, requesting denunciations of residents known to have practiced "sins and excesses."[16] In more than half of the denunciations, residents accused their neighbors of sexual immorality: concubinage, illicit relationships, "living as if married," and spouses living apart.[17] Many of those accused had a child, many children, and even adult children, suggesting that nonformalized unions were stable and often lifelong. The *devassa* also revealed that consensual partnerships and single motherhood generalized across color lines. Yet, the lessons of this and other studies of concubinage and illegitimacy are somewhat ambiguous. Nonformalized unions and the children of single mothers were certainly common and accepted features of Bahian society, but these situations could still be considered immoral by neighbors and the Church. The Church did not judge the children of "marriageable" parents and relationships between single adults as harshly as unions that could not be legitimized—adultery, for example. Where adults formed unions that could theoretically become Christian marriages someday (which could retroactively legitimize children), these community members were far from social outcasts.

Patronage ties united the various types of Bahian families, and this was most apparent in the homes of the city's well-to-do families. Families of means enjoyed the service of free and enslaved men and women who performed the majority of domestic duties and cared for children. After 1850, when many slaves were sold south, domestic service became the most common form of labor among enslaved people in Salvador. For the free poor, it was a poorly remunerated occupation. Both men and women worked in service, but it remained the dominant form of wage labor for urban women even after abolition. Poor women had few other employment options; therefore, Bahians generally understood domestic service as a female occupation. Household service was also racialized in that the majority of domestics were black and brown women, and the majority of wage-earning black and brown women worked as domestics. Domestic work signified more than a vocation; it represented a type of social, even familial, relationship between employer and employee, even for the enslaved. Typically, household domestics were part of an extended notion of family that characterized traditional forms of Brazilian patriarchalism. Domestics, even when of free status, commonly lived in the households where they worked. Naturally, domestics also had their own families, their own ties of blood, kinship, and affection beyond the families they served.

Living in complicated the separation between working hours and personal time, providing domestics little opportunity to lead independent lives. Being considered part of the patron's family was a double-edged sword; domestics faced difficult barriers to maintaining their outside relationships with their own children, partners, and relatives. Because service was such common employment for *soteropolitanas*, the wet nurses, nannies, laundresses, seamstresses, and maids who served in "respectable" households were also mothers to the majority of the city's children. If these mothers were in consensual, equal relationships, they likely shared their children with men also employed in service or men who worked as stevedores, porters, and sailors—common occupations for Bahian working men. For domestics with children, patrons held the power to decide whether or not these mothers would have sufficient time to care for them in addition to their charges—the supposed symbolic fraternity between white and black children suckled at the same breast, the "*irmãos de peito*," notwithstanding.

Despite differences in structure and linkages, all families had a lot to contend with in terms of health. The frequent experience of poverty coupled with disease and sanitation conditions exacted a heavy toll on Bahians and on the province's most vulnerable residents: the enslaved, the impoverished, and the very young. Bahians suffered from high infant mortality rates, for example. Government statistics for this period are unreliable, and physicians did not take interest in estimating infant mortality until the very end of the century. However, three hundred child deaths per one thousand births is a reasonable approximation for most of the period. Other cities, including Rio de Janeiro, São Paulo, and Recife, recorded similar tragic statistics. These numbers meant that thousands of Bahian children died annually before reaching their second birthdays.[18] Thousands more suffered through episodic or chronic illnesses, as did adults, and dealing with periods of sickness in the long and short term was an expected reality of life for families of all backgrounds.

In times of illness, most families could turn to an arsenal of home remedies, passed down through generations of experience and experimentation. Families also entrusted their health to a cadre of healers and specialists that included midwives, *curandeiros* (generalists), barber surgeons, herbalists, and spiritualists. Many were well known locally and maintained a large clientele. Among the most popular and integral healers were Brazil's traditional midwives. Known affectionately as *comadres* and pejoratively as *curiosas*, midwives attended to the health needs of women and children through pregnancy, delivery, and beyond. Their involvement with their clients extended over and above the labor itself, and the relationships formed were more intimate than clinical. Midwives offered advice and support from the earliest stages of pregnancy. In addition to technical knowledge, their work was full of mysticism, spirituality, and a sense that supernatural forces influenced birthing and revealed the outcome of pregnancies. They advised on diet, offered cures for ailments, and proscribed certain behaviors that they contended would interfere with a smooth delivery or cause a lifelong curse on the newborn. Folk midwives read signs in nature and in the body to determine whether labor would be easy or difficult and to determine the sex of the fetus. Beyond prenatal care and birthing, Brazilian families entrusted their midwives with carrying newborns to baptism and with advising mothers on their proper care. Midwives were also well known for their expertise in reproductive health, abortion, and treatment in times of illness.

The mysticism and spirituality associated with traditional midwifery eventually led physicians to label midwives as irrational and dangerous. Yet in this period, physicians' judgments held limited relevance because biomedical opinion did not dominate most families' choices on health issues and childbirth. Midwives attended the vast majority of births; physician-assisted birth was an exceptional experience in the nineteenth century.[19]

In many cases, Brazilian families preferred the expertise of popular healers over biomedical practitioners. This was not simply a matter of lack of access to the biomedically trained or of expense—though medical consultations would have been financially out of reach for most families. Biomedicine had not yet reached the heights of legitimacy and hegemony that it would occupy by the mid-twentieth century. Consequently, most Brazilians remained unconvinced that biomedical treatments were perforce superior to other traditions of healing. This would slowly change as medicine increasingly professionalized and specialized. Physicians, moreover, actively constructed a space for themselves in Brazil's twentieth-century health landscape and republican bureaucracy.

Nineteenth-century medicine was not so far differentiated from empiricism anyway. Physicians relied on trial and error and on many of the same treatments, herbs, purgatives, and teas commonly employed by healers and spiritists.[20] Brazilian physicians trained at one of two domestic institutions: the Bahia School of Medicine and its counterpart in Rio de Janeiro, both founded in 1808 after the transfer of the Portuguese monarchy. Bahia's School of Medicine remained smaller and less generously funded than the Rio de Janeiro academy. It had a reputation for being quite traditional: patronage ties were critical to success; the school had little autonomy; instruction conservatively followed French models and precedents. However, the Bahia School of Medicine offered scholarships for students in need, making the institution a vehicle of social advancement for both the petit bourgeoisie and *mulatos*. Because of this, a medical degree was often the entryway into other careers—in politics, journalism, or letters. Only a fraction of graduates later practiced medicine professionally.[21] As expected, students were almost exclusively men. Yet Bahia's School of Medicine was the first in Brazil to graduate a female physician: in 1887, Dr. Rita Lobato Velho Lopes. Whether male or female, the population of physicians remained small. Most practiced privately and made home visits to a select clientele. An even smaller contingent was regularly attached to clinical institutions like hospitals.

While the School of Medicine may have been quite orthodox, the province boasted a cadre of physicians who built an international reputation by rejecting the predominant climatic determinism thesis and championing locally produced research to address local health conditions. These physicians, the Tropicalistas, were a small group of foreign and Brazilian doctors who devoted themselves to professionalizing medical practice in Bahia. Consolidating much of their reputation during the cholera and yellow fever epidemics, they performed experiments at a time when medicine was more conservative than innovative and pioneered the introduction of new medical techniques into Brazil. The Tropicalistas saw scientific authority as the key to Brazilian progress if it could be "purged of the discordant elements of competition, politics, and religion."[22] Part of their pursuit of that authority entailed solidifying the distinction between medical and "empirical" practice. Their *Gazeta Médica da Bahia*, first published in 1866, was Brazil's first scientific medical journal. The Tropicalistas' outsider status vis-à-vis the mainstream establishment—none of them were teaching faculty at the School of Medicine—allowed more leeway for inquiry and exploration and a greater challenge to the status quo.

Local studies were rare in Bahia due to the presumed superiority of French models and the lack of clinical infrastructure to advance medical research. Hospitals in nineteenth-century Brazil, for example, were generally the last resort of the desperately poor and resourceless: slaves, prisoners, and soldiers as well as the mentally ill. In times of serious illness or injury, Brazilians of means could appeal to private family physicians. The majority, however, turned (presumably reluctantly) to hospitalization only if home treatment was ineffective or impossible. The sour reputation of the hospitals went beyond being associated with society's underclass; nineteenth-century hospitals could be quite dangerous places, notorious for inadequate facilities and unsanitary conditions and procedures. In Salvador da Bahia, options for hospitalization were extremely limited. There was the Hospital de Isolamento, created in response to the 1853 wave of yellow fever but only open during episodes of epidemic disease. For most of the century, the São Cristóvão Hospital was the city's only permanent hospital, founded and administered by the Santa Casa de Misericórdia, a Catholic lay brotherhood that is one of the oldest institutions in Brazil. São Cristóvão was the sole hospital for a population surpassing 200,000 in 1872.[23] At São Cristóvão, patients were seen free of charge as part of the Misericórdia's mission of caring for the ill, an extension of Christian charity.

For maternal and child health, the insufficiency of treatment options was further magnified. Part of this problem followed from a lack of medical expertise. Though the history of obstetrics and gynecology in Bahia is long, these academic tracks did not prepare physicians for the actual practice of assisting births until the closing years of the century. The School of Medicine curriculum first added an obstetrics course in 1818 at the specific request of the king, Dom João VI.[24] Only sixty years later, however, was practical experience added to the course, giving students the opportunity to actually witness the birthing process. The Bahia School of Medicine also offered a midwifery course for women. Like obstetrics, the early midwifery course included no practical experience or observations of births and attracted very few students. The theoretical orientation required an advanced level of prior academic study, which was unavailable to poorer women in Salvador. Only wealthier women would have had the necessary educational background, but they generally came from families that were unlikely to send their female relatives to learn a trade like midwifery.

The School of Medicine did not even maintain a facility where a teaching course could take place until 1875, when the São Cristóvão Hospital opened a birthing room. Few women were willing to give birth there, however. The appalling conditions and dreadful reputation were enough to keep pregnant women from entrusting their care to hospital physicians. Conditions improved in 1893 when the birthing room moved to the Santa Izabel Hospital in the neighborhood of Nazaré, and the number of patients slowly increased. The new hospital was the Santa Casa de Misericórdia's second clinical facility for Salvador's residents. Even with the transfer of the birthing room, only two or three births typically took place there during the entire duration of the School of Medicine's obstetric course. These numbers slowly increased at the turn of the century, according to Dr. Francisca Prageur Fróes, who recorded twenty-two births in 1902.[25] Though the School of Medicine attempted to offer specialization in gynecology and obstetrics, the lack of opportunity to train physicians and nurse-midwives in birthing compromised that effort. Without patients to observe, graduating physicians had less legitimacy as experts in birthing than did their midwife rivals. Thus, resource-poor women experiencing complications gave birth in the Misericórdia hospital alongside the ill and unlucky children who were interned with the adult population. Before the twentieth century, there were no specialized hospital facilities for Bahian children at all.

For poor families, severe illnesses in children or their caretakers could provoke a serious crisis. Many families had no other option but to relinquish custody of their children to the Santa Casa de Misericórdia in these extreme circumstances. On January 30, 1889, a nine-month-old baby named Josepha and identified as *"parda,"* or "brown," in skin tone was left in the Misericórdia's foundling wheel, for example. Through a note left with the child, the nuns of the institution learned that Josepha's mother suffered a grave illness that prevented her from being capable of caring for the child. Josepha apparently did not have a father at home, and the mother hoped to retrieve her child at some future date if her health allowed. Unfortunately, Josepha's story ended like that of many thousands of other Brazilian children. She survived four months before dying of complications related to teething. A similar tragic fate befell Francisco, another *pardo* infant, approximately one year later. When his mother fell ill in January of 1890, she also turned to the Misericórdia to provide for her five-month-old's care. No information was provided about Francisco's father. The baby survived only one month before dying of unspecified "fevers."[26] Although Josepha and Francisco arrived at the Misericórdia in an apparent state of health, many weak and ill babies were left in the wheel. Perhaps in some of these cases, the severity of illness pushed familial resources beyond their capacity, resulting in the transfer of custody to the Misericórdia. It is impossible to know with certainty whether prior illness was the determining factor, but the fact that treatment options were exceedingly limited in Salvador is unquestionable. Most of these children, whether they entered the foundling wheel in a state of health or illness, would soon fall sick and die, allowing the Misericórdia to fulfill its mission to ensure them a "good death."[27]

This lack of facilities demonstrates that prenatal, maternal, and children's medicine were neither widely practiced disciplines nor medical priorities in Bahia. "Women's medicine" did not draw much medical attention before the late 1800s, and this was in line with international trends.[28] Changing real-life conditions and intellectual concerns as the century came to a close made particular reformist ideologies attractive and paved the way for ideas to manifest into projects and institutions, representing an elemental change from the dismal state of public health of the early century. Foremost among those real and intellectual shifts was the abolition of slavery and debates over its legacy. It is difficult to identify a series of transitions that rocked Brazilian intellectualism, especially science and medicine, more fundamentally than the protracted abolition of slavery and the corresponding controversies over the impact of race on the nation. Medicalization provided a new framing of Brazilian social relations once slavery began to diminish, and the close of one century offered the potential of crafting a "better" Brazil for the next. That context and the social, political, and ideological questioning it engendered was the most crucial transformation that helped to bring health reform focused on women and children to the forefront of medical priorities.

THEORIZING RACE AND PROGRESS

The end of slavery loomed on the Brazilian horizon for a long time. By midcentury, politicians, coffee planters, and intellectuals were already debating the fallout of abolition and devising schemes to appropriately manage the transition to wage labor and (attenuated) Afro-Brazilian citizenship. In medicine, this dialogue resulted in immense treatment of race, racial origins, and racial degeneracy. Immersed in French scholarship and observing their own society, physicians determined that Brazil, like France, had demographic problems. Brazil's demographic problems were racialized in specific ways, however, as physicians read the future possibilities for their nation in light of its slaving past. Rather than the depopulation that French pronatalists feared, Brazilians worried that their nation was "underpopulated"—a disconnected hodgepodge of poor rural black and brown people too dissimilar from those of the urban coast to constitute an identifiable national race. In the opinion of many physicians and political figures, the Brazilian population suffered from a crisis of both quantity and quality. An unhealthy and unstable populace could not generate the (free) labor force necessary to fuel a potent, vigorous nation. Myriad solutions came from this general prognosis, the most dramatic of which was a grand plan to replace Brazil's enslaved and working class with immigrants from abroad. These discussions and pilot projects were well under way by the 1860s.[29]

Intellectuals surveying the nation's postabolition prospects also faced the challenge of resolving troublesome European theses of racial and climatic determinism that demeaned nations with population and environmental characteristics like those of Brazil. Determinist theories held that tropical climates and "racially inferior" populations sealed the fate of nations like Brazil and justified a Eurocentric hierarchy of nations. For proponents of climatic determinism, the struggle to master nature in the tropics prevented people in those regions from developing advanced civilizations. The energy required to survive in American and African environments compromised the intellectual capacity of "tropical" peoples. Worst of all for tropical societies hoping to "regenerate," determinist theories asserted that hot climates could cause white European people to degenerate or regress to the state of precivilization that was the assumed perpetual condition of people native to the tropics.[30]

Beyond climate, Brazil was dually condemned by European theories of racial degeneration. Degeneration theorists reserved their most vehement attacks for nations where miscegenation was widespread. The most famous proponent of this new spin on racist doctrine was the French diplomat Arthur de Gobineau, Brazil's "cordial enemy."[31] Gobineau's theories were well known among the Brazilian intelligentsia. In his notorious 1853 treatise on the hierarchy of races, Gobineau wrote:

> The word *degenerate*, when applied to a people, means ... that the people has no longer the same intrinsic value as it had before, because it no longer has the same blood in its veins, continual adulterations having gradually affected the quality of that blood ... The heterogeneous elements that henceforth prevail in [the degenerate man] give him quite a different nationality—a very original one, no doubt, but such originality is not to be envied.[32]

This was bad news for Brazilians who claimed an affinity with the Latin peoples of Europe and considered themselves inheritors of a European culture simply transferred to a tropical environment. Any Brazilian could plainly see that their population was far from the Aryan ideal that Gobineau praised, and Brazilians had been socially, culturally, and racially mixing since the sixteenth century. For Gobineau, "hybrid" people could only produce an irreconcilable hybrid civilization. He particularly condemned people of African descent, characterizing them as the lowest form of human being. Brazil was the most African nation in the hemisphere demographically, having enslaved supposedly degenerate people in a degenerating tropical environment. "No Brazilian is of pure blood," according to Gobineau, writing home from an 1869 trip to Rio de Janeiro, and this caused a terrible degeneration in "both the lowest and highest classes."[33] The author's biting words recalled those of the scientist Louis Agassiz, who penned another famous text in 1868, *Journey in Brazil*, reveling in the luxurious native flora and fauna but condemning the "mongrelization" that resulted in a people "deficient in physical and mental energy."[34] Most distressing for aspirant Brazilian intellectuals must have been Gobineau's contention that the characteristics of the disparate human races were permanent. For Gobineau, weak races were unlikely to improve, but strong races could definitely degenerate, and such degeneracy was irreversible. Brazilian intellectuals were caught between their acceptance of the concept of degeneracy, their assumptions of the superiority of French and English theories, and their hesitancy to accept their nation as a perpetual backwater.

Degeneracy and social stagnation had specific contours in Bahia. For critics, the province seemed to show signs of degeneracy on all fronts, and it certainly did not help to be the "Old Mammy" of a nation seeking progress. There was the historical problem of Bahia's long association with slavery, colonialism, and agricultural oligarchy—all signs of backwardness for degeneracy theorists. The environs of urban cities like Salvador caused degeneracy by an "excess of civilization," meaning an overemphasis on cultural pursuits and moral problems such as bachelorhood, prostitution, "denatured" motherhood, and venereal disease.[35] The overwhelming majority of Bahians were black and brown, 70 percent in 1890, and travelers commonly asserted that miscegenation was a characterizing feature of the region.[36] People of mixed ancestry were even found among the intellectual elite, particularly within the medical community. The presence of a number of *mulato* doctors should have demonstrated Brazilian social flexibility at work, but in the nineteenth century, most would agree that it was just another sign that even the best Bahians were limited by racial ancestry. Bahian physicians engaged their southern counterparts in debates over European immigration, but it was never a serious possibility in Bahia, given the local economy. There was no hope, therefore, for "counteracting" the black presence through immigration as occurred in the South.[37]

Moreover, Bahian physicians were more likely than their *carioca* colleagues to accept the miscegenation-causes-degeneracy thesis. The prevalence of articles in the *Gazeta Médica da Bahia* on the relationship between race and diseases (syphilis, tuberculosis, and leprosy) confirmed this preoccupation. Race continued to be a principal topic at the School of Medicine, which was the leading center of knowledge on racial science and legal medicine, thanks largely to the influential work of Dr. Raymundo Nina Rodrigues. Working on miscegenation, African religions, and criminology, Rodrigues conducted pioneering investigations into Afro-Brazilian culture in the 1890s, only to ultimately argue that black Brazilians were too barbarous to be held to the same criminal code as whites. He argued that miscegenation was one of the major problems facing Brazil, since the lack of "uniformity" compromised the nation's potential. Like his contemporaries, Rodrigues was well versed in European racial theory and cited both Gobineau and Agassiz in his own work.[38] The Rodrigues school of thought did have its opponents in Bahia, including the physician Manoel Bomfim, who rejected the notion of the inequality of races and charged that this rhetoric was simply a racist tool invented by Europeans and North Americans to justify their imperialist intentions in Latin America.[39]

Rodrigues's work proved highly influential in promoting a research-based approach to the nation's "racial problems," but ultimately characterizing Brazil based on strict racial types was an untenable argument. Without some modifications on the basic theme, the overt racism of degeneracy theory only served to confirm the notion of a hierarchy of nations. As the century came to a close, several theorists, including prominent intellectuals such as João Batista de Lacerda, Oliveira Vianna, and Sílvio Romero, began to argue that miscegenation was a potential cure for degeneracy rather than its cause. They argued that racial mixture elevated society through the process of whitening, or *branqueamento*. Superior white genes did not weaken through intermixture with inferior blood, as Gobineau had argued; rather, superior genes overtook inferior ones as in Mendelian genetics, successively whitening each future generation. In historical and political terms, miscegenation had prevented racial conflicts, proponents argued, sparing Brazil from the great mistake of US-style segregation. For these scholars, whitening would eliminate Brazil's African and indigenous ancestry within several generations, leaving only a native-born white population. Further integration, therefore, was an expected and hopeful consequence of abolition. *Branqueamento* implied both biological and cultural assimilation, achieving "whiteness through participation."[40] Some more extreme eugenicists clung to *mestiço* degeneracy theory, but the majority of Brazilian elites enthusiastically received this new optimistic outlook on Brazil's racial future.[41]

Intellectually, whitening theory made a nice complement to Brazilian positivism, since both philosophies were predicated on the notion of successive improvement and societal change. Positivist ideology was popular in Brazil and fundamental to the end of the monarchy in 1889 because republicans objected to its centralized nature, which they claimed confined Brazil to a preindustrial religious traditionalism. Discouraged by seigneurial rural politics, they pressed for a political system that would promote urban interests and liberal economic policies.[42] Moreover, Comtean positivism placed a strong emphasis on family and patriotism, which appealed to Brazilians favoring change but not individualism. Brazil's privileged classes were also attracted to the concept of modernization without social mobilization.[43]

Drawing on whitening, positivism, and eugenics, intellectuals and physicians across Brazil contended that the nation could "regenerate" through a series of scientific interventions. Their rejection of *mestiço* degeneracy was not unrelated to the fact that segregation by then was impossible in Brazil. None of this meant an end to racial prejudice or discrimination in the state of Bahia or elsewhere. Replacing explicitly racist views with other ways of thinking about degeneracy was a long process, as most intellectuals continued to see Brazil's racial situation as disadvantageous but not necessarily insurmountable. They continued to debate the relative significance of racial, health, and educational factors in Brazil's quest for progress well into the following century. However, physicians and intellectuals came to mostly agree that the major impediment to Brazil's becoming a modern nation was not racial backwardness but the fact that Brazilians were backward in their *habits*, which they attributed to culture and a lack of investment in health, hygiene, and education.

Thus, the medical community diagnosed the nation as in dire need of scientific intervention and professional guidance to generate a "better" Brazilian type. International dialogues and French precedents of the late century helped concretize this diagnosis into an increased emphasis on gynecology, reproduction, and children's health at both Brazilian medical schools. These were active arenas where physicians and biomedical knowledge could theoretically alter or even perfect the race of the future.[44] Conceptually, Brazilians' campaign for healthier babies and better mothers was rooted in the French theory of *puériculture*.

"*Puériculture*," originally coined by the Parisian physician Alfred Caron in 1865, referred to the improvement of the human species through infant care. Caron's theory was largely ridiculed and forgotten in medical circles until Dr. Adolphe Pinard revived it in 1899. Pinard, a leading expert on infant health, served as chair of obstetrics at the Faculty of Medicine in Paris. He defined *puériculture* as "knowledge relative to the reproduction, the conservation and the amelioration of the human species."[45] His advocacy of "conscious and responsible procreation" and its relation to the emerging science of eugenics differentiated puericulture from contemporary pronatalism.[46] That eugenic connection between reproduction, heredity, and racial improvement suggested that a child's health and character were influenced long before birth or even gestation. *Puériculture*, adopted as *"puericultura"* in Portuguese, became the rallying call for a movement to reduce infant mortality rates, provide prenatal and well-baby care, and introduce the latest scientifically approved principles of child rearing.[47]

Brazilian physicians were not simply enamored with puericulture theory because French science was fashionable. Wealthy, educated Brazilians did hold up French intellectualism and culture as a model of "civilization," but adopting and refashioning French medical ideas was not merely a form of imitation. Rather, puericulture and eugenics offered a framework for both real and imagined social conditions that were increasingly identified as national problems. These theories also fit well with homegrown ideologies of progress and reform during a period of rapid transformation as Brazil and Bahia grappled with the transitions outlined in the first section of this chapter. Where reformists adopted foreign theories, they made active interpretations based on local concerns, filtering the literature and discarding that which was untenable, impolitic, or illogical in Brazilian terms. This conditional intellectual adoption was particularly relevant for "loose" and malleable theories like eugenics. In addition to fitting into the larger climate of social reform, puericulture and eugenics—enacted through women's and children's medicine—also appealed to the medical community's desire to professionalize their practice and create a new relevance and significance for biomedicine.

It did not take long for Brazilian physicians to agree that eugenics and, later, puericulture could hold the answers to local social problems.[48] In 1876, Dr. José Francisco da Silva Lima wrote that Bahian families desperately needed the "knowledgeable intervention" of infant care specialists in order to make the best decisions for their children. Dr. Julio Pereira Leite concurred in 1893, writing that maternal health and welfare was "necessary for the future of the nation."[49] Bahian physicians fretted over families like the Lacerdas of the Largo de Piedade, who employed eighteen-year-old Aldagira Josepha da Costa, a *preta*, to nurse their infant child. They turned a disparaging eye on families like the Dutras of the Calçada do Bomfim, who entrusted their baby to Melania Joaquina Reis, their thirty-four-year-old *preta* wet nurse.[50] Yet this generation of physicians worried little over Aldagira da Costa's and Melania Reis's own children.

Medical concerns do not necessarily become public concerns, however, and all medical concerns do not have the requisite clout to spawn a welfare state. In this case, the medical community's interest in maternalism connected to the larger public through dialogues and anxieties related to national "progress." That broader anxiety about the nation's past and its future became a point of convergence between the medical community, political elites, wealthy benefactors, and civic organizations. Engineering healthier Brazilians through public health as well as healthier environments through sanitation seemed to be the keys to a national regeneration that would make Brazil more competitive and more modern. Once Brazil secured its place as the last monarchy and only remaining slave society in the Americas, these debates became even more intense. With the new century brewing, physicians and other intellectuals pronounced on what type of citizenry Brazil needed to flourish in the "modern age," and what should be done to make postabolition, postimperial Brazil a powerful, industrial, and whiter nation.

The emphasis on producing, reproducing, and generating change meant that reformists saw women as indispensable agents of Brazil's "civilization."[51] Pinard's *puériculture* provided a scheme for using targeted family intervention to effect comprehensive reform, but the rationalization and implementation responded to a context and culture that were specifically Brazilian. The gendered roles women played as mothers, midwives, health practitioners, and domestic servants were profoundly tied to reproduction and child rearing, and these roles had important class and racial implications as well. The "proper" exercise of mothering took on new significance as one of the main elements determining whether Brazil's future would be marked by progress or stagnation. For the Bahian medical community, birthing and general issues of women's and children's health, previously of marginal interest, were now (postabolition and post-empire) paramount to state and nation, and there was a surge of medical literature on these topics. The authors loaded the "problem of motherhood" with cultural assumptions and meanings, owing to family dynamics, high infant mortality rates, and the hierarchal social structure of Bahia. Color and class differentiated experiences of birthing and mothering as well, so all of these elements bore upon the medicalization of motherhood.

MEDICINE, GENDER, AND CULTURE

This final section of the chapter revisits the familial and servitude relationships that typified Bahia in the second half of the nineteenth century. But here the emphasis falls on the symbolic uses of these relationships and gendered "types" in medical discourse. Following Jane-Marie Collins, this history demonstrates the power of the household to produce social change as an "originary agent" rather than simply a reflection or refraction of outside forces.[52] Brazilian physicians recognized this fact well. They pinned their hopes for Brazil's bright future on this family-household-society articulation while casting children as the future's present-day representatives. In medical literature, the actions of their mothers and mother-figures were of utmost significance. Nineteenth-century thinkers proved largely unable to translate their rhetoric into programs or projects. That would come at the dawn of the 1900s. Yet these physicians turned their gaze to mothering and familial relationships as the crux of orchestrating Brazil's imminent reinvention as a postemancipation society and, soon thereafter, a liberal republic.

With any discursive change, it is difficult to pinpoint its exact invention and inaccurate to attribute it to a singular stream of influence. This was certainly the case for Brazilian medical discourses, which responded to diverse international and domestic theories, literatures, and circumstances. Physicians filtered foreign theories through local cultural narratives—some widely shared and some particular to the lettered and privileged—and refashioned those theories to fit Brazilian realities. In this way, the production of knowledge on women's and children's health was dynamic, an interactive process in which medical understandings and cultural ideas intertwined. Some of this exchange was intentional. Bahian physicians surveyed the Mulata Velha and saw rampant contagious disease and tragedies of childhood illness, death, and abandonment with virtually no biomedical facilities to address them. To fill the gap of nonexistent institutions, physicians actively sought to influence the beliefs and behaviors of local families. Despite the turn toward professionalization, cultural ideas about race, gender, family, and class continually informed biomedical knowledge. If improper mothering compromised Brazil's future health, it was due to the carelessness of wet nurses and nannies, the immorality of "unnatural" women, and the ineptitude of "superstitious" midwives. All of these medical cautionary tales encapsulated new and older ways of thinking about race and gender.

It would be overly simplistic and outright misleading to argue that Bahian medical literature integrated cultural images uncritically, but medicine did lend an air of scientific authority to certain popular stereotypes and biases. Iconic figures found their way into the literature where authors explored cultural truths as if they were medical facts. In a larger sense, this literature aided in defining motherhood as a technical practice—a qualitative exercise of birthing and rearing performed by women whom physicians judged to be of greater or lesser competence. By setting parameters and labeling people and practices as either legitimate or pathological, the medical community helped determine what motherhood should mean (from their perspective), how women's "nature" could be maximized scientifically, and how the experience should be delineated by race and class. Physicians were not the only voices in this process, and it is no coincidence that they latched onto *puériculture* in the late 1800s when intellectuals regularly debated race, abolition, and Brazilian identity. The literature is fascinating, but pushing beyond the pages, it is vital to recognize the connection between *ideas* about women, family, color, and class and the *strategies* employed to effect Brazilian "regeneration." The symbolic use of gendered tropes had real consequences for public health practice. Therefore, the imagined nineteenth-century "ignorant wet nurse," "denatured mother," "incompetent midwife," and "strong but benevolent father" set the stage for institutions that came into being in the early years of the next century and are explored in subsequent chapters.

The Mãe Preta

Arguably, the most enduring "mother figure" of the nineteenth century is the black Brazilian wet nurse, the *mãe preta*—whose memory varied from beloved to sinister, depending on perspective. As explained, nursing and caring for children were customary forms of paid or forced labor. In Bahia, wealthy households absolutely depended on domestic help, and those relations between patrons and female servants were common, relatable features of urban and rural life. As physicians turned their attention to maternity, they labeled female servants, particularly those who cared for children, as the "uncivilized" element within the typical Brazilian home. The medical community saw servants as "doors" through which physical and moral contagions entered respectable families.[53] Physicians assumed that wet nurses were culpable for high infant mortality rates, and this denigration of "mercenary mothers" paralleled contemporary French literature. Though Brazilian physicians integrated French concerns over wet nursing and infant mortality, local context and the racialized nature of servitude in Brazil were as important to the emergence of this topic in medical discourse. As eventual emancipation became inescapable, physicians wrote that the intimacy of black women within the traditional patriarchal home posed a danger to children and families.

The "perilous wet nurse" became a regular feature of dissertations on family health at the Bahia School of Medicine. Wet nurses, physicians contended, were irresponsible and incapable, maliciously shirking their duties or unintentionally endangering their charges with their ignorance of hygiene and proper feeding. As one editor of the *Gazeta Médica da Bahia* argued, Brazilian families' reliance on wet nurses meant the sacrifice of thousands of lives to "ignorance, negligence, and fraud."[54] Physicians debated the transmission of moral characteristics through nursing and wondered if a nurse's sexuality or personal habits could influence the type of adults their charges would one day become. And how much more so after abolition when black women's activities would become more difficult to control?

In Bahia, Dr. Joaquim Telesphoro Ferreira Lopes Vianna catalyzed this debate in 1853. Analyzing French literature on unregulated wet nursing, Vianna concluded that Brazil's situation was especially precarious. While his French counterparts gave precise prescriptions for selecting an ideal wet nurse, Vianna argued that suitable wet nurses were nearly impossible to find in Brazil. Vianna conflated race and illness, stating that most Brazilian wet nurses imparted disease along with their breast milk, "being in their majority Africans, stupid, immoral, without education, without beauty, without religion, lacking in affectionate sentiments, deformed, irascible, unclean, spiteful, careless."[55] For Vianna, black wet nurses not only harbored disease within their bodies, but their irresponsibility, African superstitions, and ignorance of hygiene endangered their charges. This emerging perspective about disease and wet nursing continued onto the pages of the *Gazeta Médica da Bahia*, where authors frequently published articles on wet nursing as a syphilis threat. In an 1866 issue, Dr. Claudemiro Caldas asserted that syphilis resulted from three sources: a punishment to lascivious men, a tragic accident of birth, or "the mercenary wet nurse . . . who transmits the fatal venom through her milk, [imparting] instead of nourishment—pain, disturbance, and death."[56] For years physicians at the School of Medicine repeated these unfortunate racist defamations of wet nurses, and the suspicion of black female servants continued to grow.

Medical discourse on the dangers of domestics was ambiguous, perhaps acknowledging the absolute centrality of wet nurses and nannies to Brazilian families. While delineating the hazards of "mercenary nursing," physicians consistently offered suggestions on how a nurse should be selected—always with the assistance of a physician. They warned families not to trust their own judgment, and much less the judgment of the lady of the house if left to her own devices. One physician wrote condescendingly that mothers put more thought into choosing a dress than into selecting the women who would nurse their children.[57] Professional examination was necessary, physicians argued, because wet nurses could have diseases that escaped the perception of untrained family members. An appearance of health might mask a hidden illness, and a pleasant disposition might obscure a dubious character. Character related to the unresolved question of the transmission of moral traits, and to physicians' assumption that wet nurses lied when asked about their age and previous illnesses. Families should treat nurses with suspicion;

only a qualified professional could see beyond their bodily and intentional deceptions.[58]

Dr. Carlos Arthur Moncorvo de Figueiredo, a pioneer in Brazilian pediatrics, endeavored to assist physicians and the state in determining the suitability of wet nurses in 1876 when he penned "Project on the Regulation of Wet Nurses" for the *Gazeta Médica da Bahia*.[59] Moncorvo's feature was the first publication on wet nurse regulation in the journal, but through the following decades, the subject inspired a lively conversation within Bahia and between the Bahian and Rio de Janeiro medical communities. In the article, the *carioca* physician spelled out a detailed methodology for the structure and functioning of a *public* department to examine wet nurses. Moncorvo proposed statutes for such an organization as well as the components of the medical exam. Thereafter, the doctor installed a small project in his own children's clinic to examine wet nurses, but the initiative quickly failed for lack of funding. Moncorvo's son, Dr. Moncorvo Filho, would later realize the wet nurse examination program in Rio de Janeiro—once again from a private clinic.[60]

Back in Salvador, and at the insistence of the local medical community, the city government attempted widespread measures to address the fear of domestic servants. In the 1880s, this meant controlling domestic labor and formalizing relations between patrons and servants as slavery rapidly diminished in the city. In 1887, the city council approved a measure that would require the official registration and certification of all domestic servants. Every "free or freed" person wishing to work in household service was to be recorded in a police registry and to receive a passbook, renewed annually at the domestic's expense.[61] The surviving records indicate that nearly eight hundred persons registered between 1887 and 1893. The registration process required domestics to provide the name and address of their current employer, presumably as documentation of a binding agreement and possibly as a tracking method should he or she need to find a new position.

The act determined special provisions and punishments related to disease. Any person determined to suffer from a contagious disease or to "cause repugnance" was denied enrollment in the registry. Any wet nurse found to have intentionally hidden a disease would be fined 20$000 milreis or sentenced to four days' imprisonment.[62] The council designated a local physician to conduct medical inspections of potential wet nurses. Though it seems that the city government never consistently carried out these inspections, the provisions demonstrated that public authorities considered disease to be a criminal issue. To reduce transmission of disease, servants, particularly those caring for children, had to be tightly controlled and subject to medical surveillance and police authority. Representatives of both medicine and law enforcement asserted authority to read the visual signs of danger on the servant body.

Registration resembled a criminal process or perhaps was reminiscent of the old inspections of the slave auction. In addition to age, marital status, and parentage, the registrars noted the characteristics of each domestic servant, including detailed physical descriptions and any suspicion of disease. They noted identifying marks such as freckles, scars, and missing teeth. In 1887, seventeen-year-old Lourença Ritta Epiphania, an *ama secca* (or dry nurse), was only given the description of having "signs of smallpox on her face." Andreza Maria da Conceição, twenty-four years old in 1893 and daughter of an *africana* called Leopoldina (no surname given to connote enslaved), worked as a *criada* and was described as "black, medium stature, long face, black eyes, sparse eyebrows, course hair, large flat nose, large mouth, with missing upper teeth." Jovita Candida Ribeiro, a twenty-nine-year-old *ama secca*, was identified as "*cabra* [brown], regular stature, oval face, black eyes, regular eyebrows, course hair, thin nose, large mouth, freckled face" and registered in April of 1887. Maria dos Praseres da Conceição, age twenty-four, was an *ama de leite*, or wet nurse: "black, tall stature, long face, large black eyes, regular eyebrows, course hair, flat nose, large mouth and white teeth." Adelaide Maria dos Prazeres, daughter of Esperança (another *africana* with no surname), enrolled in 1887 at thirty years of age, having also worked as an *ama de leite*. The registrar described Adelaide as "black, regular stature, round face, black eyes, regular eyebrows, course black hair, flat nose, regular mouth with some lower teeth missing, no unique features, does not know how to read."[63]

These detailed descriptions and codifications were meant to afford some guarantee of suitability for service. With the patron's name to verify gainful employment and "*bons costumes*" (good habits) and a physical inspection to validate a healthy appearance, the city's registry offered both a moral and a corporal guarantee. According to Walter Fraga Filho, the legislation and registry were the city's response to the *famílias baianas* who insisted on a control mechanism and an assurance of labor to replace the dying master-slave relationship. That this control was medicalized is a telling sign of shifting times, illustrating the growing influence of medicine on state policy, the entrance of public authority into private family issues, and, importantly, the overlap of these two processes with the deconstruction of slavery. The council registered hundreds of domestic servants, but Salvador was a large urban center by the 1880s. Only a small fraction of the total population of domestic laborers presented themselves for registration. Apparently, neither domestics nor their patrons judged the registration as essential to household service.

Thus, the uncertainties of emancipation spurred a preoccupation with maintaining order amid transition and promoting scientifically defined "racial" progress. Within household labor, controlled transition meant continued control over black women's bodies—their sexuality, their reproduction, and how their child-rearing expertise would be appropriated for children other than their own. Control of black women's bodies was policy inherited from a long legacy of American slavery in Brazil and elsewhere. As the century concluded, physicians coupled these old ideas with modern ideas about the need for medical and state authority to supersede patriarchal household management. They asserted that the traditional patriarchal style of social control was insufficient to address scientific problems like disease and infant mortality and incapable of placing Brazil on the path to societal advancement. When physicians argued that the *mãe preta* posed a disease threat for *famílias baianas*, they offered themselves as the most educated and rational experts for a modern society.

The Mãe Desnaturada

The notion of motherhood as the most natural, predestined, or ultimate expression of womanhood long predates the nineteenth century. To literary, folkloric, and religious understandings, ideas about motherhood as womanhood found new idioms in scientific and medical rationale in the 1800s. Physicians at both Brazilian medical schools sought to define the parameters of the healthy exercise of motherhood. Defining motherhood was an active cultural and political process for other reasons as well. Debates around the 1871 Free Womb Law, for example, politicized the question of enslaved mothers' right to cohabitation with their minor children and freed children's right to the maternal breast. Meanwhile, there was an explosion of literature narrating tragic stories of foundling children who had been rejected by their mothers, denied their birthrights, and raised without knowing their social place. The Free Womb Law and these fictitious narratives centered on the relationship between mothers and children as an integral part of social relations, legal and patriarchal structures of power, and the proper ordering or functioning of society. Far from simply a reflection of abstract theorizing or artistic creativity, the implications of the Free Womb Law had enormous impact on the lives of enslaved families.[64] At the same time, Brazil did have a serious foundling problem, as each year thousands of mothers and fathers found themselves unable or unwilling to raise their children, and most of these cases did in fact end quite tragically for those children. Novelists fictionalized this very real problem and envisioned all manner of links between slavery, race, women's honor, and child abandonment.[65]

Therefore, the stakes in these imaginings of motherhood were high, and physicians were not the only ones engaged in defining, denigrating, or defending women's roles as mothers.

The "unnatural failure" that most related to Bahia's public health system concerned the hundreds of mothers who turned over custody of their infants to the Santa Casa de Misericórdia yearly to be raised as foundlings. Brazilians used two interchangeable terms for foundlings, either *"crianças enjeitadas,"* rejected or abandoned children, or *"crianças expostas,"* which translates more closely to "foundlings," that is, children found alone and exposed to the elements. In Salvador, residents recounted terrible scenes of infants discovered in the streets, at the shore, and on the doorsteps of churches and convents. Both *"enjeitado"* and *"exposto"* connoted a broken or failed bond between mother and child. The assumption was that a mother had ejected her child from the safety of family life and social identity, refusing motherhood and defying her "nature." It is difficult to know much about the mothers or fathers whose children ended up in the custody of the Misericórdia's Foundling Home due to the anonymous process of depositing children through the infamous turning wheel. Following Portuguese traditions, Brazilian society had always attempted to protect these children but with limited success. Census data annually classified hundreds of children as foundlings in Brazil. Both the Bahian and Rio de Janeiro Foundling Homes regularly took in children, but they endured short, wretched lives more often than they survived into adulthood. In Bahia, for example, the Misericórdia "found" 58 children in 1852, of whom 24 had died by March of 1853.[66] In the first half of 1877, the Home took in 49 children, who joined a population of 248. Within those six months, 19 of the new arrivals were deceased.[67] The overall numbers are staggering; the two Misericórdias of Salvador da Bahia and Rio de Janeiro recorded a total of 50,000 foundling children between them over the course of the colonial and imperial periods.[68]

Historians have dedicated much of the research on foundlings to understanding why mothers willingly gave up custody of their children to unknown persons or to the anonymous foundling wheels. Issues of honor, illness, and poverty explain the great majority of these cases, though the "urgent need to conceal" has certainly received the most scholarly attention.[69] This was also the explanation that most contemporary observers understood to be the root of the foundling problem. Because the majority of children left in the foundling wheel in Salvador were white (50%–60%), race has been the primary evidence in histories that see issues of honor and shame as the motive for separations of infants from their birth families.[70] The maintenance of familial honor and consequences for its erosion fell disproportionately on women. Families of means carefully guarded the chastity, morality, and sexuality of women, and individual women's behaviors were considered to reflect on the honor of an entire family. Enforcing female honor, through social convention or violence, was one way that elites distinguished between common folk and *gente decente*. It is certainly imaginable, therefore, that women of status would resort to leaving a child in the foundling wheel rather than endure the repercussions of having an illegitimate child.

This explanation, however, supposes that white skin and wealth were synonymous in eighteenth- and nineteenth-century Brazil, which they were not—highly correlated, undoubtedly, but not synonymous. It also presumes that the absence of children of color reflected a lesser significance placed on honor among the majority population. Rather, in chapter 3, I argue that mothers of color were less likely to turn to the Misericórdia until the dawn of the twentieth century because of the persistence of slavery. Brazilian newspapers commonly carried scandalous stories of foundlings who, though free by law, were fostered to dishonest caretaker families and later sold as slaves. Bahian newspapers of the period attest to the sale of newborns and infants. Thus, free black mothers understood the real possibility that their children could be enslaved, and they likely were reluctant to turn to this option to protect their children. When children of color were left in the foundling wheel, they were at times accompanied by notes testifying to their "free" status or, in some cases, explicitly certifying that the child was white. Therefore, it is important to contextualize issues of honor and shame in terms of class and the diversity of life experiences that befell women in nineteenth-century Salvador. The ideal of the secluded Christian mother was merely that. The vast majority of Brazilian women, regardless of color, did not conform to the expectations of the elite class, and this was common knowledge.

Physicians charged the mothers of foundlings with immorality, adultery, and irresponsibility and had comparatively little to say about the fathers. Contemporary observers concurred that any mother who willingly left her child "abandoned" or "exposed" placed no value on the child's life and did so to unburden herself of a "problematic" birth, leaving the child to endure a solitary life on the margins of society. For nineteenth-century physicians, anonymous abandonment was a necessary evil. Society needed such a system to protect the honor of disgraced women and their families. By leaving the child to religious charity, both mother and baby could be saved from social death and infanticide, respectively. At the School of Medicine, physicians largely agreed that these children were "the products of error" whose secrecy should be safeguarded so as to maintain family honor—the basis of Bahian society.[71]

The crux of their discourse was an attempt to draw together an idealized and medicalized prescription for motherhood as a practice with the needs and expectations of a changing society. Physicians agreed with their contemporaries in the political and literary worlds that there was something about the relationship between mothers and children, and the rearing of children in general, that was or should provide stability amid change. Where women did not conform "appropriately" to the role of mother or refused it outright, physicians saw pathology. They redefined the failure to mother as a medical problem, an internal deficiency. The "denatured mother" was a failed woman; failing was not an action but a characteristic. Ultimately, physicians and reformists understood mothering—birthing, breast-feeding, and rearing—to be an innate attribute of healthy womanhood. Women who did not breast-feed or raise their children refused their duty as women, rejecting "the supreme and most noble sentiments that the Creator implanted in their hearts."[72] According to this logic, only "true mothers" completed their function through the care and nurturing they provided; those who did not were simply "half mothers."

This explanation of mothers and foundlings serves to distinguish the actual complex history of this issue from its cultural and medical imaginary. "Denatured mothers" and their natural children played a critical role in the development of public health strategies. In many ways, Bahian *puericultores* saw their objective as one of repairing the damaged relationships between these mothers and children to the greater good of their families and society at large. Ideologically, reformists encouraged a specific vision of dutiful motherhood primarily in the form of maternal nursing; distrusting the advice of midwives, servants, and others outside the biomedical community; and prioritizing the bond between mother and child over all other interests or responsibilities.

The Curiosa

In Brazil, as in most places, female midwives were the authorities on birthing in the nineteenth century, and there is really nothing curious about that. Bahian women trusted in their expertise, and women who sought out physicians often did so only upon the appearance of complications. Hospitalization options were restricted and undesirable. Birthing at home with a midwife to assist was customary, even for families of means. Biomedical assistance often was a subsequent or final alternative. Bahian midwives typically saw their profession as a spiritual calling. Prayer and invocation to the saints were common responses to difficult births and integral elements of the practice. By fulfilling these spiritual and health functions, midwives were cherished community members who were not easily displaced from their roles. Thus, women, and women of color in particular, had power over the world of healing.[73] In Bahia, midwives tended to be poor *mulata* women who were recognized in the streets by their black clothing and mantillas.[74] A few white, immigrant midwives belonged to the "professional" sector, but no single individual had as much prominence as Madame Durocher in Rio de Janeiro, for example.[75] What Bahia did have was a long-established tradition of spiritual healing and female authority in the *terreiros*—an authority that included birthing but was not limited to it. Within the world of healing, hierarchies of color, class, religious orthodoxy, and gender were perhaps not completely overturned but were at least fundamentally challenged.

Like wet nurses, midwives became the focus of much medical concern in nineteenth-century Bahia. Also like wet nursing, midwifery was nothing new when physicians took notice. Brazilian physicians collectively had little direct experience with birthing and tended to believe foreign travelers' assertions that "tropical women," both Africans and Indians, gave birth more easily than Europeans and did not require assistance. Supposedly, "civilization" and lives of luxury and ease caused women to experience painful and difficult labors. Given these stereotypes, the Brazilian medical community saw nothing of interest in the birthing process and made few attempts to compete with midwives until the second half of the century.[76]

Midwifery, then, took on new meanings, which drew medical attention. Physicians charged that the reliance on midwifery signified Bahian backwardness. For them, midwives were incompetent and treacherous, like wet nurses, but midwives were also worrisome because they practiced independently rather than attached to households under the regular supervision of male patrons. Midwives posed the greatest competition for influence over women's and children's health and became symbolic of the conquest of "scientific rationality" over "charlatanism." The popularity of local midwives presented a formidable obstacle to Bahian physicians who hoped to become the predominant health-care providers for pregnant women, mothers, and children. This was a worldwide trend by the late 1800s as male physicians gradually replaced female midwives in providing birthing assistance and women's health care. Competing with midwives formed part of the professionalization of biomedicine in general—that is, the formal specialization among physicians, surgeons, and pharmacists and the more rigid distinction from competing traditions of treating the body. In this climate where the nation's future depended on the health and number of its citizens, according to many, these issues were not to be left to popular cures, religious authorities, and "uneducated" women.

In the 1850s, Bahia's Tropicalista School attempted to seize birthing from the traditional realm of midwifery. For the Tropicalistas, medical professionalization would involve secularization, experimentation, and specialization—all bolstered by replacing "superstition" with reason. Consequently, these physicians saw folk midwives as representing everything wrong in Brazilian medicine, given their lack of biomedical training, the recognized authority of women in matters of health and well-being, and the spiritual and religious nature of their practices. The Tropicalistas decried this situation in their *Gazeta Médica da Bahia*, asserting that midwives' techniques caused infection, injury, and death in cases where biomedicine would have offered cures. Folk midwives, Tropicalistas wrote, were responsible for the high incidence of stillbirth and maternal fatalities during labor. Beyond incompetence, they also accused midwives of practicing abortions and assisting with infanticide. Some went as far as to label midwives "angel-makers," presuming that midwifery cost infant lives.[77] In fact, medical literature attributed abortions to two sources: midwives and practitioners of Candomblé, "*feiticeiros; mães e pães de terreiros*."[78] For physicians, it was in the *terreiro*, where debauchery and sinister African practices reigned, that all manner of crimes were planned and committed to the beat of the *batuque*.

As with the wet nurse, with the "superstitious midwife," Bahian physicians struck at larger societal problems—as they conceived them. For critics, inferior and treacherous birthing practices were simply symptomatic of a disordered and backward society. Poor women, women of color, and women's knowledge—characterized as literally life threatening and symbolically impeding national development—were entry points for effecting a widespread reordering. Though the medical profession was growing in prestige, Bahian women were hardly likely to turn to clinical birth simply because physicians insisted on it. Furthermore, unlike the government of Rio de Janeiro, the Bahian provincial government did not allocate resources or implement surveillance measures to combat midwifery.[79] Thus, the Tropicalistas represented a bit of a vanguard, urging a transition to biomedical birthing long before any institutional apparatus existed to support the change.

The Pai dos Pobres

All of these female tropes demonstrate an attempt to explicitly define the boundaries of proper and improper motherhood in relation to society and to classify motherhood and child rearing as objects for medical study and intervention. These discussions of motherhood also reconceptualized masculinity, patriarchy, and men's roles in modern families. In many maternalist debates, the relationship between women, fathers, and male heads of household was implicit or assumed. If anything, physicians' notions of scientific family dynamics undermined cultural understandings of patriarchy; physicians advocated for inserting themselves and the state over the traditional rights exercised by men and men of means in particular. However, in this society, patriarchy—like motherhood—was not a given. Some members of society had always enjoyed the right to exercise patriarchy or maternity in full, and others saw their rights mitigated or denied outright by class or legal status. So there were complex gendered variables at play in these debates. Ultimately, the modern version of motherhood, though it took an accusatory tone toward many women, led to dramatic changes in Bahia's public health infrastructure. These transitions created a vastly different institutional landscape in the twentieth century than that of the mid-1800s, when health institutions were few and far between and those catering specifically to women and children were nonexistent.

Patriarchy politics and nationalism became most salient in the Getúlio Vargas administration (1930–1945), a symbolic and functional union of working families with the "Father of the Poor." Vargas promoted a working-class patriarchy that did not fit neatly into Bahian maternalism. Nevertheless, President Vargas's "politics of the working man" reinforced the indispensable element of institutional and individual patronage of the cause of family welfare. As Brazil's welfare state grew, so did opportunities for public cooperation with influential private benefactors. These partnerships were already a reality in Bahian maternalism and had been for decades. Federal interest in poor fatherhood and poor families brought Bahian maternalist programs and their spokespeople into a national network. Patronage ties solidified local and national organizations and helped procure funding for public health and welfare services. Brazil's blend of public and private patronage muddied the waters between a formalized, institutionalized welfare state and acts of charity by the wealthy and powerful few.

THE CAST OF FEMALE AND MALE CHARACTERS THAT populated medical discourse of the nineteenth century illustrated Bahia's struggle with persistence and change. Health and sanitation conditions were still precarious, infant mortality was still high, no children's or women's clinical facilities existed other than a small birthing room, and the government devoted few resources to public health. Meanwhile, families continued to depend on household domestics, midwives delivered most babies, and the nuns at the Santa Casa de Misericórdia took in hundreds of foundling children. However, these persistent characteristics of life for Brazil's "Old Mammy" increasingly appeared unacceptable to those who desired family dynamics and local infrastructure to reflect a more evident break between imperial society and the modern republic on the horizon. Yet physicians only conceived of social change within acceptable boundaries, and older ideas and assumptions around race, gender, and class largely mitigated those boundaries. Therefore, medical and cultural biases intertwined in the construction of these symbolic gendered characters. These gendered characters also provide a starting point for analyzing the actual experiences of families, particularly women and children, in health and welfare institutions. Although reformers may have catered their intentions to imaginary women, the construction of institutions and women's roles in that process were multifaceted and complex.

In sum, thinking about wet nurses, midwives, unnatural mothers, patriarchs, and the "modernizing" state opens many threads to follow. As argued here, international, especially French, medical dialogues helped inspire concern with Brazilian mothers and babies. However, maternalism in medicine and the cultural imaginary was rooted in Brazilian realities—though not a mirror reflection of them. Mothers and children, understood as a type of shorthand for discussing the population and national identity in general, were wrapped up in anxieties about political and social change in the wake of liberalism, abolition, and republicanism. Slavery, abolition, race, and degeneracy dominated social ideas of the period, and social medicine proved no exception. Medicalization of the family offered a new conceptualization of society's past and its future. Moving beyond the symbolic, maternalism resulted in the creation of myriad institutions and programs in Bahia and across Brazil at the dawn of the twentieth century, once medical interest met financial resources (mostly in the form of elite patronage) and political will. Having established the intellectualism and cultural imaginings behind the maternalist movement, I now move on to the early years of the republic to explore family and professional experiences in the public health system, the medicalization of society, the changing nature of the state, and the enduring importance of race and gender in modern welfare policy.

CHAPTER TWO

Domestic Health Care

THE *MÃE PRETA*

INETEENTH-CENTURY BRAZILIAN PHYSICIANS COUN-seled against the dangers of black maternity in servitude. They worried over the alleged incapacities of the *mãe preta*, in particular, and the risks she posed to the health of privileged children. The term *"mãe preta"* is close in meaning to the English "mammy." It literally translates to "black mother," referring to female domestics' role in nursing and raising their patrons' children as well as the assumed bond of affection between "black mother" and "white child."[1] By the opening decades of the twentieth century, black maternity began to take on new meanings in the popular imagination and in medicine. New cultural ideas placed the symbolic black wet nurse as a positive element in Brazil's national family history, while Bahian medicine targeted black maternity/popular maternity as the key site for improving the well-being of local children. Even in everyday discourse, the *mãe preta* became increasingly politicized, such that one scholar has characterized the popular literature of the period through the appearance and elevation of the beloved mammy.[2] The common thread among these reimaginings of black maternity is that the mothering activities of women of color held a special relevance to society at large. Furthermore, the folkloric view, with all its patronizing and reductionist tone, continued to associate women of color with domestic service because the real-life contemporary connection between black maternity and servitude was inescapable. Social hierarchies, limited educational and economic opportunities, and inequalities of race and gender ensured that women of color overwhelmingly labored in household service long after abolition. In this chapter, I argue that the institutionalization of maternalism, while connected to international dialogues, revealed expanding federal directives, local socioeconomic realities, and Bahia's racialized cultural politics. The shifts and stagnations in international, national, and local political terrains directly bore upon the creation of maternal and child services and helped frame the experiences of mothers of color (the *mães pretas*) and their families.

This chapter picks up where the previous one closed, with the early years of the republic and the ascension of poor motherhood into both a nationally debated problem and a springboard for the institutionalization of family health and welfare services. It ends in the 1930s, by which time the Bahian maternalist movement had fully institutionalized. Though the analysis begins in 1904 when the first maternalist organization opened, three anecdotes from the tail end of the period help situate the transformations and continuities that brought maternalism into the twentieth century. These episodes from 1933 evidence how older patterns intensified in the new century while others were rigorously challenged. First and most widely known, the sociologist Gilberto Freyre penned his celebrated *Casa-grande e senzala* in 1933, translated as *The Masters and the Slaves*. *The Masters and the Slaves* was an extensive exploration of the roots of the Brazilian "character," which Freyre located in the historical experience of master-slave relations on the colonial and imperial plantation. Condensing a complex text into a few lines, Freyre asserted that Portuguese culture and the (forcible) incorporation of Indians and Africans made Brazil particularly open to developing a new type of society. Unlike the race-based violence and segregation plaguing the United States, of which Freyre was a firsthand witness, Brazil had escaped the long-term negative effects of slavery by blending diverse elements into one. Each "original race" made its own indispensable contribution, and the resultant biological, social, and cultural fusion produced all that was unique and authentic in Brazilian society. All of this gave Brazilians a fundamental commonality and created a distinctive type of democracy.

Freyre's notion of a raceless Brazilian nationalism distorted both history and reality, and the author remained openly skeptical of the ability of the poor to participate fully as citizens. The extremely influential concept of racial democracy has had its many critics over the years, and rightfully so. It is the process Freyre formulated to explain Brazil's distinctive miscegenation that relates to this chapter, however. Freyre wrote, "Miscegenation, widely practiced here, corrected the social distance that would have been enormous otherwise between the big house and the tropical forest, between the big house and the slave quarters."[3] Brazil's very nature was conceived in intimate relations between masters and slaves, the most significant of which were sexual and matriarchal, according to the author. Sexual relations between male masters and female domestic slaves, on the one hand, and the intense attachment between white children and black wet nurses (the *mães pretas*), on the other, "corrected the social distance" and made Brazil's *mestiço* society possible. As that corrective bridge, black and brown women's bodies played an essential role in crafting society, though mainly through coercion, as Freyre acknowledged. The *mãe preta* was particularly suited to her station in the author's view: "Brazilian tradition leaves us in no doubt . . . when it comes to a wet nurse, there is none like a Negro woman."[4] Freyre did not invent these ideas out of whole cloth; this articulation of the black wet nurse as the elemental unifier in Brazilian nationality predated *The Masters and the Slaves*. Yet he was the most prominent and remembered member of a generation of scholars and artists who valorized Afro-Brazilian, indigenous, and popular culture.

In that same year of 1933, Brazil's intellectual community was engaged in contemporary issues facing mothers and children. At the Second National Child Protection Conference, physicians, jurists, and educators debated a range of topics related to children, from prenatal health to adolescent delinquency. Four physicians composed the Bahian delegation, including the state's most illustrious *puericultores*, Dr. Martagão Gesteira and Dr. Álvaro Bahia. The doctors' presence reflected their distinguished reputations and the fact that Bahian physicians had participated in international conferences of this type for decades. Brazil, however, was only recently in the business of hosting congresses on topics related to children, a result of growing interest in healthy children for a stronger nation. Since the advent of Brazil's republican government, public health, sanitation, and hygiene had received unprecedented institutional and bureaucratic attention. The Bahian doctors well represented how physicians saw these issues in their home state as they emphasized reducing childhood mortality through preventative medicine and directed welfare programs.

Dr. Gesteira spoke about the disastrous institutionalization experiences that befell Brazil's large population of foundling children and the need to mobilize to prevent the separation of mothers and children due to familial poverty. For his contribution, Dr. Bahia presented the importance of medically supervised free milk dispensaries. These services could facilitate maternal nursing by assisting working mothers who often simply did not have the time to stay at home and breast-feed. Mothers' milk was the linchpin of the problem, the solution to impoverished children's deprivation and high mortality rates. It was even the key to the foundling problem, according to the doctors, because mothers with help to stay at home were less likely to need the institutional option. In sum, Bahia's delegation put poor mothers at the center of their arguments and proposals. And as everyone was well aware, this population had a color. As one Bahian physician in attendance argued, "The *mestiço* population . . . and the black population constitute the great majority of the poor classes, the most destitute of comforts and of hygiene, and therefore, the most plagued by misery, ignorance, and sickness."[5] Black and brown mothers must be the priority of health and welfare reforms, physicians asserted, and ensuring that they could breast-feed their children should be a major initiative.

As Freyre, Gesteira, and others theorized about mothers real and symbolic, twenty-year-old Marciana Maria Conceição and twenty-four-year-old Maria Silva made their first visits to the prenatal clinic at the Third Health Post in Salvador. In that same month of December 1933, twenty-seven-year-old Francisca Pereira de Sousa made the same decision, and Francisca brought along her two-year-old daughter, Nilza, for a well-baby visit.[6] All three women lived in the working-class "Lower City" neighborhoods of Salvador. By 1933, preventative consultations for expectant mothers and young children were not such exceptional experiences. Dozens of mothers walked into these clinics daily to take advantage of free health-care options. More than seven thousand expectant mothers used the clinics in 1933, in fact. Like many prenatal clients and mothers of well babies, Marciana Conceição, Maria Silva, and Francisca Sousa were *mães pretas* in a double sense. They helped support their families by serving in the households of others, as did tens of thousands of Bahian women: preparing meals, cleaning, running errands, and caring for children. However, these women had their own familial responsibilities and their own children waiting at home. They likely had a different perspective on domestic labor and servant-patron relations than did Gilberto Freyre.

Certainly, Conceição, Silva, and Sousa were too young to have memories of slavery, but Freyre argued that patriarchal relations, inherited from the *casa-grande/senzala* complex, continued to anchor Brazilian social relations. What Freyre could not have known in 1933 was how profoundly influential his "social democracy" would become. While Freyre argued for the historical importance of the *mãe preta*, physicians like Gesteira and Bahia argued for the significance of black and brown mothers to Brazil's present and its future. Both versions of black motherhood were presumptuous and patronizing, but they were elements of an ideological and institutional shift that opened opportunities for families that would not have been available when Marciana Conceição's, Maria Silva's, and Francisca Sousa's mothers were raising children.

Although Brazilian society had not undergone a radical reshuffling, something fundamental had changed in the decades since the close of the nineteenth century, and intellectuals, physicians, and everyday families all played a part. New ideas brought increased support, and physicians were finally able to manifest their concerns in concrete programs. There was a growing consensus beyond medicine that "bettering" the average citizen could revitalize the nation. This consensus over population reform brought financial support, media attention, scientific and sanitary missions, and new legislation. The federal policies and projects born out of that context are an essential legacy of the First Republic. Medical interest in mothers and children led to an unparalleled institutionalization of Brazilian health and welfare services beginning in the 1890s and continuing well into the 1940s. Interestingly, in Bahia, as the infant and maternal health and welfare movement grew, the targets for reform were the female domestics who had been so vilified in the medical literature of the previous century. Poor women's status had not changed with abolition and republicanism, as poverty, racial prejudice, and gender-role constraints ensured that women of color found few employment opportunities beyond domestic service and informal market activities. This time, however, physicians acknowledged poor women as mothers rather than focusing exclusively on their duties as caretakers to their charges.

Brazil's "Old Black Mammy" exemplified a few different trends at once, some in the world of ideas and others that were grounded in day-to-day realities. This chapter plays with two concepts of black maternity, using them to describe an underlying tension between the lingering notion of black maternity as servitude and the new emphasis on poor mothers' health and welfare. Linking the two was mothers' milk, adding more irony to the *mãe preta* as wet nurse versus the *mãe preta* as domestic servant with her own infants to feed at home. In Brazil, the topic of wet nursing was full of cultural, historical, and ideological baggage; thus it proves impossible to disentangle the interwoven threads of race, gender, servitude, and nation within the quest for healthier mothers and babies. While the double entendre frames the discussion, this chapter explains the nuts and bolts of health institutions: their trajectory, staff, patients, and programs. To explicate the institutionalization of maternalism in Brazil and to place poor families at the center of these developments requires an initial turn to the intellectual and political context of the early republic.

A VAST HOSPITAL: NEW IDEAS FOR A NEW CENTURY

Contemplating the end of monarchy and both promising directions and worrisome alternatives for restructuring society encouraged a proliferation of new ideas at the dawn of the new century. These ideologies helped set the stage for women's and children's health and welfare to be institutionalized. As reformists increasingly agreed that racial composition was not the nation's primary "obstacle," they turned their attention to environmental problems like public health. Rather than refute foreign accusations of backwardness head-on, Brazilian reformists redefined the cause. Illness became a defining feature of "authentic" Brazilianness, in fact. Brazil was a "vast hospital" in the infamous words of Miguel Pereira of the Rio de Janeiro School of Medicine, but systematic, government-led interventions held the promise of curing the entire nation. The federalism of the First Republic challenged these grand visions of state intervention in public health. Nonetheless, this period solidified the transition from a nineteenth-century explicit discourse on race to a twentieth-century one emphasizing public health and education as cooperative missions of state and society.

Despite the turning tide, this conception of health retained a number of elements from the older discourse of race. Like race, reformers conceived of health as an inheritable quality, a generational familial truth expressed as either sound (among the privileged) or defective (among the marginal). Health was a quality to be preserved and protected from deleterious influence. Brazilian eugenics also supported this perspective. Like most Latin American eugenicists, Brazilians generally subscribed to a French-style eugenics based on the theories of the biologist Jean-Baptiste Pierre Antoine de Monet, the Chevalier of Lamarck. Neo-Lamarckian eugenics held that traits acquired during the human life span could become hereditary, and therefore, individual behaviors and bodily conditions could influence successive generations of the bloodline. More than a specific set of theories, eugenics became an overarching conception in Brazil. As an illustration of this ambiguity, "eugenics" was often conflated with "hygiene," "sanitation," or "preventative medicine." Consequently, individual and community health, like race in an older conception, could impact the nation as a whole; health thus played a prominent role in defining Brazil itself.

In some ways, therefore, one may understand health in this context as a reinvention or reimagining of race. Health became another framework through which to theorize the nation, its history, and its inhabitants, but there were two crucial differences. First, according to eugenicists, health was malleable and could be improved though successive generations. Racial thinking pushed forward in this direction as well. This focus on improvement meant localized health issues were social problems, and health experts, social engineers. Second, health concerns could easily be translated into concrete arenas for institutional action—at least on paper. As a result, the turn of the century witnessed an unparalleled creation of public institutions devoted to poor women and children as a starting point for effecting widespread generational social change. These were the first tangible manifestations of the maternalist movement.

These ideological shifts occurred within a political climate in which the responsibilities of the state to its citizenry were being redefined. Prior to the republic, local and federal governments, when not completely absent, represented primarily an agent of coercion for the majority of Brazilians. Where the state was meant to provide services, such as sanitation and arbitration, it was notoriously inadequate. With the decentralized federation and the promulgation of the 1891 Constitution, Brazilian states took responsibility for many functions, including public health, while navigating the complication of constitutionally guaranteed municipal autonomy. Federalism, a conquest of the First Republic's liberal instigators, further entrenched regional discrepancies between wealthy and poor states, sparsely populated and highly populous states, strong economies and weaker ones, and states with the infrastructure and political capital to carry out public projects and those with neither. This last point proved especially impactful for public health. Throughout the republic, health care and social assistance remained a mix of private and charitable initiatives under state authority, partially funded by governmental subventions. The republican context saw the rise of new partnerships and agendas, such as medicalization and maternalism, reflecting and reinforcing the larger consensus on the exigency of population reform.

Bahian public health reform began in earnest with Governor Joaquim Manoel Rodrigues Lima (a physician), who administered the state from 1892 to 1896, and his successors Luiz Vianna (1896–1900) and Severino Vieira (1900–1904). All three inaugurated new institutions and restructured old entities. Nevertheless, Bahian public health and sanitation efforts suffered from redundancy, inefficiency, and inter-institutional jockeying between state and municipal jurisdictions.[7] By the end of Vieira's tenure in 1904, Bahian maternalism bore the first fruits of institutionalization. Over the subsequent decades of the republic, Bahia transformed from a state with no specialized facilities to the home of a number of prenatal, well-baby, and children's health and welfare programs. That average people could extract benefits from their government was a watershed change from the oppressive slave society that had existed a few decades prior. At no point were services sufficient to meet the health and welfare necessities of all those in need, but the programs that did exist filled an essential void.

As the century opened and progressed, the Bahian maternalist movement expanded to regard maternal health on a grand scale. Different from the literature of the 1800s, physicians no longer wrote of black maternity primarily as wet nursing—as irresponsible, untrustworthy, and African servitude. Rather they regarded poor women as mothers in their own right, raising their own children as their first priority. From reformists' perspective, the national significance of these women was not in their being domestic workers, but mothers, because Brazil needed healthy families and health progeny of all classes. This included the poorest classes, whose children would eventually make up Brazil's agricultural and industrial workforce. Physicians still held poor women liable for the illnesses and early deaths of their own children, similar to the accusations leveled at the wet nurses of the previous century. However, physicians and their bureaucratic allies charged themselves with creating institutions that would improve the health of poor families. While Freyre "rescued" the "black mother" of old, the Bahian health system connected to mothers of the modern period. The dangerous mammy of the nineteenth century became the mother-client of the early twentieth whose child-rearing efforts were offered as a service to the nation. Slippage still occurred between the "mammy" and the "mother," so even the new conception did not completely break with the past. Yet these changing concepts had vital real-life consequences for how average people, particularly poor black and brown families, were incorporated into the private and state-funded clinical institutions. This was the context families confronted when they chose to seek medical assistance at the new institutions.

BAHIA'S FIRST MATERNALIST PROGRAMS, 1904–1935

The emergence of Bahia's maternalist organizations fell in line with trends in Brazil's other center of medicine, the federal capital of Rio de Janeiro. In both cities, small groups of well-known and indefatigable physicians concretized their concerns over maternal and child health, epitomizing a version of "medical philanthropy" typical of the early century.[8] In Rio, Dr. Carlos Arthur Moncorvo Filho founded the Childhood Protection and Assistance Institute, or Instituto de Protecção e Assistencia á Infancia (IPAI) in 1889, and it became a model institution with affiliates across Brazil. Moncorvo Filho was the son of Dr. Carlos Arthur Moncorvo, the "Father of Brazilian Pediatrics," who had established a general children's clinic in 1880, likely the first of its kind in the nation. The junior Moncorvo trained in his father's polyclinic, as did Arthur Fernandes Figueira, and the two became leading names in mothers', children's, and familial health. Rio de Janeiro gained additional services shortly after the IPAI opened, with the opening of the Polyclinic at Botafogo (founded in 1899 by Luiz Barbosa, another student of Carlos Moncorvo), the Laranjeiras Maternity Center (1904), and the Children's Polyclinic at the Santa Casa de Misericórdia do Rio de Janeiro (founded in 1909 by Fernandes Figueira). Laranjeiras warrants an additional note; it was established under the auspices of Minister of Justice and the Interior José Joaquim Seabra, who became governor of Bahia eight years later.

The IPAI was the most comprehensive, offering free health services but maintaining more of a focus on treatment rather than prevention. It opened before Pinard defined *"puériculture"* in France, but through the years, the IPAI incorporated trademark puericulture programs such as wet nurse registration, healthy baby contests, and the *gotta de leite*, or milk depot.[9] In fact, its timeline demonstrates that child protection had become an international issue, thanks largely to nineteenth-century reformers, even before the scientific community developed theories such as puericulture to advance it. Although the *carioca* IPAI and the later Bahian one did incorporate well-baby care, both institutions performed more treatments than consultations and worked with older children, not restricting themselves to prenatal and infant care as puericulture programs generally did.

A group of Bahian physicians was motivated to re-create the IPAI after a local newspaper published a series of biting critiques in March 1903 about the lack of such programs in the state. Within three months, its author, Dr. Joaquim Tanajura; the renowned pediatrician Dr. Alfredo Ferreira de Magalhães; and other colleagues wrote the statutes for a Bahian branch of the IPAI. The founders lamented the dearth of children's health institutions and the lack of governmental attention, much less funding, for this matter. Magalhães assumed the directorship and ultimately would be remembered as a founding father of Bahian children's medicine. Tanajura left Bahia soon thereafter to tackle the integration of the hinterlands, family health's twin in the population reform projects of the First Republic. He became medical director of the Rondon Commission, a military mission charged with constructing telegraph lines and contacting indigenous peoples in the Amazon.[10] Back in Salvador da Bahia, the IPAI pledged to "protect the poor, sick, defective, morally mistreated, abandoned, etc., children of this capital."[11] Like Moncorvo Filho's institute, the Bahian chapter hoped to encourage breast-feeding and regulate wet nursing; investigate living conditions; offer hygiene education; regulate women's employment outside the home; and promote the establishment of maternity wards, daycares, and parks.

The IPAI's Children's Clinic opened its doors on May 13, 1904. Within the first two years of service, hundreds of Bahian families sought medical attention for their sick children as the clinic served more than two thousand children. Service was free of charge, thus the majority of these children came from Bahia's poorer families. Clinical staff attended to children of all ages, and those under two composed approximately 40 percent of the patients. Most families would learn that their sons and daughters suffered from digestive disturbances—the most common diagnosis made at the clinic, followed by respiratory infections. Physicians generally attributed children's poor nourishment to parental "ignorance" rather than habitual poverty, unsanitary milk, and Salvador's lack of sewers and treated water. The IPAI also distributed thousands of free medications, over ten thousand in its first decade.[12] This distribution was undoubtedly a vital resource for many families. Several years later, Dr. Martagão Gesteira of the Bahian League against Infant Mortality complained that families came to his clinic primarily to request medications. While his Liga intended to provide well-baby care exclusively, most families arrived seeking medications and treatment as well. There was continuity, therefore, in the ways that Bahian families utilized the health resources available to them. Unsurprisingly, well-baby care was not the first priority for poor families, given the formidable odds they faced in just ensuring their young children's survival.

In Rio de Janeiro and Bahia, much more was at stake with the institutionalization of maternalism than simply providing fodder for reformists' lofty imaginations or relevance for a medical specialization seeking its due. Physicians and families mobilized to combat infant mortality because it continued to be a catastrophic problem. In 1904, the same year in which the IPAI was founded, the state recorded 2,337 births, while another 975 children died before reaching age one. Though reliability is questionable with early-century statistics, this number does not seem too far off, as the historian Dain Borges estimated a 300/1,000 infant mortality rate for this period. Bahian sources suggest a 30–40 percent infant mortality rate was also typical for Rio de Janeiro and São Paulo. To contextualize these rates, French sources documented a 150/1,000 infant mortality rate at the turn of the century. In the United States, infant mortality rates varied widely depending on the region, with the lowest rates in the Northeast and West and rates approaching Brazilian statistics in the South. In 1900, the US Department of the Interior registered 170/1,000 for New York City and 136/1,000 for San Francisco, compared to 232/1,000 for Washington, DC; 299/1,000 for Savannah; and 322/1,000 for Charleston. Back in Bahia, stillbirth rates caused concern as well. In the same year of 1904, 118 stillbirths were recorded per 1,000 live births, more than double what physicians recorded for US cities such as New York, Philadelphia, and Boston.[13] When Bahian physicians analyzed infant mortality, they typically included comparative figures to confirm that Salvador's statistics were similar to other Brazilian capitals and that all of Brazil was behind more "civilized" nations. Statistical data, while informative, may veil the human stories behind these events. For poor Bahian women like Marciana Conceição, Maria Silva, and Francisca Sousa from the opening story of this chapter, losing a child was an all too common tragedy. If none of these women had suffered the death of a child, they undoubtedly had relatives, neighbors, or friends who had.

Like many institutions, the IPAI partnered with women's auxiliaries to support patient families. These organizations assisted in ways socially suitable for women of the higher classes, continuing a long legacy of women's charitable assistance work.[14] The IPAI benefited from the support of the Sociedade Beneficente Bello Sexo—the Fairer Sex Beneficent Society—a society of *"mães de família,"* to use Alfredo Ferreira de Magalhães's words, which offered an in-home assistance and birthing program (catering exclusively to *married* poor women) and a clothing program for newborns called "Protecting the Cradle." Sociedade members took responsibility for providing clothing, linens, and supplies for expectant mothers and newborns. Their support allowed the IPAI to expand its reach into family welfare. However, these were comparatively minor aspects of the IPAI's mission, as the institution concentrated on clinical work with children beyond the infancy stage.

Magalhães created a women's auxiliary specifically to aid the IPAI as well. The Damas de Assistencia á Infancia, or Childhood Assistance Ladies, also provided clothing for the mothers and children who used the institute's services. They held Christmas and São João parties for impoverished children and sponsored fund-raising banquets and bazaars. The Damas also maintained an Escola do Lar, a Homemaking School, where they instructed girls of eight to eighteen years of age from the poorest sectors of society. The Escola organizers expected the "advice of sensible, educated *senhoras,* the taste and neatness gained through company with well-educated young women, along with the teacher's lessons, to bring great benefits to the young girls of the *povo.*"[15] This approach to female domestic education was in accord with maternalist objectives in general, which were to "remedy the errors" committed by poor women in child-rearing. On the other end of the spectrum, the Damas were never afforded their own space in the IPAI's journal *O Petiz* or in institutional reports to represent their own work. Dr. Magalhães and the organization itself appear as protagonists, not the women who led the Escola and organized women's charitable contributions. Yet the patriarchal hierarchy and elitist language should not completely negate the positive consequences of their efforts. The Damas' fund-raising was fundamental to Magalhães's dream to open a children's hospital in Bahia—a reality that, unfortunately, would not come to fruition for several decades.[16]

Despite these early precedents, the years between the World Wars truly represented a highpoint in the establishment of maternal and infant institutions. This was due to both local and international factors. Brazil, like several nations, mobilized in the wake of the conflicts and became swept up in what was both a global and a Pan-American campaign to better children's health.[17] Within Brazil, international awareness only reinforced "modernization" efforts that had already been identified as public priorities. Paralleling its efforts to medicalize motherhood, the First Republic levied federal and even international resources to invest in urban rejuvenation, sanitation infrastructure, and disease eradication—all considered eugenic imperatives. The Federal District benefited first from the zeal of spatial beautification (1902) and then from yellow fever eradication (1904). Rural interior Brazil proved the next great frontier for intervention in the republic's second decade.

The backlands, or *sertão*, took on enormous significance during the republic as the locus of authentic Brazilianness, for better or worse. For coastal Brazilians, the *sertão* had long represented backwardness and lethargy. Bahia was particularly condemned by these stereotypes after the journalist Euclides da Cunha published his popular report on the Canudos War of 1896—a bloody conflict pitting the federal army against a rural Bahian community that politicians considered dangerously separatist and fanatical.[18] Scientific research missions in the second decade of the century, headed by the federal Oswaldo Cruz Institute, added "diseased" to the stereotype of the "interior man." Doctors Arthur Neiva and Belisário Penna led the most famous of these missions in 1912, traversing much of the rural Northeast and documenting social, economic, and disease conditions. Their findings alarmed the urban residents of the littoral. Neiva and Penna reported that the average *sertanejo* was shockingly ignorant and primitive, lacking any identification with the nation and riddled with hookworm, malaria, and Chagas disease (which Neiva questionably estimated affected as many as 70% of inhabitants in certain regions). The physicians equivocated on whether the *caboclos* and *mestiços* of the interior were somehow racially inferior, but they blamed the lack of sanitation and high incidence of disease on governmental failures and issued a strong call for the federal government to address what they saw as extensive and generational health deficiencies.[19]

Bahia received special attention in these sanitation-as-civilization missions. Beginning in 1916, Bahian public health took on an international dimension following the first Rockefeller Foundation surveys. The Rockefeller Foundation's International Health Board set out to combat hookworm, malaria, and yellow fever and remained in Brazil working collaboratively with local physicians and politicians (though not without recurring conflicts) for nearly three decades. Perhaps surprisingly, Brazilian projects received the greatest share of the foundation's Latin American budget, and much of it was destined for the backlands of states like Bahia. Salvador, moreover, was a major center of the yellow fever eradication effort because the foundation pursued a strategy of exclusive focus on large cities.[20] Many projects organized by the Oswaldo Cruz Institute were also under way in the interior. Public health schemes of broad national scope were the order of the day in the Old Republic. Despite federalism, these were action areas in which the federal government sought to centralize their efforts.

Bahia's interwar years were dramatic—the continuation of a trend that began with the declaration of the republic. Political competition provided almost constant intrigue, periodic episodes of violence, and repeated federal interventions. Governor José Joaquim Seabra (1912–1916 and 1920–1924), one of the winners of Bahia's contested political space, spearheaded an ambitious campaign of urban renewal. Seabra had previously served as minister of justice and interior affairs under President Alves during the modernization of Rio de Janeiro. The governor was keen to add Salvador to the list of state capitals, such as São Paulo, Belém, Porto Alegre, Fortaleza, and Recife, with large-scale urban projects under way. As in many places, modernization of the city meant creation, beautification, and demolition. The governor ordered the construction of aesthetic avenues, contemporary bureaucratic offices, and new health facilities as well as the destruction of older churches and colonial mansions that had been divided up into small private residences.[21] For many prominent Bahians, modernization was a health *and* a population reform issue, as they associated disease and poor sanitation with urban poverty and chaos. By this logic, sanitation problems like the lack of water and sewer disposal were facets of the disordered reality of the poor. The "disruptive" and "uncivilized" presence of the urban poor, in contrast to Seabra's aspirant modernization, was a favorite topic of the local press. Ultimately, the demolitions and commercial expansion into residential buildings plunged Salvador into a housing crisis and worsened conditions for a poor population already experiencing decline. An outbreak of Spanish flu from late 1918 through 1919 exacerbated that crisis; the flu reached epidemic proportions, flourishing amid the state's insufficient sanitary infrastructure.[22]

Bahia also suffered economically due to disrupted European markets for textiles. The textile industry was comparatively small, but along with food production, it was the most significant form of manufacturing in Bahia. During the war, the textile industry endured periods of overproduction and rising costs of inputs. Laborers faced job insecurity, depressed wages, and worsening conditions. Conditions were already depressed for women, who typically earned half of men's wages, and for children, who often worked in exchange for food, clothing, and the opportunity to learn a trade with no remuneration at all. This situation repeated in garment manufacture—where the majority of employees were female—and in construction. Added to the falling wages was the rising cost of basic necessities as well as the flu epidemic that affected all families. Bahian teachers were the first to strike in March of 1918, followed by a paralyzing general strike on June 2, 1919. Porters from the docks, streetcar operators, and construction workers building the new public library and treasury headquarters joined the textile and garment producers. That strike ended with significant gains for labor, but textile workers stopped production again soon thereafter in September 1919. Large-scale strikes took place in 1920 and 1921 in the Bahian Recôncavo, and finally Bahia's railway laborers halted work in May 1927. In general, the political ruptures within the elite provided an opportunity for working people to actively push their interests onto the public agenda.[23] Worker agitation and a maturing intellectual and scientific focus on the masses created a new atmosphere. Given these circumstances of economic decline and worker mobilization, the interwar years provided the right local context for the institutionalization of public health focused on the poor. The emphasis on *family* came from the presumed utility of health interventions to engineer a productive and manageable postabolition, "modern" working class.

With increasing attention to public health and its infrastructure, the IPAI continued its services, attending to thousands of children. But by the 1920s, the IPAI was eclipsed in absolute numbers of clients and in local prominence by the Liga Bahiana contra a Mortalidade Infantil, the Bahian League against Infant Mortality (Liga). The Liga differed from the IPAI in that its creators maintained a deliberate focus on *puericultura*, meaning pregnant women, nursing mothers, and children up to two years of age. *Puericultores* and eugenicists recognized the importance of treatment but agreed that treatment did not hold the same promise of effecting enduring societal change. They also recognized that the most severe crises of mortality and morbidity occurred in children within the first twenty-four months of life. The Liga also differed fundamentally from the IPAI due to its complicated relationship with the state government. Even more than the IPAI, the genesis of the Liga helps explain how maternalism moved from the realm of private philanthropy to state-mandated public health and welfare. The institutionalization of maternalism in Bahia has a unique history, owing to the collaboration of federal, state, and private interests in the 1920s.

During this period, the federal government was deeply involved in disease eradication in the Bahian *sertão*, as has been mentioned. In 1921, the federal government actually took control of Bahian public health services, subordinating state-level programs to federal ones by asserting that epidemic disease posed a threat that superseded state authority. Despite the federalism of the republic, the federal state could insert itself legally in Bahia because the Sanitary Code of 1920 gave Dr. Carlos Chagas, national director of public health, the prerogative to intervene in state-level services under such circumstances. Through Chagas, the Federal Department of Public Health replaced the state of Bahia in a cooperative agreement with the Rockefeller Foundation. Thus, the federal government became an additional partner under the umbrella of the Rural Sanitary Service, whose director, the Rural Health Inspector, was also named director of the Federal Sanitary Service of Bahia. This reorganization meant more funding, literally, in the form of a 1922 budget allocation that was nearly twenty times greater than the entire federal budget for sanitation in 1917.[24] Though primarily directed at disease, the federal government's involvement meant funding for other public health projects in Bahia as well as federal supervision. Maternal and child hygiene programs were part of the agreement, since a Children's Hygiene Inspection Office already existed in Rio de Janeiro, directed by Dr. Fernandes Figueira, who extended services during the "federal occupation" of Bahian public health. By 1923, the Sanitary Service established the Bahian Children's Hygiene Service, which was quickly reorganized in 1925 as the Directory of Infant and School-Age Hygiene. Governor Goés Calmon created the Sub-Secretariat of Health and Public Assistance in 1925 (including the Infant and School-Age Hygiene Office) and named Dr. Barros Barreto, a federal health inspector and director of the Rockefeller Commission in Bahia, as Bahian secretary of public health. It is obvious, therefore, that organization of maternal and child hygiene in Bahia was a strange and convoluted mix of federal interventions and local administration right from the beginning.[25]

Further complicating this picture was the Bahian League against Infant Mortality, or Liga, founded by Dr. Joaquim Martagão Gesteira and colleagues from the School of Medicine. According to Dr. Gesteira (Liga president from 1923 to 1936), he had long maintained an interest in founding an organization devoted to reducing infant mortality and saw an opportunity with the federal intervention into Bahian public health. Gesteira reasoned that this type of private institution could only be successful in partnership with a public agency. Thus, Gesteira, Dr. Álvaro Bahia (the Liga's second president, 1936–1964), and five colleagues founded their institution in 1923 as the federal effort was under way, taking the name from the Parisian Ligue contre la Mortalité Infantile—founded in 1902 by the celebrated pronatalists Paul Strauss, Théophile Roussel, and Pierre Budin. Gesteira stressed that the Bahian Liga would address the ignorance and misery that produced an "avalanche of tiny coffins" every year.[26] The doctor's disturbing tone signaled a grave reality; infant mortality in Bahia (under age one) remained around 300 per 1,000.[27] Quoting Paul Strauss, Gesteira argued that Brazil's high infant mortality rates constituted "the greatest shame of a superior civilization."[28] Like its French predecessor, the Liga focused on prevention, often imprecisely called "hygiene." In Gesteira's words, the "maximum diffusion of *puericultura* and intensive propaganda in basic notions of infant hygiene" would make the greatest contribution to reducing infant mortality, justifying the emphasis on preventative medicine and well-baby care.[29]

The Liga inaugurated its first well-baby clinic, Regina Helena, that same year of 1923 in conjunction with the inauguration of the federal services so the clinic pertained jointly to both institutions. In other words, the Liga administered the infant hygiene services, which were cosponsored with federal

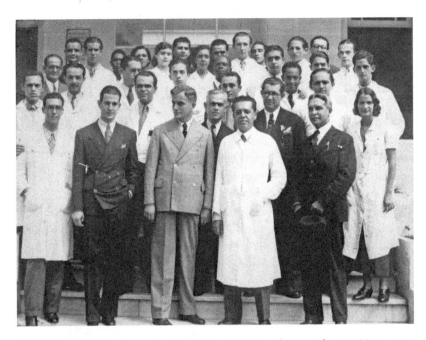

Staff of the Bahian League against Infant Mortality. Founding president Dr. Martagão Gesteira stands in the front in the white coat. To his left stands a special guest, Dr. Clementino Fraga, Bahian senator and director of the National Health Department. Over Fraga's left shoulder stands Dr. Álvaro Bahia, second president of the Liga. (Archives of the Liga Álvaro Bahia contra a Mortalidade Infantil)

funding. Gesteira himself was a hygiene inspector for the Rural Sanitary Service and became head of the Infant Hygiene Service in 1923 while simultaneously directing the Liga. In this way, the institutionalization of maternalism actually resulted from a three-pronged partnership uniting the state government, the federal government, and the Liga. Gesteira guessed correctly about attaching his organization to the bourgeoning state apparatus, as both the public and private wings of this new structure espoused similar missions. The Bahian Infant and School-Age Hygiene Office, for example, tasked itself with the formidable objective of attending to "all that is in the interest of the lives of children."[30] Apparently, this mission involved (1) establishing puericulture and prenatal clinics; (2) conducting home visits; (3) examining children in well-baby clinics, institutions, and impoverished households; (4) conducting wet nurse examinations; (5) teaching infant hygiene and nutrition; and (6) preventing contagious disease. The Infant and School-Age Hygiene Office was the first of several permutations of state institutions dedicated to children's health and welfare. The Bahian public health system stayed in an almost constant state of reform and reorganization in the early century, meaning that women's and children's services moved from one bureaucratic department to the next. Collaboration between the state's programs, under whatever name, and the Liga as well as the religious confraternity, the Santa Casa de Misericórdia, soon thereafter remained a constant. The Liga and the Misericórdia also brought the financial resources of their donors to the mission.

The Liga and the Infant Hygiene Service quickly went about opening a number of free specialized clinics in Salvador, and these endeavors opened to great fanfare and press coverage.[31] The Regina Helena Clinic was founded on October 12, 1923, and named in honor of the daughter of the newspaper owner and benefactor Ernesto Simões Filho. The clinic served well babies exclusively and offered puericulture education for local mothers. The Liga's private benefactors largely subsidized the Infant Hygiene Service during these early years, even though the Federal Department of Public Health appointed the members of Dr. Gesteira's small staff. No school existed in Bahia in 1923 to train nursing assistants and visiting sanitary nurses, so the Liga trained its own staff, twenty nurses in the first year of service. Fellow founders Drs. Álvaro Rocha and Hélio Ribeiro were the attending physicians, along with Gesteira and Bahia. Over the years, the Liga also partnered with the School of Medicine to provide training and internship for students of pediatrics.

From the outset, the small Regina Helena Clinic saw more than twenty children daily, most with digestive disturbances and respiratory infections—common ailments, as the IPAI had previously confirmed. Within three months, the clinic had seen over one thousand babies. Despite Gesteira's hope for an exclusive preventative hygiene, puericulture, and education service, the high occurrence of illness and disease made this goal impossible. He also claimed that working mothers resisted bringing healthy children to the clinics and avoided services until their babies fell ill. As babies who arrived at the clinics were often already ailing, physicians and nurses distributed medications and attended the sick in addition to their preventative programs. Regardless of the intention to serve healthy babies as Budin's well-baby model suggested, hygiene clinics were often treatment centers. Little by little, mothers began to bring their healthy children to the clinic for examination, particularly if the infant had previously been treated there for an illness.

The year of 1924 was an important one for the Infant Hygiene Service, as they added five new clinics to Salvador's growing children's health infrastructure. The state-Liga partnership expanded in the summer of 1924 with two "mixed" clinics designed to serve both infants and preschool children. The Adriano Gordilho Clinic, inaugurated on May 14, was attached to two textile factories, Boa Viagem and Fábrica Luiz Tarquínio, and attended to the children of female employees. The second mixed clinic, situated next to the Misericórdia's Santa Izabel Hospital, opened on July 6. All of these clinics specialized in vaccination, and the Service opened two prenatal clinics: the first was inaugurated on May 14 and the second on November 5 in the Climério de Oliveira Maternity Center.

Beyond the clinics, the Liga maintained a range of services that took staff members into the neighborhoods and homes of their patients and potential ones. In addition to "educational" visits to expectant mothers, Infant Hygiene Service nurses made home visits across Salvador to supervise the sanitary conditions of poor households with babies. Dr. Álvaro Bahia oversaw this service, and the staff secured the civil registry from the Secretariat of the Interior in order to systemize their work. The Liga's staff was ambitious; nurses attempted to visit all families with newborns in the city. Upon finding the infant in an affluent home, they offered pamphlets on puericulture. Taking advantage of visits to wealthy families, the pamphlets doubled as donation requests, detailing the good work under way for the benefit of the poor. For families of a lower station, nurses made regular visits to persuade parents to register their infants in one of the well-baby clinics. Nurses also inspected orphanages and public daycares, particularly those attached to factories such as the Villa Operaria's daycare at the Fábrica Luiz Tarquínio. The Service founded its own daycare on October 12, 1924: the Creche Fernandes Figueira, named in honor of the federal inspector of Infant Hygiene, which was for domestic servants who did not have the opportunity to take their infants to a factory daycare. In lieu of bottle-feeding, the Fernandes Figueira daycare hired wet nurses (after rigorous medical examination) to nourish the infants of mothers whose employers would not allow them to leave during work hours to nurse at the daycare. With the daycare, the Liga extended its mission beyond strictly health and into social assistance. This distinction is actually an anachronism because Bahian maternalist advocates did not separate questions of children's health from their familial well-being. Advocates argued that free daycare centers could reduce infant mortality and morbidity by protecting children from "incompetent" caregivers and unsterilized animal milk.[32]

The maternalist movement continued its rapid institutionalization through the late 1920s and into the 1930s. The Liga opened one of its largest clinics in 1928: the Instituto Baptista Machado, named for the father of its benefactor Alice Machado Catharino, who, along with her husband Álvaro, were among Salvador's wealthiest families. The Regina Helena Clinic and Fernandes Figueira daycare relocated to the new building. The Liga also rented one floor to the Secretariat of Health for a new public clinic. The Instituto would also become home to the state's Children's Department (1935),

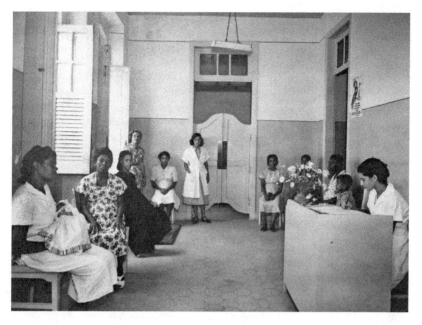

Waiting room at the Puericulture Post in the neighborhood of Brotas. (Archives of the Liga Álvaro Bahia contra a Mortalidade Infantil)

a division of the Department of Public Health and Assistance. By the time of its creation, Bahia no longer had cooperative agreements with the federal government, as President Washington Luiz disbanded the Federal Inspectorate of Children's Hygiene back in 1930. This provided an opening for the Bahian state to develop more autonomy in the local health system. Dr. Gesteira and his colleagues heralded the support of Bahian Appointed Governor Juracy Magalhães in establishing the new organization, which was Brazil's first state-administered Children's Department. Naturally, Gesteira was named director, and the Children's Department was not sufficiently funded to exist separately from the Liga. In addition to renting the floor in the Instituto Baptista Machado, the department utilized all of the Liga staff. By the end of the decade, the Children's Department oversaw puericulture services in six public clinics. Some slightly predated the Children's Department and others were added in its inaugural year: the Sanitary Center on Rua Dr. Seabra (1932), the Mario Andréa Sanitary Center at Calçada (1932), the Abrigo dos Filhos do Povo clinic at the Misericórdia (1933), the Health Post at Estrada de Liberdade (1935), and the Health Post at Rio Vermelho (1935), plus the Suburban Maternal and Children's Hygiene Service, which was an ambulatory care program. The puericulture services at Rio Vermelho, Estrada de Liberdade, and the Santa Izabel Hospital were joint efforts of the state and the Liga. The state administered the others directly.[33]

By the end of the 1930s, the state of Bahia had attained more independence from the Liga, mainly because by then the state managed more health posts in general where maternal and child programs could be added to the roster of services. State health posts maintained their own staff and served thousands of children and pregnant women annually. Prenatal and child health care represented only one service, but they did offer both preventative care and treatment at some locations. Treatment services included dental care, otorhinolaryngology, medication distribution, and follow-up for children and adults infected with syphilis and tuberculosis. Visiting nurses associated with the public clinics made tens of thousands of home visits, just as Liga nurses did, distributing information about prenatal and children's health and encouraging families to bring sick infants into treatment clinics. Following the commitment to nutrition and welfare, some of the clinics also maintained milk depots and maternal cantinas where women were served free daily meals. In sum, by the century's third decade, the state of Bahia was firmly on board with the ideologies and methodologies of maternalism in both its preventative and treatment branches.[34]

The critical issue concerning the complicated establishment of these public health services is that prior to 1923, the state government maintained no specialized facilities of any kind dedicated to prevention or treatment for women and children. At the end of the period analyzed in this book, there were dozens of free public and private facilities scattered across Salvador and into the neighboring smaller towns, serving the poorest residents. Furthermore, institutionalization matched the modernizing spirit of the republic and only intensified in the Vargas era that followed Brazil's Revolution of 1930. Even with all of these programs, the maternalist movement could not fully meet all of the health and welfare needs in Bahia. It was a valiant effort against a structural tide of inequality, racism, poverty, and poor health. And the state of Bahia undoubtedly stood as a leader and an innovator in the larger Brazilian movement for healthier mothers and babies. When President Getúlio Vargas made "protection of mothers and children" a priority of his family policy in the 1930s, his administration encouraged states across the nation to adopt programs identical to those that had existed in Bahia for decades.

THE CLIENTELE: *MÃES PRETAS* (AND *PARDAS*)

The institutionalization of family health and welfare did not occur in a cultural vacuum. As much as public health, disease eradication, and eugenic sanitation campaigns pressed the necessity of the masses to the nation's future, this era also witnessed a new cultural agitation in favor of celebrating and incorporating at least the symbols of the racial inclusiveness Brazil claimed. Intellectual movements such as São Paulo Modern Art Week are familiar to historians of Brazil, but this reclaiming of Brazil's multiracial "roots" occurred in popular politics as well. In September 1929, for example, the fifty-eighth anniversary of Brazil's Free Womb Law, black leaders of Salvador hosted a "Mãe Preta Day" in celebration of wet nurses' contributions to the formation of "the race." *Soteropolitanos* of all skin tones paid tribute to the *mãe preta* through special masses, marches, and speeches. The Bahian community of color was well represented in the street processions in particular, since an Afro-Bahian workers' association, Centro Operário, organized the event.[35] The Historic and Geographic Institute proudly displayed Bahian artist Presciliano Silva's reproduction of the painting *Mãe preta* by Lucílio de Albuquerque (1912), and students of Salvador's Institute of Music sang an original piece, called "Hymn to the Mãe Preta."[36] However, the representations commemorated on Mãe Preta Day either confined black maternity to a long-suffering past or relegated black women to a pacifying postabolition force through their continued work in household service. The daily *Diário de Noticias* best expressed the latter idea. "The facts [of the *mãe preta*'s loyalty] demonstrate that, upon the extinction of slavery, the slaves integrated into the family. They did not separate from that attachment to the home because of the bond of fidelity, an entrenched part of their character."[37] Both problematic and patronizing, Mãe Preta Day appropriated black maternity and black women's bodies as the folkloric manifestation of authentic Brazilianness and an indispensable link to the supposedly benign racial politics of the present.

Meanwhile, in the very concrete realm of modern family life, black and brown mothers and mothers-to-be crisscrossed the city to find prenatal, well-baby, and children's services. Who were the women who registered themselves and their children for Bahia's new preventative medical services? In Bahia, the racial composition of the poor meant that the target population for free maternal and child services was obvious. Although race was not always explicit in documents, it is abundantly apparent that the Bahian maternal and child health movement centered around women of color and their children. Playing with terminology here, it is also apparent that the majority of these mothers worked in domestic service. Though comprehensive and chronological data no longer exist, a few examples establish that black and brown domestics and their children were the overwhelming majority of clients for public health services. In 1926, for example, 766 women sought prenatal examinations in two clinics run jointly by the Infant Hygiene Service and the Liga. The records identified 84 percent of patients as black or brown in skin tone (*preta* or *parda*) and 69 percent as employed in domestic service. Similarly, *mães pretas* (and *pardas*) brought their young children to the clinics in impressive numbers. That same year, 2,332 children were examined at three public clinics offering well-baby and medical care: Regina Helena, Adriano Gordilho, and Santa Izabel Hospital. Ninety-two percent of their mothers worked as domestics (including laundresses, seamstresses, and specialized servants), and 75 percent of the children were classified as *pardo* or *preto* in skin tone.[38] These same patterns are clear in other clinics when racial and employment data were recorded. The mother clientele was not exclusively *mães pretas*, but nearly so.

Racial and other data from these records contribute much to establishing a general profile of participant families and beginning to uncover their histories. The records from the well-baby and maternal clinics can be quite rich, providing solid evidence about typical Bahian families of the twentieth century. Thousands of expectant mothers and small children frequented these institutions in their early years. Because these were preventative medicine clinics, staff members attempted to create long-term relationships with their clients as well as a means of tracking them over time. All patients were asked to register, and clinical records traced both new registrations and the overall number of clients served. Many mothers and babies made repeated visits to the clinic. In fact, it was not unusual for some of the infants to visit weekly, thus fulfilling the expectations of the proponents of puericulture. In addition to providing developmental tracking, well-baby visits were convenient for vaccinations and unspecified "minor treatments." Vaccination and tracking were also major components of prenatal care. Additionally, the prenatal visit often included the administration of the Wassermann reaction to detect syphilis. Finally, "maternal education" was one of the most emphasized elements of well-baby and prenatal visits as is described later in this chapter.

As the number of facilities increased through the 1930s, so did the total number of families who sought preventative care. As evidence, parents and children helped celebrate the Liga's one-hundred-thousandth preventative consultation in April of 1932. Both the private and public clinics saw dozens of women and children daily. At the Third Health Post, for example, it was common for physicians and nurses to see twenty to thirty newly registered and repeat patients in a single afternoon. On January 2, 1934, six expectant mothers and twenty-six children under two years of age visited the clinic. Among those seeking their first prenatal consultation that day were thirty-nine-year-old Prima Maria Graciliana, twenty-three-year-old Valdeliz Pinho Mello, and twenty-year-old Maria Francisca de Jesus. All three were native Bahians who worked as household servants, and all three were typical representatives of the clinic's general patient population. Between June 1933

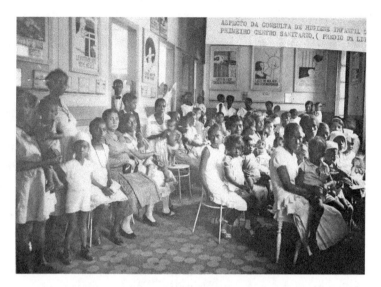

Well-baby consultation waiting room, Liga services at the First Health Post. (Archives of the Liga Álvaro Bahia contra a Mortalidade Infantil)

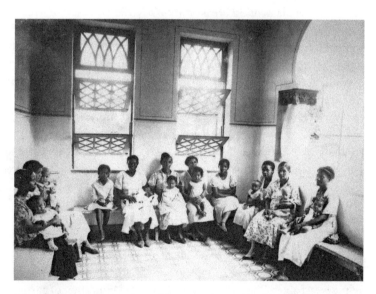

Waiting room at the Fourth Health Post in the neighborhood of Rio Vermelho. (Archives of the Liga Álvaro Bahia contra a Mortalidade Infantil)

and January 1934, 284 new prenatal patients registered at the Third Health Post. Eighty-one percent of these mothers-to-be were *mestiças, morenas, pardas,* and *pretas,* and ninety-five percent worked as domestics.[39] Maria Francisca de Jesus was also representative in that she lived in the outlying suburbs of Salvador. Since there were no maternal clinics in those areas, expectant mothers and mothers seeking well-baby care traveled into the heart of the city for services.

Clinical records also help elucidate other facets of family life. *Mães pretas* (and *pardas*) juggled work in domestic service with the responsibilities of motherhood. Only a minority of prenatal patients, for example, were experiencing their first pregnancy. Most women who frequented the clinic already had one or more children at home. These mothers elected biomedical prenatal care for subsequent pregnancies after their first. By selecting the clinical experience, they either experimented with puericulture or already valued that approach alongside, or even as a substitute for, the expertise of a traditional midwife. As must have been common for working moms, these mothers tended to nourish their infants using some combination of breast milk and "artificial" nourishments, much to the disappointment of the clinical staff. Supplementing breast milk was often done out of necessity, since baby formulas were not yet as popular and available as they would become in the 1950s, and animal milk (cow's milk and goat's milk) was notoriously dangerous, given Bahia's uneven sanitation oversight. Combating the use of "mixed" feeding regimes was the primary focus of the clinics' educational mission. If the use of supplements was indeed a consequence of working mothers' demanding schedules, this serves as another reminder that families relied heavily on relatives, older children, friends, or even paid caregivers for daily child care. Balancing strenuous physical work such as domestic service with raising a family could only have been possible within these bonds of community. Unlike the city's wealthiest homes, these households would have depended on the pooling of resources—both in time and in milreis—in order to provide for children during their parents' working hours.

This public health movement had an almost exclusive focus on mothers and children, the "mother-child binary" to use the contemporary language. In the early years, however, some information was collected about the fathers of the well babies. The 1920s records give some indication of partnership and family patterns as related to men, and family patterns were likely largely similar in the 1930s. About half of the women who visited the clinics reported being married; we can assume that most of the remaining mothers shared their children with consensual partners. Many of the young patients were categorized as "natural children," also suggesting parents bonded by consensual partnerships. Undoubtedly, some of these children were born of more casual unions. Most families lived in individual homes rather than shared dwellings, and that was typical of urban Salvador compared to São Paulo's tenement housing, for example. Similar to their partners, the vast majority of fathers were Brazilians, although there were more immigrants among the fathers than the mothers, primarily Portuguese and Spaniards. Men had a greater diversity of employment opportunities available than did women, even among the working classes. Fathers whose children enrolled in the well-baby clinics worked as artisans, porters, unspecified "laborers," streetcar operators, soldiers, and factory workers, among many other occupations. On the whole, these men, like their female companions, carried out all the labor that made life in Bahia possible for everyone; and also like their partners, they earned low to average wages. Moving into the 1930s, maternalist agencies recorded fathers' information with less frequency. Nothing suggests that these fathers were absent from the lives of their partners and children; rather, the recording methods increasingly marginalized them from the process.[40]

As expected, most of the city's poor mothers reported having delivered their babies with the help of folk midwives. In this context, this reality is actually suggestive of mothers' approach to family health care in general. Presumably, the midwives who delivered these thousands of infants could also have offered healing treatments. Bahian midwives could easily have been consulted for prenatal care. The fact that many mothers sought out biomedicine is a telling choice, therefore. It demonstrates that the well-baby and prenatal clinics attracted mothers with other health-care options rather quickly. Physicians may have expected even greater turnout in their first decade, but clinical care caught on with many thousands of families almost immediately. The clinics' own outreach work must have influenced many families as well; visiting nurses canvased neighborhoods all around Salvador and deliberately searched for pregnant women and mothers of newborns. Even if one of these visits prompted a family to try the local clinic, mothers must also have held some expectation that the clinic was a viable medical option. And the visiting nurses were not the only source of information; word spread quickly within neighborhoods once local mothers had their own firsthand experiences in the clinics. On August 7, 1933, next-door-neighbors thirty-two-year-old Eulina de Araujo and twenty-two-year-old Stellita Souza likely traveled together from their homes on São Paulo Avenue in the Japão neighborhood to the Third Health Post to request their first prenatal exams. Lindaura Magalhães Castro, age twenty-two, and America Magalhães Rosa, age twenty-six, were next-door neighbors living in the neighborhood of São Lourenço who also shared the experience on January 20, 1934.[41] All four of these expectant mothers worked as domestic servants, so scheduling to travel together must have required careful planning. The use of these services does not necessarily mean that families definitively rejected their midwives and healers. Perhaps these mothers utilized the local clinic in addition to consulting with a midwife.

Dr. Hosannah de Oliveira, pediatrician, director of the School of Medicine, and attendant IPAI physician, also provides some evidence on this issue. Oliveira served as sometime informant and occasional tour guide for the American anthropologist Ruth Landes in 1938. Landes's primary research interest was the Afro-Brazilian religion of Candomblé, and she interviewed the doctor in that context. Dr. Oliveira complained to Landes that expectant and nursing mothers visited medical clinics only after consulting with their *mãe de santo*, or spiritual leader. If the *mãe de santo* advised a medical consultation, mothers would oblige, but they often used clinical prescriptions alongside "herbs and magical formulas." Like Landes, Oliveira had a deep interest in Candomblé, but the physician spoke condescendingly about what he considered women's unfailing obedience to and reverence for the female leaders of their *terreiros* compared to a fickle commitment to their local physician. Oliveira charged that mothers were "too ignorant to understand and take advantage" of medical treatments and resorted to that with which they were more familiar.[42] Despite physicians' insistence, there was really no impediment to families using any and all options available to them simultaneously, but the use of these new medical services does provide clues about growing favorable attitudes toward clinical care.

Unfortunately, institutional records do not provide much evidence for seeing how women and families considered and compared their health-care options. Their actions, however, help expose both the absolute need for free medical care and women's own commitment to utilizing these services to raise healthy children. Despite physicians' assertions that poor women were too traditional, too premodern to understand the benefits of biomedical care, pregnant women and women with young children filled the waiting rooms at the clinics. The thousands who sought maternal and child services during the first decades of the century suggest that women's interest was a function of the availability of medical care rather than a fear or aversion to "modern" medicine. Often mothers sought out more than one service in a single visit, requesting prenatal exams for themselves and well-baby or child-hygiene consultations for their children. Expectant mother Expedita da Cruz visited the Third Health Post on October 16, 1933, for a prenatal exam while also seeking a well-baby assessment for her sixteen-month-old son Annibal.[43] Again, this efficiency would have been necessary, given the scheduling challenges facing women working in household service who had to carve out time to attend to their own needs and those of their children.

While poor women were eager to access care, their responses to certain services prompted changes in administration. For example, women initially rejected the preventative approach of "child hygiene" and insisted that sick children be treated in free clinics, as previously mentioned. This illustrates the high incidence of childhood illness in Bahia and the fact that mothers did not initially comply with the call to monitor their rearing of healthy children. Puericulture held the expectation of medical intervention *before* illness as one of its fundamental tenets. Dr. Gesteira regretted that preventative clinics were initially unsuccessful in convincing mothers to bring in healthy infants despite the rigorous propaganda campaign undertaken by their brigade of visiting nurses. Gesteira admitted that attending to well babies exclusively was impossible, given the lack of medical facilities in Salvador as well as mothers' reluctance to bring in healthy children. According to Gesteira, many adhered to the old adage that "children who are weighed do not grow nor prosper."[44] He cited medication distribution as the major attraction to the clinic and charged Bahian families with being uneducated and unprepared for preventative services.

Clinical records attest to the fact that the staff did spend quite a bit of time distributing medications. In fact, the well-baby clinics attended more sick infants than "well" ones for their first few years. To keep up with demand, the Liga solicited local pharmacies for donations due to the sheer volume of requests from women with sick children who visited Regina Helena daily. These women's choices suggest continuity in the tradition of familial control over infant health rather than ceding complete control to the physician, which would have been the result of using the clinic for preventative visits only. Mothers depended on physicians' expertise, but seeking medications meant that healing sick children would be performed at home, likely in conjunction with other customs that may have included particular foods and other remedies. Mothering and healing continued to be closely linked to religious beliefs, as Nancy Scheper-Hughes argued for rural Pernambuco.[45] Home remedies had always been an integral part of women's general understandings of health, illness, spirituality, and family and were likely used in combination with biochemical medications obtained at the clinic.

Their willingness to seek medications and the number of registrants certainly demonstrate that women trusted in clinical practice. This would not necessarily have been the case in the nineteenth century and illustrates a much larger trend of the expansion of biomedicine across the globe in the early twentieth. The comparative lack of resistance to prenatal services may be due to the fact that the idea of prenatal care was not really new. Midwives had always prescribed and proscribed certain behaviors and diets for expectant mothers. Well-baby care did begin to catch on in Bahia within the first five years. Perhaps women's preference for using the clinic only as a treatment facility was a rejection of the intrusion into their family lives required for enrollment in the well-baby program. A visit to the clinic did not only entail babies being weighed and measured. Upon enrollment, mothers were asked to provide a great deal of personal information about their family histories and living situations. In addition to basic identification data, clinical staff asked mothers about the condition of the homes in which they lived, the cost of their rent, and the names of all residents. They asked about mothers' and fathers' places of employment, including questions on their salaries and hours worked per day. Mothers were asked to list the number of living and deceased children they had given birth to, the number of miscarriages, and the causes of death for each of their deceased children. Finally, staff asked mothers to state the legitimacy of the child, to report the person who assisted the birth, and to explain why they did not breast-feed if applicable.[46] In a hierarchal social system like that which existed in early 1900s Bahia, one can imagine that it was an extremely uncomfortable situation for a poor black or brown woman to have her family life investigated by a clinical staff member, who was often a state employee.

The right to a private familial domain without supervision and intrusion may have held particular significance in this context, causing some to initially avoid the experience of entering the clinic unless children were in need of treatment. This idea parallels Teresa Meade's arguments about mandatory smallpox vaccination in Rio de Janeiro in 1904. Meade argued that the citywide riots following the introduction of this policy reflected a widespread popular discontent with the priorities and methods of urbanization projects, which disproportionally impacted the poor, rather than a lower-class fear of modern health care.[47] A similar process likely took place in the well-baby clinics. Certainly, the modernization projects under way in Salvador would have made families skeptical that the state actually had the interests of the poor in mind. And Dr. Gesteira's and Dr. Oliveira's own biases were evident when they accused mothers of being too superstitious and uneducated to agree to preventative care. It seems contradictory to argue that families actively sought "modern" medicines but were too "backward" to allow their children to be examined by a physician. Perhaps women were reluctant to open their family lives to medical scrutiny, particularly in a culture where questions of such a private nature would never have been asked of well-to-do families. As their actions demonstrated, thousands of poor mothers in Bahia took full advantage of medical services and were the first advocates for the health and welfare of their own children.

For mothers living beyond the center of Salvador, however, finding treatment facilities or well-baby care proved more problematic. Biomedical facilities were an option for many families in the center of town, perhaps even for the majority by the 1940s. Though a number of organizations provided services, they did little to no work in the suburbs, where the need for medical care and assistance was acute. In fact, suburban residents lived in the most extreme levels of poverty in the urban region. Health conditions there were precarious, and no medical services existed for infants or children. In 1937, the state created a roving medical center for suburban residents, designed to offer evaluations and treatments to neighborhoods as far out as Pirajá. The Ambulatory Medical Social Assistance Service was a new division of the Children's Department, headed by the Liga physician Dr. Eliezer Audíface. December 15 marked the first day of service, and as the van made stops in Fazenda Grande, São Caetano, and Pirajá, dozens of mothers met the staff with their young children who needed examinations, medications, and food. That inaugural day, staff members examined hundreds of children and distributed badly needed provisions. The immediate appearance of crowds of local families evidenced both the necessity and the demand for more health services in suburban neighborhoods. Unfortunately, the suburban service was habitually underfunded, preventing vehicle repairs and causing the service to operate irregularly. Permanent suburban posts for the care of women and children did not appear until the following decade when the Social Assistance Council constructed a small (twenty-bed) maternity center to serve the communities of Periperi and Paripe in 1943. Beyond these efforts, the suburban population remained largely ignored, and mothers had to travel into the center of the city for prenatal care or for medical services for their children.[48]

Families living in the interior of Bahia had even fewer resources, though physicians repeatedly pleaded with the government to expand services beyond Salvador. The rural areas were clearly the most neglected, and health conditions were dire even in the Recôncavo region, which is relatively close to the state capital. In the city of Santo Amaro, for example, childhood deaths outnumbered births according to municipal records.[49] There was likely a great deal of undercounting in public records, but it is clear that childhood mortality was a serious issue. As explained, disease eradication efforts in the interior had been under way since 1920, but women's and children's services were slow to follow. Families could access treatment and vaccination services at one of several health posts, thanks to the federal health intervention. Health posts existed in Alagoinhas, Cachoeira, Santo Antônio de Jesus, Jequié, Ilhéus, Caravelas, Caetité, Senhor do Bonfim, Juazeiro, Barra, and Bom Jesus da Lapa; and smaller "subposts" in Itaberaba, Cipó, and Santarém. These posts served Bahia's most populous areas outside of the capital city. However, Bahia was home to 4,265,074 residents according to the 1936 census, fewer than 9 percent of whom lived in Salvador where services were concentrated. Though local families counted on the health posts during times of illness, these centers did not provide preventative medicine (other than vaccination) for mothers and babies.

As in Salvador, private *puericultura* institutions attempted to fill this gap where the state was absent. In 1936, Martagão Gesteira, as director of the state Children's Department, identified Castro Alves, Itabuna, Santo Amaro, and Alagoinhas as the most appropriate sites for extending services beyond Salvador. The small town of Castro Alves already had a privately run maternity center, opened that same year by a Dr. Jayme Coelho, and its own Liga Castroalvense contra a Mortalidade Infantil, so it seemed the logical choice for the first interior Puericulture Post. *Castroalvense* families also visited the Lactário Lavinia Magalhães for free distribution of sterilized milk. The Lactário, a joint effort of the state and the Liga Castroalvense, was named for the first lady of the state and was the first milk depot outside of Salvador. The Children's Department moved quickly to establish posts in other cities where private services already existed. Itabuna and Santo Amaro also had child welfare organizations, and Santo Amaro had a Liga Santoamarense contra a Mortalidade Infantil that supported a small maternity center.[50] In the following decade, Santo Amaro became home to the first foster care center in the nation.[51]

These Puericulture Posts were an important resource for Bahian families, being the only "hygiene" clinics beyond Salvador for several years. In 1944, a national women's organization called the Brazilian Assistance Legion (LBA) launched a campaign to "redeem the Brazilian child," which involved opening well-baby clinics and milk dispensaries across Brail. The LBA selected São Felix, Bahia, as home to their first Puericulture Post. The LBA's activities are described in detail in chapter 5 on the Estado Novo, but the relevant point here is that puericulture clinics were few and far between in the Bahian interior well into the 1940s. Despite the explosion of concern for Bahian mothers and children, little actual practice spilled beyond the borders of the capital city. In fact, other than Itabuna, which is about 250 miles from Salvador, all of these towns with designated well-baby and prenatal services were relatively close to the capital—within 100 miles. These were close distances in a state extending over 200,000 square miles. So the public extension into the interior, though significant, largely did not reach Bahians beyond Salvador's immediate vicinity. Mothers and children living in the more remote rural areas of the state were not served. This unequal development of Bahian maternalism was unfortunate and ironic, given that the initial federal funding that made preventative medicine possible came from the *Rural* Hygiene Service.

For many of Bahia's *mães pretas* (and *pardas*), caring for the health of their families had taken on new possibilities in the first decades of the twentieth century. Some were immediately drawn to preventative care, and some would be among the tens of thousands who chose to use the clinics in the 1930s and 1940s. Just as family life had a new biomedical dimension for many, Bahia's bureaucracy had also transformed in personnel and in responsibilities, linking itself in new ways to private organizations. Poor families were right at the heart of those crucial changes. Brazilian medicine had fundamentally changed with the "modern" politics of the new century, and the *mães pretas* and their children had become a medical priority. Because the free health-care system reflected Bahia's socioeconomic and racial realities, it must have been obvious to any observer that maternal and child programs served primarily black and brown domestics and their families, even when race was not recorded. In Bahia, "domestic," "wet nurse," and "impoverished mother" were not racially neutral terms anyway. Within the maternalist movement, a clear dichotomy existed between a white, educated elite (both male and female) who advocated for health reforms and the poor working women of color who accessed public services. It is impossible to understand the development of the public health system without taking the racialized nature of Brazil's social structure seriously. Though much had changed, there were also key continuities. Racial ideologies were lurking beneath the surface when Gesteira charged Bahian mothers with being "superstitious," when countless physicians referred to their supposed "ignorance," and when clinical staff endeavored to educate poor women in "proper" child rearing. Many of these assumptions about the literal *mães pretas* (and *pardas*) were exactly the same as those leveled at the symbolic *mãe preta* of nineteenth-century medical literature.

REFORMING POOR MOTHERS

Mothers sought out medical assistance for the well-being of their families. What they may not have known before their first visit was the emphasis maternalist advocates placed on influencing poor families' childrearing practices. While physicians and nurses attempted to usher as many clients as possible into the clinics, one of their major goals was to influence mothers to adopt new procedures for raising their children. Maternal education was a major objective of the puericulture movement when working with poor families. Impoverished children suffered the most from disease and premature death, so the increased medical attention was of critical importance to many families. Clinical staff were explicit in the intention to use preventative visits to change families' behaviors at home. As their advertisements stated, "At the Infant Hygiene clinics, a physician is available daily to attend to poor mothers, advising them in the best methods to raise their children."[52]

Clinical and home visits included minilessons on child care and hygiene.

When visiting nurses made their rounds, they came armed with flyers and literally distributed tens of thousands of pieces of material annually. Staff members hoped to influence the process of mothering from marriage partner selection all the way through children's development, and this was in accord with the eugenic principle that healthy procreation began before conception and continued through adolescence. Visiting nurses flyers' contained various messages, all sharing the title "For the Good of Children." On premarital medical certification, the flyers stated, "Failure to consult a physician before marriage is the cause of a great number of illnesses and the most serious ones among children."[53] Premarital certification was a favorite topic among eugenicists in Brazil and around the world. Brazilian eugenicists hoped medical examinations would encourage partners with "defective" backgrounds to voluntarily refrain from marrying and producing children. The premarital warning was an interesting choice for this propaganda, however, since visiting nurses intentionally sought out expectant and new mothers, not young people who were yet to have children. The inclusion of this topic suggests that local *puericultores* hoped to diffuse this warning broadly, even to those for whom the message might not directly apply, and within the poor community in particular.

Puericulture propaganda had other critical messages to impart as well. On prenatal health, flyers encouraged expectant mothers to avoid physical activity during pregnancy—a tall order for women who labored daily in household service to support their families. "The pregnant woman, who thinks of the happiness and health of her future child, makes the sacrifice of spending the pregnancy in tranquility. Resting 40 days prior to the birth will benefit the child." At the conclusion of a healthy pregnancy, the flyers alerted women to the dangers of midwifery. "How desirable it would be if all births were attended by competent persons! Lacking such a person, at least protect the newborn by inserting a solution into the eyes that protects against one of the most serious diseases." The second line referred to neonatal conjunctivitis, ophthalmia neonatorum, which can cause blindness in newborns. Physicians regularly warned that midwives were inattentive to hygiene in their immediate postnatal procedures. Interestingly, one version of the prenatal flyer slightly altered the closing line, informing that the clinic's physician attended to "poor, pregnant *senhoras*, providing advice and the indicated medications." The reference to medications reinforced the distinction between clinical prenatal care and that provided by a midwife. By referring to their target clients as married "*senhoras*," it also contained a suggestion of respectability that would have been immediately recognized.

More than any other message, *puericultores* promoted maternal breast-feeding. Breast-feeding was mothers' best weapon against childhood illnesses, which clinicians explained were largely the result of poor hygiene and therefore preventable. A variety of print and visual materials drove this message home. The visiting nurses instructed, "The child who is breast-fed exclusively until six months of age has enviable development and better resistance against contracting illnesses than other children. Avoid them and let us all continue with wisdom." Mothers were also urged to "do everything possible to raise your child on the breast." This last flyer accompanied a much longer twenty-three-point pamphlet entitled "Useful Advice for Mothers and Wet Nurses" with a litany of suggestions for hygiene and feeding. This was an updated version of a similar pamphlet, "To Young Mothers," created during the Liga's first year of service. Both versions emphasized that nursing, coupled with rigorous adherence to domestic hygiene, was advantageous to both mother and child.[54]

Given that the majority of Bahians were illiterate, flyers were only one strategy employed. At the Liga, wall posters lined the waiting rooms, bearing illustrations and messages that could be inferred without reading. Two prominent ones at the Instituto Baptista Machado reminded mothers of the superiority of breast milk. The first depicted a sickly cow next to a large glass of milk infested with menacing-looking insects. The short caption read, "Cow's Milk: Full of Microorganisms." In the second poster, a woman held a clean and pure glass of milk up to the sun above the caption, "Woman's Milk: Does Not Contain Microorganisms." Regardless of method, the message was the same: mothers of healthy children consulted medical professionals at every stage and rigorously observed their instructions. The primary instruction was to privilege exclusive maternal breast-feeding above all child-rearing duties. Healthy childhood did not happen by chance, but rather resulted from the choices that mothers made every day.

It is difficult to ascertain how women responded to these messages. Obviously, there is no record that can provide a true look into families' behaviors in their own homes. One can assume these mothers were well aware that their working situations placed significant constraints on whether and how they could breast-feed their infants. Getting to the clinic during service hours must have been challenging for many, not to mention the difficulty posed by having other children in tow. In the early years, the well-baby clinics were only open for half days, with the exception of Regina Helena, and the prenatal clinic was only open from 8 a.m. to 10 a.m. Local *puericultores* had an idealized and somewhat naive view of the ease with which mothers could balance full-time work and breast-feeding. The clinical literature reminded women that employers were required by law to allow short breaks for nursing. Of course, working women knew firsthand that these laws were regularly ignored in practice, and they only applied to women with formal employment in registered businesses at any rate. Most women worked in domestic service and therefore had no legal protections or guarantees. The brochures went on to explain that nursing during a short work break was a simple endeavor. After nursing, the child becomes quickly satisfied and falls into "a sweet sleep . . . The mother returns to work. She has completed her mission."[55] Any mother with actual experience would have known this was a romanticized picture that downplayed the effort involved in combining exhaustive work with the equally exhaustive task of caring for an infant. In time, *puericultores* came to realize that "completing the mission" was often not simply a matter of choice, and that mothers' failure to breast-feed exclusively was not merely a function of their "ignorance." Perhaps the mothers who utilized the clinics educated the staff because by the 1940s, physicians were heavily involved in more ample welfare programs that assisted poor mothers in new ways. These programs also evidenced the double meaning of the term "*mãe preta*," since maternalist advocates urged the state to provide welfare support so poor mothers could be "the wet nurses of their own children."[56]

After ten years of distributing propaganda and holding individual maternal consultations, the Liga borrowed a more systematic model for spreading the message of "modern" child rearing: the Better Baby Contest, Concurso de Robustez. The Better Baby Contest originated in the United States at the 1911 Iowa State Fair. Two concerned mothers, one of whom was a physician, designed the contest as an experiment to determine whether a competitive event at the fair would encourage Americans to invest in "bettering" the human breed similar to the way that such competitions had improved the quality of livestock. Popularized through women's magazines and linked to state fairs across the country, Better Baby or Eugenic Contests drew attention to the US race betterment movement. Thus, the organizers sought a nationalist ideal, the "perfection of American babyhood."[57] Evaluating baby health, organizers used these events to inform parents of how and why their children failed to reflect the exemplar of human development. The difference in the Brazilian version was that the impetus for organizing this type of event came from the medical community; it was not the result of women's mobilizations as occurred in the United States. And certainly, Brazilian Better Baby Contests were not explicitly racially segregated as they were in the United States.

Bahia held its first Better Baby Contest in 1933, a joint effort of the Liga, the Bahian Press Association, and the local chapter of the Rotary Club. The initial contest was open to all babies regardless of socioeconomic background, maintaining the structure of its American predecessor. Including babies of all social classes did not really embody the educational goals of the Liga, however. With the founding of Children's Week in 1936, the Better Baby Contest became an annual event, open only to the city's poor children. The inspiration for Children's Week came from an earlier academic event of the same name. Bahia had been host to Brazil's first Children's Week, December 5–11 of 1927—a weeklong conference hosted by the Liga in partnership with several prestigious medical organizations, including the Medical and Surgical Society of Bahia, the Hospital Medical Society of Bahia, and the Bahian delegation to the first Pan-American Child Congress taking place that same week in Cuba.[58] The 1927 Children's Week provided a forum to discuss medicine as well as education, sociology, psychology, and legislation related to children. By 1936, Liga physicians decided that Children's Week would have more significance as a popular event rather than a medico-legal conference.

That October, the Liga revived Children's Week as a citywide celebration of children and preventative medicine. The commemoration included a variety of events for different audiences, and thereby sought to incorporate a large swath of Salvador's population. The event sponsored play days in local parks, toy distributions for institutionalized children, screenings of educational films for mothers along with children's movies, presentations on hygiene and parenting to aspiring teachers at the Normal School, and lectures at the local clinics for both general and medical audiences. Additionally, the Foundling Home, hygiene clinics, and free daycares offered open houses and tours so wealthy residents could examine the modern medical facilities available for impoverished families. With the cooperation of the Bahian Press Association, Children's Week received a great deal of media coverage throughout the 1930s and 1940s, highlighting the latest institutions and services, providing a space for medical and social debates about mothers and children, and, of course, advertising the Better Baby Contest.[59]

The Better Baby Contest became the hallmark event of Children's Week. Enrollment in a local well-baby clinic was a prerequisite, providing an added incentive for families to enroll their children and reinforcing the organizers' goals of using the contest to bring more poor families into the well-baby movement. All babies between three months and one year of age were eligible, and eventually children up to two years of age could also compete. Volunteer judges meticulously examined all baby contestants. The medical evaluation centered on weighing, measuring, and performing developmental assessments in order to compare babies to established norms for their ages. The contest qualification was a serious medical exam, in fact. Mothers must have watched with interest as physicians measured the circumference of their children's craniums and throats and asserted that those rankings had some relation to the overall status of their babies' health and heredity. Some must have responded with surprise upon hearing how their children's bones, organs, nervous systems, and motor skills compared to those of the "best babies."

Meanwhile, the contest staff also investigated the mothers' histories and child-care practices. Much like the enrollment process at the well-baby clinic, contest staff recorded the state of health of each contestant's parents, along with the number of healthy births, stillbirths, and miscarried pregnancies experienced by their mothers. Additionally, they asked about living and deceased siblings, including the causes of death of the latter. All of these data were considered to establish a generational pattern of health or illness, in eugenic terms. One of the most important pieces of the background investigation was questioning mothers about how and when they fed their children—how long they breast-fed (if at all) and whether they rigorously observed a feeding schedule. Conversations with mothers over the results of the medical examination afforded staff the opportunity to "correct" familial habits, particularly as related to feeding. Thus, for the organizers, the contest was as much an evaluation of Better Mothers as it was of Better Babies.

Families who registered their children in the Better Baby Contest could expect information, goods, and even cash awards. Every child brought for evaluation received a toy and a baby layette. Organizers reserved prizes and medals for infants whose mothers could confirm that they had breast-fed exclusively for a minimum of three months and continued to breast-feed even with supplements for an additional three months. Moreover, babies were only eligible for the "health award" if they had been enrolled in their clinic from the age of two months or younger. One can assume that contest staff did not really expect parents to register their children with the clinic simply for eligibility in two years of Better Baby Contests, but making early well-baby enrollment a distinction between "good" and "better" babies further emphasized preventative medicine as a fundamental expectation of healthy infancy. In addition to the baby layette, the children medaled as "healthy" received a deposit in the National Bank worth either 50$000 or 100$000 milreis, depending on the level of their award: gold, silver, or bronze. Gold-medalist babies often had their pictures taken for the Children's Week spread in the local paper. In 1937, this honor went to three-month-old Walter Tapuz Ramos and his mother, Lindaura, who had their picture taken with Gustavo Capanema, federal minister of education and health, who was in Bahia examining the state's maternal and child assistance programs. Provocatively, Walter's father, Joaquim, was not pictured alongside his family in the newspaper article.[60] It is clear, however, that the quest for better babies warranted the attention of the nation's highest authorities.

RETURNING TO THE EPISODES DESCRIBED AT THE OUTset of this chapter, the real and symbolic *mães pretas* (and *pardas*) of 1933 signify a crucial piece of a larger story. The year 1933 was distinctive in some sense due to Gilberto Freyre's iconic publication, the Child Protection Conference, and Bahia's first Better Baby Contest. All of these events exemplified new trends in thinking about Brazilian families, even poor ones, and their relationship to both the nation and the national imaginary. On the other hand, that year was just one in a decade marked by a thriving movement in favor of poor women's and children's health and welfare, a movement that drew upon international, national, and local intellectual currents, cultural trends, and financial resources. Brazilian institutions undoubtedly took inspiration from French and US models. Well-baby clinics, maternal stipends, milk depositories, and free daycares for working mothers were inventions of the late-nineteenth-century French pronatalist movement. Though the Brazilian campaign re-created certain aspects of the US child welfare movement, the latter was characterized by the mobilization of women as institutional leaders, such as in the US Children's Bureau. Female advocacy was fundamental to institutional development in Brazil as well, but there were few examples of medical organizations led by female physicians.[61]

Despite some key similarities, the Brazilian welfare state developed in a manner distinct from the US and European models that have been so thoroughly analyzed. In Brazil, it combined a high degree of state intervention, as in the French model, with an absolute dependence on private organizations and charities, as in the United States. Though Brazilian governments of the twentieth century were basically authoritarian in their administrations, they placed a relatively high priority on health and social welfare. However, the state lacked the resources and the reach to enact its policies without the cooperation of local institutions and wealthy philanthropists. The dependence on "charity" ensured that old modes of patronage persisted even as the modern progressive working mother continued to serve in the households of these same patrons.

In Bahia, more programs and institutions were established to aid mothers and their children than ever before. These campaigns, though intense and institutional by the 1930s, were the continuation of nineteenth-century medical concerns. Within the "modernizing" spirit of the new century, that concern emphasized the poor as a means of "bettering" the Brazilian race. After all, they were an indispensable element in Brazil's history and "proof" of its social democracy. Medically, black women were central to anxieties about mothering, and had been since the 1800s. Succeeding generations of physicians, however, realized that black women were mothers themselves and not just wet nurses, or at least primarily nurses to their own children. Accordingly, the medical community placed a high priority on black maternity. For its part, the state government of Bahia gave poor families a great deal of rhetorical attention and backed that up with a fair amount of funding. Though insufficient, it represented unquestionably more funding than in any prior period. On these issues, Bahian medicine and its bureaucratic partnerships were pioneering, and thus Bahia's welfare policy was born.

Bahia was home to hundreds of thousands of poor *mães pretas* (and *pardas*), whose integration was essential to the success of any society-wide health effort. But the medical community saw them in specific ways. Though top-down, the emphasis on preventative medicine was admirable and badly needed, even as it characterized the movement as an oft-repeated battle against poor mothers' "ignorance" and "misery." Within the movement, the distinction between the *mãe preta* as servant and *mãe preta* as mom was completely murky. In reality, the vast majority of these mothers *were* servants; Brazil's unequal society closed other alternatives to them. As women, their expected service to the modern nation was in birthing, breast-feeding, and rearing healthy children as well. "Modernization" meant a healthy and sound majority with "civilized" habits, even if that majority was impoverished. For the *mães pretas*, there was an added element in that even their milk could be used as a public service—as described in chapter 3. Thus, the new institutions also recycled some old ideas. Despite problematic assumptions, family health was a real and serious issue. As services expanded, Bahia's poor mothers maximized the resources at hand to assist their families. They visited the clinics annually by the thousands, enrolled their children in the Better Baby Contests, fully engaged in the medical community's maternalist campaign, and guided that community in forming a more realistic view of their families' needs and challenges.

CHAPTER THREE

Foundling Care and Family Welfare

THE MÃE DESNATURADA

O N FEBRUARY 23, 1937, MARIA DO CARMO DA CONCEI-
ção gave birth to a son, José Augusto, at the free maternity
clinic in Salvador da Bahia. After José was born, Maria and her son relocated
to the Maternal Shelter on the campus of the Santa Casa de Misericórdia as
part of a welfare program that provided temporary housing and a monthly
stipend for mothers with newborns. Participating in the program gave Maria the opportunity to live with and care for José full-time, but it came
with the expectation that she breast-feed her infant. The shelter was one
of a host of new structures and services the Misericórdia had recently undertaken through a major renovation initiative in partnership with the Bahian League against Infant Mortality and the state government. By November, Maria could no longer nurse and was compelled to leave her son at the
Misericórdia's Foundling Home due to an "absolute lack of resources" to care
for him.[1] Although the Liga's reformist physicians devised the welfare program with the intention of keeping babies out of the foundling system, José
Augusto ended up there anyway. Maria had her son baptized on November 7
at the Igreja da Vitória with his godparents, Clarita and Clemente Mariani,
standing witness, and then she took her son to the registration desk at the
Foundling Home.

When Maria enrolled José, she elected to formally register her child, leaving her name and contact information. Like many mothers of foundlings in
the late 1930s, Maria opted for open registration rather than the anonymous
process of placing her child in the notorious foundling wheel. By that decade, the colonial foundling wheel, *roda dos expostos*, had become a scandalous symbol of abandoned and forgotten babies, permanently separated from
their mothers and their surnames and destined for early graves. By selecting
registration, Maria kept viable her option to return for José. And the reno-

vation and modernization of the Foundling Home had greatly improved the odds that children like José would survive their institutionalization. Fortunately for both mother and son, Maria was able to return for and retrieve her baby just three months after his enrollment.

Mothers like Maria do Carmo da Conceição had typically borne the brunt of medical and cultural disapproval for the serious problem of abandoned and foundling children.[2] According to cultural wisdom, foundlings were the unfortunate children born of "sinful" unwed or adulterous parents. For many Brazilians, detachment from a family name represented a type of social death—the denial of an identity, a birthright, and the protection of a community. Thus, the assumption was that foundlings were doomed to an ambiguous and unstable social place. And this was without considering the abysmal survival rates for institutionalized children that are detailed in this chapter. Social death was often the precursor to an imminent physical death. Though it is impossible to elucidate parents' motivations for relinquishing guardianship in every case, familial poverty as well as the weight of constructs of honor/shame underlay most of these situations, particularly in the colonial and imperial periods. Leaving an infant to the care of a foundling institution may seem an extreme measure, but many Brazilian families faced extreme circumstances, motivating them to relinquish custody of their children. The blame for "abandoning" children fell disproportionately on their mothers due to unequal constructions of female sexual honor and also the normalizing of motherhood and female domesticity in general. Both medically and culturally, mothers who did not raise their children were "*desnaturadas*," disgraced and unnatural women.

But Maria do Carmo da Conceição lived in a different context than her nineteenth-century counterparts; for Conceição's generation, medicalization and reformism helped define the parameters of "appropriate" motherhood. The Foundling Home's modernization and the dismantling of the turning wheel were examples of that. By the 1930s and 1940s, physicians such as those at the helm of the Liga advanced a social and structural understanding of motherhood that was somewhat diminished in moralizing, though poor women of color occupied a specific place in those articulations, reflecting the continued presence of the ghosts of Brazilian slavery.

The Bahian state physician Dr. Almeida Gouveia best expressed these emerging concepts of social maternalism and their contradictions by arguing for the separation of motherhood into two distinct phases: an involuntary biological process and a psychological or sociological transformation. For Gouveia, the female body was passive during the impregnation and gestation stages of motherhood, merely hosting the growing and imposing fetus. By contrast, "Motherhood," which the author distinguished with a capital *M*, required choice, intention, and sacrifice. The "Mothering" female body became active and deliberate, dedicated to nurturing an interdependent relationship of "affection and dedication" with her child that was both "spiritual and divine."[3] For Gouveia, the act of raising the child transformed the birth mother into a "*Mãe.*"

Gouveia's notions of a sociology of motherhood fit well with the campaigns spearheaded by the Liga. Their rhetoric and initiatives followed from structural conditions reformists identified as preventing impoverished mothers from making that transition from biological host to "*Mãe.*" Departing from an earlier discourse on the mothers of foundlings, Liga physicians argued that mothers like Maria do Carmo da Conceição were not "unnatural women," "*desnaturadas,*" but rather loving mothers besieged by poverty and need compelling them to relinquish their children to the Foundling Home. These were women with the desire and intention of practicing "Motherhood," but the harsh realities of living in poverty and surviving on low wages from domestic service made those maternal intentions nearly impossible to realize. Moreover, the Liga coupled that understanding of impoverished maternity with a narrative on single motherhood. They assumed mothers of foundlings had been abandoned by "seducers"; thus, for reformists, poverty and single motherhood were two sides of the same coin. Foundlings were fatherless children, and their mothers, rejected and desperate women. State and private organizations could step into the breach created by lack of resources and "absent" fathers, mitigating or even preventing the need for mothers to leave their children at the Misericórdia's Foundling Home.

Child rearing had a dual meaning for reformists, however. Maintaining custody and caregiving were only one aspect of solving familial separations due to the insecurities of living in poverty and illegitimacy. In Brazilian Portuguese, "to raise" a child, "*criar,*" was also a synonym for "to breast-feed"— shorthand for the phrase "to raise a child at the breast." When reformists envisioned restoring the *mães desnaturadas* to their natural state, they had child rearing *and* breast-feeding in mind. Maternal breast-feeding was also an integral tenet of *puericultura.* To Dr. Gouveia, for example, breast-feeding was "maternity at its highest expression"; the intimate contact, sustenance, and socialization turned mothers and their children into a "social unit."[4] Other contemporaries, such as the leaders of the Liga, referred to this as the "mother-child binary." From both perspectives, the active election to rear *and* to breast-feed defined motherhood. In 1930s Bahia, moreover, commercial milk was often dangerous, so there was a real risk for infant health. Maternal breast-feeding was one of the few realms where medical instructions were the same for all mothers regardless of social class. But, for Afro-Bahian women, mothering and nursing continued to be connected to the long-standing expectation that these women could or should provide breast milk for children other than their own. Rearing and nursing, therefore, were the starting points for integrated welfare projects in the late 1930s that aimed to keep mothers and babies together and away from the gates of the Foundling Home. These were collaborative efforts uniting private and public resources as reformists attempted to ensure that mothers like Maria do Carmo da Conceição could *"criar seus filhos"* in both senses of the phrase.

The mother-child binary and maternal breast-feeding became twin poles of a medicalized concept of "preventative abandonment," that is, keeping infants with their families rather than in the Foundling Home. In theory, welfare support in the form of small stipends would assist and encourage impoverished mothers to stay out of the labor market and at home breast-feeding their newborns. With this stipend program, medical reformists certainly acknowledged that breast-feeding and child rearing were forms of labor, and this is unsurprising, given Brazilians' long tradition of relying on domestic slaves or free poor wet nurses and nannies to care for children. Within the maternalism-as-modernization model, the urgent need for optimal children and "progressive" medicalized family practices warranted direct remuneration for reproductive labor because that labor and those transformations were keys to national regeneration. Thus, the reproductive labor of breast-feeding that Bahia's fledgling welfare programs acknowledged perpetuated the assumption that poor women nourish children in addition to their own and for a larger purpose, a burden that Brazilian women of color had shouldered for centuries.

MOTHERLESS CHILDREN AND BRAZILIAN MATERNALISM

Doctors like Gouveia used sociological Motherhood to communicate the need to keep mothers and babies together. Medicalizing and modernizing foundling care also made sense within the larger picture of ideological, political, and economic change (or lack thereof). Beyond the relatively closed confines of medical journals, *puericultura* profited from a new intellectual and political emphasis on the working poor and their contributions to developing the nation. This connection provided greater significance to maternal and child health and gave meaning to collaborative partnerships between private philanthropy and the state. The denigration of native labor that emerged in the waning years of slavery had subsided by the 1930s as a generation of artists, intellectuals, and labor activists reclaimed the historical roles and untapped potential of Brazilians in building the nation. They advocated for pro-Brazilian labor and cultural policies. Competition and conflicts between Brazilian and foreign labor had never affected Bahia directly, since there was no immigration boom there, but this did not mean that Bahians were disengaged from that national dialogue about the "fitness" of Brazil's working classes.

That consistent rhetorical thread in the 1930s placed new value on Brazil's multiethnic laboring bodies and the potential of those bodies to produce progress. No one questioned that Brazilian bodies had been well suited for bonded labor under unrelenting supervision and violent coercion. The demands of the modern age could also be carried on the backs of those bodies, but ensuring their peak capacity would require scientific, and particularly medical, intervention. As argued previously, these narratives of national progress through the working classes linked directly to the emergence of the maternalist movement. And the medicalization of foundling care developed in that same wider context. To claim that reformists' interest in saving foundling children's lives was only a functional calculation of their economic "worth" would be a crass exaggeration. Physicians and family advocates did not see poor babies as simple commodities, but they certainly did recognize the children of the popular classes as "human capital" whose labor would pay dividends in an imagined industrial future. Outside of Salvador, no one would characterize Bahia as particularly industrial anyway, but the spirit of preparing for the rigors of Brazilian modernization only buoyed the maternalist movement. Perhaps time and investment could bring Bahia up to par with the rapidly industrializing South; but in the meantime, state efforts could at least be directed toward maximizing the local population. Through various initiatives, that pursuit of "race betterment" targeted the health and welfare of poor mothers and their babies, who all too often ended up in the Foundling Home.

Brazil's major cities such as Salvador and Rio de Janeiro had large populations of foundling children. Tens of thousands of children were left anonymously to religious charity in those cities between the colonial period and the advent of the First Republic. In both cities, the governing councils partnered with their local branches of the Santa Casa de Misericórdia to care for foundlings, and this had been the case since the early days of the colony. Few institutions were as closely associated with the colonial past as the Santa Casa de Misericórdia—a confraternity that arrived in Brazil shortly after the Portuguese made landfall in the early sixteenth century. By updating the Misericórdia's Foundling Home, modernizers truly inserted themselves into the most traditional of child-care practices and institutions and demonstrated that maternalist concerns could even be applied to motherless children. The history of the rocky but cooperative state-Misericórdia partnership is long and helps contextualize the 1920s–1930s campaign against the *roda* and in favor of renovating the Foundling Home; the blending of private charity with public welfare; and the experiences of mothers, fathers, and their children who found new opportunities and adopted new strategies in their use of the Misericórdia's resources by the twentieth century—even if their opportunities were constricted by certain problematic assumptions within the reformist agenda.

The Santa Casa de Misericórdia, the lay Brotherhood of Our Lady, Mother of God, Virgin Mary of Mercy, dates back to fifteenth-century Lisbon. Dedicated to charitable assistance, the Santa Casa de Misericórdia da Bahia was founded in 1552 and is best known for constructing and administering the city's only hospital in the colonial period. The Misericórdia and the municipal government of Salvador shared responsibility for caring for foundlings in the sixteenth and seventeenth centuries until this duty was formally turned over to the brotherhood in 1726. Caring for foundlings was a typical mission of the various Misericórdia brotherhoods across the Portuguese Empire, who saw the extension of charity as a means to earthly repentance. By law, all municipal governments in the empire officially held responsibility for caring for foundlings. This entailed paying a small stipend to temporary families, "*famílias criadeiras*," who agreed to care for a child found in the streets or left on a doorstep. Families were eligible to receive the stipend until the death of the child or the age of seven (whichever came first) in hopes that caretaker families would bond with and retain the child until the age of majority. In some cases that occurred; in others, seven-year-olds were returned and institutionalized until another solution could be found. For Catholics, taking in a foundling was an act of Christian charity, and many families did so as an expression of their faith. Unfortunately, foundlings were also a source of cheap labor, and many were exploited as servants and slaves. The Misericórdia continued this circulation procedure in the eighteenth century, placing foundlings with wet nurses for three years in exchange for a small stipend. As is to be expected, most were free poor women of color. After three years, children were placed up for adoption, which often eventually entailed domestic service work for girls and apprenticeship or military service for boys.

The foundling issue in Bahia reached a tragic crisis point in the early eighteenth century when municipal funding was no longer available and the Misericórdia could not afford to care for these children. While municipal authorities and the Misericórdia's board bickered over funding, innocent babies were left abandoned in the streets, at the shore, and on the doorsteps of churches and convents. Not surprisingly, many died of starvation, animal attacks, and exposure; the gruesome presence of dead infant bodies in the city's streets caused a public scandal. After a contentious battle in 1726, the municipal government agreed to make an annual contribution to the cost of rearing foundlings at the Misericórdia. The institution was also granted the right to maintain a butcher shop, providing another source of income. The Misericórdia still relied on private charity to offset costs, which often exceeded income, leaving the institution indebted to the wet nurses who cared for foundlings.[5]

Part of the 1726 negotiations between the Misericórdia, local administrators, and the viceroy included the establishment of a foundling wheel—opened in 1734. The foundling wheel or *roda dos expostos*, was a revolving compartment on a street-facing façade of one of the buildings within the Misericórdia's complex. A medieval invention used across Southern Europe, the "turning wheel" was first established at the Hospital of the Holy Spirit in Rome in 1198.[6] When an infant was placed inside the *roda dos expostos* at the Misericórdia da Bahia, the entire compartment could be rotated to face the inside of the institution, allowing caregivers inside to retrieve the child without ever seeing the face of the person who deposited him or her there. According to the institution's board, they established the foundling wheel "to prevent the horror and inhumanity that some ungrateful and unloving mothers practice upon their newborns."[7]

Secrecy was paramount for the brotherhood, which sought at all costs to protect the anonymity of those leaving children on the institution's doorstep. The commitment to secrecy intended to protect the honor of those depositing children and serve as a preventative measure against infanticide, which many believed to be the common recourse of women facing potential threats to familial honor. For the historian Renato Pinto Venâncio, there was an ambiguity in Brazilians' social understanding of child abandonment. Though many saw foundlings as the fruits of immoral parents, born of mothers unworthy of the title, there was also the common sentiment that these children were blameless and should be protected and baptized. Foundlings suffered from social stigma and were assumed to be born criminals and prostitutes, but many Brazilians also felt they were innocent victims of their circumstances.

Before the twentieth century, the Misericórdia da Bahia was not a child-rearing institution; rather, the members of the confraternity saw their mission as primarily spiritual. In fact, the Foundling Home, called the Asilo dos Expostos or Casa da Roda, was not a "home" at all before 1847, but rather an area inside the hospital where infants were kept until leaving for their wet nurses' homes. Instead of housing children, the brotherhood's principal goal was to ensure abandoned children received the baptism sacrament before death. Like most *irmandades*, the Misericórdia sought to provide a "good death" for members and for foundlings entrusted to its care.[8] Members immediately baptized all children left in the wheel if there was no note indicating that the sacrament had already been performed. Unnamed children received the name of the saint for the day of baptism whenever possible. One of the brothers served as godfather, giving the child his own last name. All children were also given the last name Mattos in honor of João de Mattos de Aguiar, a former *provedor*, or chief administrator, and one of the first benefactors of the Misericórdia da Bahia. Mattos was even added to the surname of children who had already received the baptism sacrament before entry. All children who passed through the Foundling Home continued to receive the Mattos surname at registration, regardless of their length of stay, even after the system was reorganized in 1934. Therefore, somewhat ironically, Bahia's "anonymous" children all gained a new identity directly related to being severed from their family names.

Immediate baptism was absolutely necessary to fulfill the Misericórdia's spiritual mission because most children who entered the Foundling Home died within months or even weeks of their arrival. For most foundlings, the social death of anonymity and the "good death" ensured by the *irmandade* were preceded by a short and painful life. Admittance to the Foundling Home was almost tantamount to a death sentence for thousands of Brazilian children. The institutional records reveal the enormity of the tragic fate of these infants and young children. Between 1758 and 1870, the average annual mortality rate at the Misericórdia da Bahia was 649 per 1,000 children admitted, and a similar situation existed in Rio de Janeiro.[9] Foundlings had higher mortality rates than any other population in colonial and imperial Brazil. Unfortunately, administrators did not systematically record causes of death until late in the nineteenth century, but the most common causes for the brief period for which data exist were digestive problems, respiratory disease, and tuberculosis. Additionally, administrators' social prejudices were evident when they attributed high mortality rates to hereditary weakness due to degenerate parents and the supposed ineptitude of the poor women of color who served as the children's caregivers.

The Misericórdia did attempt to fulfill a patriarchal role for foundlings who survived past infancy, particularly for young girls, who tended to outnumber the boys.[10] Girls stayed in the institution until adoption, placement in domestic service with "tutors," marriage, or reaching their majority at twenty years of age. João de Mattos de Aguiar specifically designated his 80,000-cruzado legacy in 1700 for the construction of a lay spiritual home—the Recolhimento do Santo Nome de Jesus—for "honorable" women and orphaned girls and for their upkeep and dowries. After the Recolhimento was completed in 1716, small numbers of older foundlings—above the minimum of seven years of age—lived there in seclusion with the other residents.

In some cases, women who had reached their majority left the Misericór-dia to live on their own. In the case of marriage, the Misericórdia provided a 400-milreis dowry (in 1863), clothing, towels, sheets, and a wedding dress. Adult women and their suitors often negotiated marriages directly with the administration, which received requests from local men for marriageable foundlings. The French sisterhood, the Irmãs de Caridade de São Vicente de Paulo, administered both the Recolhimento and the Foundling Home start-ing in the mid-nineteenth century.[11]

Boys had fewer options; one was the Casa Pia e Colégio de Órfãos de São Joaquim orphanage founded at the end of the eighteenth century. The Mi-sericórdia tried to get boys apprenticed or enrolled in military training pro-grams. Bahian society considered foundling boys to be precriminals, so pro-viding them with structure or a trade was a key objective. Protecting boys from dishonor or abuse apparently was not as imperative a goal as it was for young girls. Like the girls, boys could be sent to work for a tutor or a fam-ily, receiving a salary if they were above twelve years of age, which should have been kept for them and turned over at majority. Sadly, too many young boys were considered difficult to place—particularly as they entered adoles-cence. If these boys fell through the cracks and managed to get beyond the Misericórdia's care, they were left to fend for themselves at a young age.

The fate of older and adult foundlings was a minority issue for many de-cades due to the appalling mortality rates at the Foundling Home. This lam-entable situation remained relatively consistent throughout the eighteenth and nineteenth centuries. In Bahia, the inner workings of the Foundling Home did not attract public attention; few members of the community were aware that foundling infants had such remote odds of reaching early child-hood. Two elements of this history point to the fact that foundling mortality rates were little known outside the institution itself. First, at times mothers left their infants in the wheel with identifying objects and notes indicating their intention to return for the child at some future date. Retrieving a child would have been nearly impossible, given the mortality rates in the Found-ling Home. The shroud of secrecy around the turning wheel seems to have obscured the reality of childhood deaths from public view. On November 25, 1889, for example, an unknown person deposited an hours-old newborn girl in the *roda* with a note declaring that the child had "no mother or father." The note also indicated that the depositor intended to return to reclaim the baby "as soon as I can." The child was baptized Leonória de Mattos, and she survived just three months.[12] Older foundlings generally fared better than newborns, but certainly not always. A two-month-old baby named Oralino, and rebaptized Vicente, was left in the *roda* on September 27, 1889. Oralino's note also indicated that he would be "sought after."[13] The child died after one month in the Misericórdia's custody. It is impossible to know whether or not these notes represented a serious commitment to retrieve these children, but the overwhelming majority of children were left with no notes at all. One may assume that in the few instances when notes, ribbons, and identifying clothing were left with children placed in the foundling wheel, those items did hold significance and were meant to communicate some information or intention.

The second clue that Bahian society was generally unaware of the catastrophic death rates of foundlings was the public reaction to the League against Infant Mortality's campaign against the turning wheel in the mid-1920s. Liga president Martagão Gesteira spent years decrying the "barbarity" of anonymous abandonment; his anti-*roda* campaign actually began when the organization was founded, but it took years to bear fruit. Thus, Bahian maternalism incorporated the plight of motherless children right from its inception. As a consequence, Gesteira regularly spoke of foundling children and their mothers during lecture appearances and in interviews in the popular press. The crux of the problem was twofold in his opinion: the turning wheel itself and the unhygienic conditions awaiting children on the other side of it. In a 1924 interview just a year after the Liga was founded, Gesteira called the foundling wheel "antiquated," "pernicious," and "counterproductive," generating mortality rates of "shameful" proportions.[14] His successor, Dr. Álvaro Bahia, later referred to the Foundling Home as a "cadaver factory."[15] Across Brazil, physicians like Gesteira and Bahia noted that annual mortality rates in the nation's Foundling Homes had not changed much with the turn of the century and consistently exceeded 50 percent. In years of epidemic disease, mortality often surpassed 70 percent.[16]

Changing this serious and long-standing situation at the Foundling Home was a conflict-ridden process pitting the Liga against the Misericórdia's administration in what was essentially a debate over the ideological underpinnings of foundling care and the Home's role in the larger community. The Misericórdia's board saw its role as primarily religious, protecting familial honor by keeping "unwanted" births secret and saving the souls of abandoned children. The Liga, and Gesteira in particular, crusaded to transform the Foundling Home into a model puericulture institution attending to both the "social problem" of foundlings and the health needs of poor mothers and children in general. Gesteira and other reformists held up the Foundling Home as the institutional epitome of dangerous and outdated child-rearing procedures, the antithesis of scientific motherhood.

The Liga's approach resonated with contemporary medical condemnations of turning wheels across Brazil. Reformists departed from the traditional depiction of foundlings' mothers as "ungrateful and unloving." For

Gesteira, for example, the much-lamented saga of clandestine pregnancies was not the backstory in the majority of cases of "abandoned" infants.
Rather, "single motherhood and misery" propelled the foundling problem,
causing permanent separations of mothers from their children. Yet these two
explanatory factors were interconnected; Gesteira's chief argument was that
mothers typically relinquished custody of their children due to a paucity of
financial resources, the need to work outside the home, and a lack of familial
support. Similar to Gouveia's sociological Motherhood, Gesteira conceptualized the problem of foundling children as a social not a moral one. Also, in
the true spirit of maternalism, Gesteira contended that improving the lot of
foundling children was a crucial step toward Brazilian progress.

> In nearly all the foundling homes in our Nation, in nearly all the Bra-
> zilian establishments dedicated to housing these unfortunate little
> ones for whom the cruelty of fate and human malice have condemned
> from birth to the deprivation of a home, of a name, and of maternal af-
> fection, there exists a horrible and nefarious institution of the Middle
> Ages that . . . must be definitively abolished in the name of humanity,
> of progress, and of science.[17]

The "horrible and nefarious institution" was the wheel itself, which became the symbol for the larger problems of foundling mortality and broken
family ties. In fact, the *roda* was technically illegal in Brazil, having been out-
lawed by the Children's Hygiene Inspectorate of 1923 and the Código de Menores (Juvenile Code) of 1926. The legal prohibitions, however, proved ineffective, and Misericórdias and other institutions across Brazil continued the
practice. In his condemnations of the *roda*, Gesteira refuted the common argument that turning wheels were a necessary evil, safeguarding honor and
preventing infanticide by providing an alternative for unwanted children.
First, he argued that secrecy was not a major cause of abandonment, since
only a minority of babies were left within the first days of birth. Second, according to Gesteira, all the health and child-care providers involved knew exactly who the parents of each child were and why the baby was being abandoned. Secrecy had little to do with the *roda*. The historian Muriel Nazzari
has made similar assertions about the foundling wheel, noting that priests,
family members, neighbors, and friends often colluded in the illusion that
certain women had not been pregnant and given birth.[18] Thus, secrecy did
not actually mean absolute privacy but rather that leaving a child to be raised
as a foundling resolved the taint of dishonor and fulfilled societal expectations, thus demonstrating both the flexibility and complexity of Brazil's culture of honor. Finally, Gesteira challenged all those who maintained that the

foundling wheel prevented infanticide by explaining that most babies left there died anyway. If the survival and well-being of foundlings justified the existence of the wheel, then much more needed to be done to save those unfortunate children from a wretched fate.

Gesteira and his supporters argued vehemently for the Foundling Home to abandon the anonymous wheel, which they believed permanently and unnecessarily separated mothers and children and posed an imminent danger to children's chances of survival. The Misericórdia should work to maintain what *puericultores* called the "mother-child binary" in every possible situation. Rather than anonymous abandonment, Gesteira recommended an open enrollment system, an *escritorio aberto*, where incoming foundlings would be registered and their parents' names recorded. An open system would allow mothers in desperate situations to temporarily leave their children but return when financial resources or other circumstances improved. Impoverished mothers and children did not have to be permanently separated if provisions allowed mothers to maintain contact with their institutionalized children and reclaim them at a later date. Based on international literature, Gesteira posited that women were often discouraged from definitively severing their relationship with their children when offered an alternative like retrieval or free daycare. An open system would likely result in *fewer* permanent abandonments (rather than *more* as the officials at the Misericórdia worried), and fewer children would be denied their right to the maternal breast and heart, condemned to death or a life of obscurity.[19]

Because Gesteira and Álvaro Bahia simultaneously served in bureaucratic positions while heading the Bahian League against Infant Mortality, as state inspector of Children's Hygiene and state physician respectively, they could draw upon their formal mandates to sanction the Foundling Home in an official capacity. In 1924, Gesteira sent Bahia to observe the Foundling Home and report on conditions there as required by the National Department of Public Health. Following Bahia's report, Gesteira composed a detailed and disturbing letter to the *provedor* of the Misericórdia, urging him to make several procedural reforms and relating just how dire conditions were in the Foundling Home. Among the worst evidence to come out of Bahia's report were the charges that children were improperly fed; basic rules of hygiene went unobserved; and children with serious illnesses shared facilities with healthy children, leading to the rapid spread of contagious diseases. Gesteira accused the Home of experiencing a 90 percent mortality rate for children left in the *roda* in 1923.[20] All of these observations and Gesteira's recommendations for reform were detailed in the local press.

The press quickly incorporated the tone of Gesteira's admonishments. Between 1924 and 1925, the local daily *A Tarde* ran a series detailing the debate between Gesteira and the administrator of the Foundling Home in response to Dr. Bahia's report. The headlines demonstrated sympathy with Gesteira's cause and perhaps sought to inflame readers with descriptions of the foundling wheel's little-known dark side. A November 20, 1924, article decried, "Terrifying statistics: Of the children who pass through the *roda*, 90% do not survive!" Two weeks later, the paper reassured its readers that "Progress trumps routine: The *roda*'s days are numbered." And the following year, on November 26, *A Tarde* reminded the public of the "sinister wheel" by asking, "Why do the children at the Foundling Home die?" [21] By following Gesteira's lead, local papers established their timeliness and relevance to social issues by supposedly uncovering the horrors of foundling mortality.

Provedor Isaias de Carvalho Santos did not welcome Gesteira's very public criticisms and recommendations. Gesteira recommended that the Foundling Home institute scientific feeding methods, avoid nourishing infants with animal milk, and contract wet nurses (who had been checked for syphilis) whenever possible or use sterilization methods when breast milk was unavailable. He advised the institution to establish separate facilities for children with infectious disease and make provisions for the disinfection of the children's clothing by installing a stove for hot-water laundry. Gesteira urged the administration to establish cleaner facilities to help combat the Home's fly problem. Ultimately, the suggestions regarding feeding, hygiene, and isolation were completely consistent with general puericulture concerns. Eventually Santos agreed to convene a junta to discuss the physician's suggestions, but a full year passed before the *provedor* made a public response in *A Tarde*. Responding in detail to each of Gesteira's comments, Santos assured the public that the Misericórdia was already aware of several of the issues Gesteira highlighted and had been working since the reform of 1916–1918 to address problems related to the Foundling Home. During those earlier reforms, they identified various causes of death: the "miserable" state of health in which children entered the Home, lack of access to breast milk or sterilized cow's milk, lack of trained staff, failure to disinfect clothing and other materials, and finally, aging and unhygienic facilities that required children to mix in close proximity and made transmission of disease unavoidable. Milk sterilization and scientific feeding methods were in place, though the *provedor* admitted that the resident physician was not permanently on-site and therefore it was impossible to know if food quantities were distributed according to the latest medical guidelines. The Home had attempted wet nursing on several occasions but abandoned the idea due to the difficulty of finding nurses. On the issue of nurses, Santos failed to cite the absolute catastrophe of 1836–1837 when the Misericórdia made its first attempt to house infants on-site rather than send them out to wet nurses. Of the seventy-five children admitted, sixty-eight died within the year due to a lack of sterilized milk to feed them.[22]

What Santos could not articulate in his dialogue with the Liga president was the Misericórdia's own ideological investment in the concept of anonymity. The initial resistance to closing the wheel and discarding the anonymity expectation should be contextualized within a broader analysis of the brotherhood's sources of authority and relevance in their local community and in Brazil in general. Understandably, Provedor Santos's argument against eliminating anonymity was that women's and infants' lives and family reputations were at stake, and this was certainly true. Thinking beyond the most apparent rationale, the Santa Casa de Misericórdia had a certain ownership of the "foundling problem" that was central to how the confraternity defined its societal mission, and guarding their right to that problem must have also propelled resistance to changing the system. By taking in and baptizing anonymous and abandoned children, the institution occupied a distinct and essential role in the Brazilian honor/shame complex. These activities were a source of spiritual fortification *and* local power. Opening the system to registration instead of perpetuating the ecclesiastical mysteries of a closed structure could undermine the Misericórdia's authority, and it did not help that the intervention of a secular private organization would mean divesting foundling adoption of its religious meanings. Therefore, anonymity was not simply an element in the admission procedures; it was integral to the social and cultural position of the Foundling Home. By retaining the custom of (re)christening children with the Mattos surname, for example, the Misericórdia held on to their practice of marking foundlings by name, connecting to a longer tradition of claiming them and "child saving." Furthermore, open enrollment implied a fundamental change, since the brotherhood's typical role as patriarch would be challenged if foundlings were simultaneously wards and members of families. With open enrollment, the Misericórdia's historic role in "child saving" would become ambiguous or at least diluted.

Thus, despite Gesteira's passionate arguments, the *provedor* countered that discontinuing the *roda* was an impossibility, given the need for secrecy in infant abandonment. He explained that thirty children had been left in the *roda* in the months immediately preceding Gesteira's campaign. What would have become of them if the *roda* were not an option? Like many, the *provedor* assumed that the wheel was primarily utilized by mothers who did not want their children. Santos did concede that an open registration system could be established if the Misericórdia leadership agreed to change their statutes, but open registration would only operate in tandem with the traditional anonymous foundling wheel, not as a replacement for it. The open enrollment al-

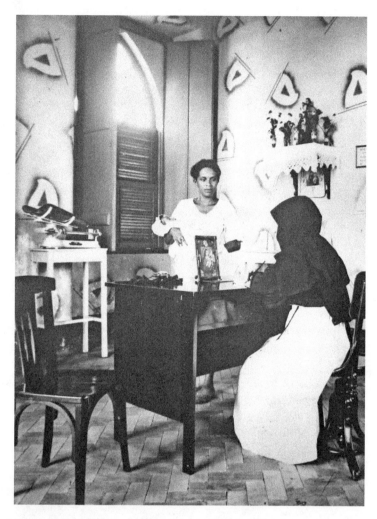

Open enrollment desk at the Foundling Home of the Santa Casa de Miseri-córdia da Bahia. (Archives of the Liga Álvaro Bahia contra a Mortalidade Infantil)

ternative became a reality in 1934, a decade after Dr. Bahia's inspection. Meanwhile, Gesteira nationalized his crusade to abolish the *roda* outright by securing letters of support from well-known *puericultores*; he unsuccessfully appealed to the Department of Public Health to enforce the prohibition against the wheel, and used his speaking engagements and the medical press to win support for his cause. In 1933, speaking before the Recife Rotary Club, Gesteira urged members to collaborate with him in the effort to eradicate the foundling wheel. Supporting that cause could be another manifestation of their commitment of service to God, he said, adding that "to serve the cause of abandoned children is to serve humanity and the patria as well as the civilization and greatness of Brazil."[23]

While no consensus could be reached on the wheel, the Liga did contract with the Misericórdia to oversee structural improvements on the campus and establish new services. In order for the open system that the Liga championed to make any impact, the Foundling Home had to first improve the health and life expectancy of their children. Thus, the two institutions agreed to a comprehensive overhaul of substandard procedures, services, and infrastructure. Interestingly, introducing open enrollment and solving the hygienic problems at the Foundling Home did not weaken the fervent calls for the closure of the turning wheel. As Gesteira repeated on several occasions, the worst horror of the foundling wheel for a *puericultor* was the separation of mothers and children. Even medically sanctioned facilities were no substitute for the loss of a mother. Again, the puericulture movement prioritized not just the physical health of children but a medicalized significance of the relationship between mother and child.

Open enrollment immediately became the preferred option for transferring children to the guardianship of the Foundling Home, once it was established. Between the first day of service on August 9, 1934, and July of 1937, only 9 children were left in the *roda* compared to 264 infants who were enrolled through the registration process.[24] This undoubtedly made a significant difference in the administration of the Home and in the lives and experiences of the children living there. The foundling wheel was eventually abolished in 1937 after falling into disuse, eclipsed by the greater popularity of open registration.

OPEN ENROLLMENT AND THE FOUNDLING HOME AS PUBLIC HEALTH CENTER

One of the critical outcomes of the open enrollment system when it was finally introduced was the ability to collect data on the children left at the Foundling Home and the families to which they pertained. For the Liga staff, data provided by open registration allowed for a more accurate, albeit incomplete, understanding of the circumstances motivating families to turn to the Foundling Home in the first place. Ultimately, the Liga's goal was to develop strategies that could aid families in keeping their children at home. The Foundling Home, therefore, was integrated into a larger scheme of social aid, designed as short-term fixes for families in need, especially mothers with infant children. Under this plan, families could freely register their children as foundlings for a limited period of time and return for those children when circumstances improved. The root problem with this approach was that poverty often was not a temporary complication, and it frequently took years or decades for foundlings to be reunited with their families even under open enrollment. Moreover, the combined resources of the state, the Liga, and the Misericórdia were always insufficient to fund the holistic familial program that reformists envisioned, so the Foundling Home often continued to be the most realistic option for families who could not afford to care for their children.

Certainly, open registration helped confirm that financial need drove most families to leave their young children to the care of the Foundling Home. Staff members created an identification file on each entering child that could include family status as well as the circumstances that had prompted the child's admission. The choice to leave any information at all was left totally to the election of the individual depositing the child. According to the Juvenile Code, it was illegal for private institutions to turn away children simply because the depositor declined to identify them.[25] The option to keep familial circumstances private was always available, and in fact, the majority of children continued to be registered as foundlings without any explanation. Maintaining the secrecy option even within the open system perhaps addressed lingering fears that without some means of anonymous abandonment, "unwanted" infants might have been left to a fate worse than institutionalization. Any child under six months of age could be registered without justification; incoming children over the age of one were always the rare exceptions. Of the records that did list parents' motives, lack of financial resources to raise the child appeared most often as families' primary obstacle.

For families who lived at the margins, the birth of a child, illness, or the death of a parent could easily leave them without means to support the entire household. Such was the case for twenty-seven-year-old Ermita de Almeida, who took her five-year-old daughter, Waldete, and newborn, Maria Luci, to the Foundling Home in October 1941. Like many of the mothers of Bahia's foundling children, Almeida had delivered Maria Luci at the Climério de Oliveira Maternity Center, an institution that provided birthing assistance free of charge to impoverished women. Almeida's husband, João, had recently died, and she was left in a dire position, surviving on her earnings as a laundress. The foundling registry provides no information of what ultimately happened to Waldete, but Maria Luci lived in the Home for one year before dying of pneumonia.[26] Though there were several cases of mothers left without resources due to death or flight of a partner, fathers also turned to the Foundling Home in desperation after the death of their infant's mother. Pedro Victor da Silva lost his partner, Santina Francisca de Jesus, just three months after the birth of their son José on New Year's Day, 1936. Silva, who worked as a gardener at the Hospital de Valença, was left to care for three children in addition to the infant. Silva had José baptized the day after his mother's passing and took him to the Foundling Home the following month. José was raised at the Misericórdia and eventually transferred to the Escola São Geraldo probably at the age of eight.[27] After José's transfer, the Foundling Home made no further updates to his record.

Both of the families above, like all those mentioned in this chapter, were Afro-Brazilians, and the preponderance of families of color in the records reflected the changing racial demographics of the foundling population and a shift in the socioeconomic background of the families leaving their children to the Misericórdia's care. By the early twentieth century, the Foundling Home had ceased to be a refuge for hiding "socially unacceptable" children and had become an institution for housing impoverished children, and this change began just after the abolition of slavery in 1889. In the two years following abolition, the number of white foundlings admitted to the Misericórdia da Bahia fell to 6 percent from a nineteenth-century average of 60 percent.[28] This was likely due to the extraordinary difficulties families of color faced during the immediate postemancipation period as well as their seeing the Foundling Home as a viable option, once foundlings of color no longer faced the real danger of falling into enslavement. Moreover, white mothers may have ceased to turn to the wheel to resolve threats to familial honor, once the Misericórdia had become so closely associated with poverty and desperation. In the first years of the First Republic, the numbers of white foundlings began to recover but only rose to a proportion commensurate with the overall population of whites in the city. It would never again reach the majority percentage that was typical of the colonial and imperial periods.[29] Based on a sample of four hundred records covering 1934–1942, the children living in the Foundling Home were overwhelmingly classified as *"pardo"* in color: 63 percent. Of the remaining children, 29 percent were classified as white, and 8 percent as *"preto."*[30] If familial honor continued to drive some portion of mothers to admit their children, these cases were obscured by the numerous stories of poverty, illness, and death. If honor continued as a motive, it was hidden in anonymity, just as poverty had been obscured by race in earlier centuries.

By the time the Bahian League against Infant Mortality created the open enrollment system, foundling children were overwhelmingly Afro-Brazilian from families immersed in financial and other crises. Mothers who were too ill to care for their families or in need of hospitalization often admitted their

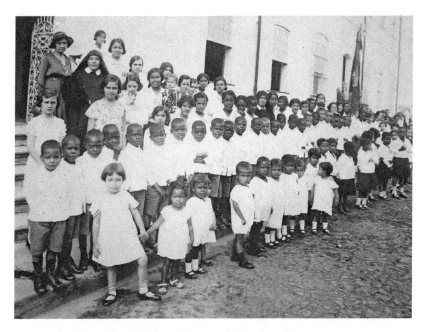

Foundling children at the Santa Casa de Misericórdia da Bahia. (Archives of the Liga Álvaro Bahia contra a Mortalidade Infantil)

children to the Foundling Home, for example. In September of 1940, Margarida dos Santos admitted her five-month-old son, Djalma. Santos was severely ill with tuberculosis, and her partner, Pedro Alexandrina da Anunciação, lived somewhere out of state. Until September, Santos's mother (who had previously suffered "insanity") had cared for both her daughter and grandson along with Santos's eight-year-old. Trapped in an unstable and grievous situation, Santos turned to the Foundling Home. Djalma was raised there until the age of thirteen, when an aunt removed him from the Misericórdia's care.[31]

The families mentioned in this chapter were among the few who elected to describe the circumstances that brought them to the Foundling Home's registration desk. The records they left behind elucidate details of their complicated and difficult situations. In these cases, child care and financial crises were evident. In most instances, however, the records are much shallower, offering little more than single words and simple phrases like "poverty" or "lack of resources" as the background storyline to these children's institutionalization—in the limited instances where the records reveal anything at all. Although open enrollment provided more information than the occasional notes pinned to children left in the turning wheel, profound gaps still remained that problematize any attempt to gain a full understanding of the separation of young children from their families of birth. Before the advent of open registration, in the absence of names and voices, observers, critics, and caretakers could ascribe any causation narrative that made sense culturally. Foundlings were the children of disgraced, unfaithful, and selfish women who callously rejected their children to hide their own shame. Anonymity may have afforded protection, but it also conferred power on outsiders to fill in a missing justification and an unspoken narrative for what seemed deviant and negligent behavior.

Even with open enrollment, reformists retained a certain power over the narrative of "abandonment." It is important to leave room for the possibility that families' responses fulfilled the reformists' own expectations. Given the context, it is hardly surprising that families who elected to "explain" their presence at the registration desk located their child-rearing crisis in poverty, illness, or the death of a parent. Impoverishment was a culturally acceptable rationale for leaving children to the Foundling Home. Perhaps this was even a simplification of a complex and multifaceted series of decisions and reactions to difficult circumstances. Other ways to read the evidence on children's circulation through the Foundling Home, for example, would be to see the mothers as exerting limited control over their reproductive, breast-feeding, and child-rearing labor; making decisions about how to constitute and manage their families; or even as preserving inadequate resources for themselves and for older children. At the desk, these types of negotiations may have been hiding behind the articulated explanations. Perhaps mothers and fathers weighed the well-being and chances of survival for their entire family and even recalled the circumstances surrounding the births and deaths of their deceased children. Medical reformists tended to imagine their female clients as if they were mothers to one newborn with no other children, but the reality was that many mothers carried both their present-day child-rearing experiences as well as the memories of their already deceased children. Furthermore, a less sentimental reading of the foundling issue might divest it of the maternal instinct assumption. Such a reading might acknowledge that some babies were unwanted or "inopportune"; perhaps the honor/shame complex was still in full force. And with the end of slavery, more poor women of color may have accessed similar honor constructs as their wealthier counterparts, knowing their foundling children would not fall into bondage. A combination of factors or none of these at all may contain the real causations behind separations of babies from their families, but the silent families and simplified records yield space for unstated possibilities.

Thus, despite opening the system, medical reformists remained in charge of the dominant "script." A prevailing narrative, inscribed in the

Misericórdia's foundling registries and its blank entry lines, continued to obscure familial complexities, negotiations, strategies, or even choices. Just like the assumed sexual immorality of "unnatural mothers," the "single, miserable mother" was also a projection of power—a reaffirmation of the reformists' own project and logic. These paradigms rendered the harsh realities and complicated calculations behind the institutionalization of infants more legible and palpable.

Returning to the example of Margarida, Pedro, Djalma, and their extended family, their experiences also illustrate an important point about foundling children and their kinship ties. Having kinship ties did not preclude poor children from entering the system, but in many cases, those ties did mean children were reunited with their families after some length of time as a ward of the Misericórdia. Kinship ties provide another clue to the socioeconomic situation of foundlings' birth families as well. Enrollment records indicate that most foundlings did have direct family ties; yet those relationships did not prevent children from being institutionalized, further supporting the argument that most pertained to impoverished families. Not surprisingly, the number of foundlings specifically listed as "legitimate" is low, approximately 18 percent of the sample.[32] In another 14 percent of the cases, however, the admissions registry recorded the names of both mother and father. Because consensual unions were more common than formal marriages among the poor, the presence of a father's name in the registry is a better indicator of whether or not the child came from a maternal-headed household. Though fathers' names cannot be taken as definitive evidence that these men were active caretakers of their children, it is suggestive because most foundlings were admitted as children of single mothers. Many foundlings also had godparents and extended families. About 30 percent of children arrived at the Home having already been baptized in their local parish. For the majority, their godparents' names—and at times their addresses—were listed in their admissions records. Other relatives, such as grandparents and aunts and uncles, appeared but less frequently. All of this demonstrates that the vast majority of foundlings had families and loved ones; they were not "abandoned children" rejected by callous mothers. And, as the example of Margarida, Pedro, and Djalma suggests, children from families in desperate situations may have circulated through the homes of extended family members before spending some period of time at the Home, later to be retrieved by parents or other relatives.

Dr. Gesteira and his colleagues were correct that families would return for their institutionalized children if the system were modernized and anonymity abandoned. Between 1934 and 1942, 177 children out of 453 were removed from the Foundling Home. In the majority of these cases (61%), families or godparents returned for their children and removed them from the institution's custody.[33] The ability of birth families to retrieve children was not a completely new phenomenon after the addition of open enrollment, but it had been much less common beforehand. In the nineteenth century, approximately 16 percent of foundlings were eventually collected by their families. Most children who left the Foundling Home's care had been wards for less than one month. These were likely cases in which mothers or other family members changed their minds and decided to retrieve newborns, or cases in which a child was placed in the turning wheel to cloud his or her parentage and then quickly retrieved by a birth parent under the guise of adopting a foundling child.

The sample of records from the first years of the open system reveals a very different picture. Only a small number of children who were eventually removed from the Foundling Home left within a year of their arrival. Most were wards of the Home for more than five years, and 38 percent of them had been under the institution's care between ten and nineteen years before their families returned for them. This was an astonishing change, as many twentieth-century children lived out their entire childhoods in the custody of the institution and returned to their families as adolescents. In March of 1941, for example, seventeen-year-old Zulmira Santiago admitted her infant daughter, Regina Lucia. Santiago worked as a domestic and had managed to take care of her daughter for three months, keeping Regina Lucia in good health. The child was raised as a ward of the Foundling Home until Santiago returned to take custody of her daughter in 1955 when Regina Lucia had reached fourteen years of age. Boys had better odds of leaving the Foundling Home sooner than did girls, probably because boys could be put to work at a younger age. Margarida Souza Paraiso and Crispiniano da Conceição admitted their infant son, Juarez, just a month after his birth. Paraiso returned for her child in May of 1951 when Juarez was eleven years old. These examples and dozens like them demonstrate that the enrollment system allowed families to maintain ties with their institutionalized children even if it is impossible to establish how many of these children were visited regularly. Far from forgetting or rejecting their children, the families of foundlings maintained the desire to bring them home over several years or even for more than a decade. They presumably waited for their children to reach an age when their daily care was less of an expense on limited resources. Teenage children could certainly have contributed some amount of income to their families in urban Salvador, and this fact likely made the difference as to whether an impoverished family could afford to have their children living in the household.

As all of these stories evidence, the Foundling Home was often a solution for mothers and families in desperate situations. Thousands of families turned to the Foundling Home when financial despair left little choice, using the institution as a permanent, short-term, or long-term solution. The circulation of children through the modern Home suggests that the old cultural assumption equating the foundling experience with social death was overstated. For many children, the turn of the wheel did signal a permanent rupture from their pasts. But for many others, enrollment as a foundling was a reflection of their family dynamics rather than the termination of them. These children likely knew exactly who they were and to what surname they pertained. For these children and families, the Foundling Home was a community institution, another aspect of the social world in which they lived, where real-life stories played out, not a Greek tragedy of mistaken identities.

Despite the revised open procedures, both the Liga and the Misericórdia administration hoped to convince parents to seek alternatives whenever possible. For reformists, registration was preferable to anonymity, but the best-case scenario was to avoid the system altogether and keep children at home. Signs placed prominently at the reception desk pleaded with mothers to "Think carefully before abandoning your child. By handing him over to the shelter or depositing him in the foundling wheel, you definitively lose all rights to the child"; "An abandoned child is a lost child."[34] Staff members at the desk asked each mother whether a little assistance, "*um jeito ao caso*," in the form of a space in the free daycare or medical treatment could help keep the child at home.

Renato Pinto Venâncio has argued that the only option for Brazilian families confronted with serious situations of poverty and illness was to give up custody of their children. But turning over custody was not the *only* option available to Bahian families by the 1930s as the maternalist movement expanded and spawned new health and welfare programs. Even in Salvador, however, relinquishing custody was one of very limited options and often the only alternative that could make a substantive difference for extended or enduring conditions of financial insecurity. While the signs in the registration waiting room seemed to represent familial separations as moral issues, the actual circumstances prompting families to enroll their children in the Home were both structural and widespread. The Liga leaders did recognize that fact, likely as a result of tutelage from real mothers using the prenatal and well-baby programs. With the Liga's urging and aid, the Misericórdia conceded to address those structural circumstances by attempting to offer alternatives to families at risk of transferring guardianship of their children to the Foundling Home. To fulfill these new expectations, the Misericórdia would have to cast its net beyond the individual families who appeared on the institution's steps to encompass the much larger problem of the general state of Bahian public health and social welfare.

"A MODEL PRO-PUERICULTURE INSTITUTION"

With the Bahian League against Infant Mortality's leadership, the Misericórdia underwent a wholesale renovation in the 1930s, not only in infrastructure but in purpose. This new mission turned the Misericórdia into an integrated complex of specialized women's and children's health and welfare services, expanding the community health role that the institution had occupied since the colonial period through its management of the Santa Izabel Hospital. The Liga agreed to provide free services to foundling children in exchange for the Misericórdia's agreement to make several changes that could theoretically ameliorate those structural problems that left working mothers with small children without financial, nutritional, or health resources and without daytime caretakers. In principle, these new sources of support would reduce the foundling population and help more families keep their children at home. The new programs were actually three-party partnerships uniting the Misericórdia, the Liga (and its benefactors), and the state of Bahia. On paper at least, it was a reformist's dream, allowing the Liga to put a number of puericulture tenets into practice by providing better hygienic, medical, and social assistance to foundling children and to those at risk of being "abandoned." With the renovation, the Liga was finally able to institute the recommendations made back in 1924 when the organization first publicized the appalling conditions within the Foundling Home.

For the Liga, "abandonment prevention" was just like preventative medicine: it required a holistic approach that began with birthing. Since 1910, Salvador had been home to a free birthing clinic: the Climério de Oliveira Maternity Center. But reformists realized that, for many women, having a safe place to give birth was just the tip of the iceberg. To maintain themselves and their families, many new mothers needed to return to work immediately but often did not have child care for their newborns. This was the type of crisis that could lead a mother with a baby in arms to the registration desk at the Foundling Home. Thus, one of the first modern installations in the integrated "preventative abandonment" plan was a Maternal Shelter, Abrigo Maternal, later renamed the Pavilhão Martagão Gesteira in honor of the Liga's founder. Constructed in 1934, the shelter was the central element in the plan to reduce the foundling population at the Misericórdia. The shelter provided temporary housing for women who had just given birth at Climério de Oliveira, who were recommended by one of the city's free clinics, or who requested admission due to lack of resources. Liga physicians and their partners intended the Maternal Shelter to be a refuge for new mothers, but this temporary support could not account for mothers with older children still waiting at home.

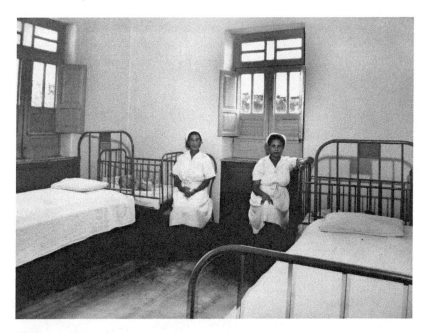

Mothers and their infants in the Nutrizes' *(Wet Nurses') Room, Maternal Shelter at the Santa Casa de Misericórdia da Bahia. (Archives of the Liga Álvaro Bahia contra a Mortalidade Infantil)*

In the Maternal Shelter, mothers shared accommodations with their infant children. Internal documents often referred to them as *"nutrizes,"* or "wet nurses," since living in the shelter came with the expectation that all women would breast-feed their babies and even donate breast milk to other needy children. In 1937, Maria Joanna Nascimento, Ester Barreto, and Maria America Gomes were among the many women who spent several weeks with their newborns living in the shelter.[35] Acceptance to reside there came with clothing, meals, and a $30-cruzeiro stipend paid upon discharge from the facility. But a temporary stay in the shelter was just that, and in extreme situations, some mothers could not afford to take their babies home after their residency ended. When Ester Barreto became too sick to continue nursing her four-month-old son, Almiro, and with no means to take him home, she registered him as a foundling, and the unfortunate child survived less than a month.[36] In addition to room, board, and a stipend, the Liga provided mothers in the Maternal Shelter with instruction in the "proper" care of their infants. The School of Medicine contributed a small museum on infant mortality, prenatal hygiene, and childhood development to assist in the effort. As argued in chapter 2, the medical community regularly accused Bahia's mothers of color of endangering their infants through "ignorant" child-care practices. These assumptions and the language in which they were expressed carried the full baggage of Brazilian racism and a general distrust, suspicion, and fear of the poor.

The second step in turning the Misericórdia into a "model pro-puericulture institution,"[37] in Dr. Bahia's words, was improving access to safe nutrition for infants and children. Upon being awarded a state Social Assistance Council subsidy in 1934, the Misericórdia made another addition to its campus: a milk dispensary serving the entire city, called the Julia de Carvalho Lactário. The Lactário weekly provided thousands of liters of sterilized milk and other nutrients suitable for babies (such as coconut milk and porridges) for distribution via the state's free health centers. This milk was also vital for nourishing sick infants in the on-site daycare. Sterilization was a life-or-death issue because the state government had always been unsuccessful in enforcing safety guidelines for commercial milk, making digestive disease a primary cause of infant mortality. In addition to sterilization and distribution services, the Lactário also dispensed breast milk purchased from mothers living in the shelter and from other poor local women.

As the Maternal Shelter and Dispensary demonstrate, the Liga was successful in convincing the Misericórdia board to extend the confraternity's radius of action to include services for poor children and their families beyond the confines of the Foundling Home. The new campus additions joined a modern, fully equipped children's medical center. The Arnaldo Baptista Marques Polyclinic opened in November of 1930 alongside the state's Fifth Health Post. State involvement brought money, and the Liga's roster of private benefactors generated a large donation from a wealthy old-money family who named the clinic in honor of their deceased son.

The logic behind having both clinics side by side was to give impoverished families an option for treatment if their children were too sick to stay at home and enrolling them as foundlings seemed the only means of obtaining medical assistance. Perhaps this assumption proved correct because the majority of children entering the Foundling Home were deemed healthy upon arrival, according to the 1930s sample. Nearly 70 percent of children were admitted in an apparent state of health, and among the sick, only 5 percent were "gravely ill" or "near death." Another 2 percent of the ill were listed as sick due to "need," a reference to children in a state of starvation and deprivation.[38] Therefore, it is likely that the free clinics helped reduce the number of children who were enrolled as foundlings when illness outstripped their families' capacity to care for them. The polyclinic offered specialized services, including simple surgeries, laboratory testing, eye and dental care as well as otorhinolaryngology. The number of children served at the polyclinic increased steadily throughout its first decade; by the 1940s, the clinic saw an average of 3,636 patients per year.[39]

Even with the "abandonment prevention" strategy, the Santa Casa de Misericórdia still had a foundling population in urgent need of better conditions within the institution. According to the terms of their 1930 agreement, the Liga took over responsibility for children under two years of age and provided all medical care for sick children up to eight years of age. The Misericórdia enacted various architectural reforms in the Foundling Home, providing for better isolation of sick children from healthy ones, a modern laundry facility for properly cleaning their clothing, and verandas to provide ventilation in the buildings where children lived.[40] Under the new procedures, all incoming children spent thirty days in a separate observation room before being transferred to live among the general population in an attempt to prevent the spread of contagious disease.

Reformers understood that the deplorable mortality rates were not due to contagious disease alone; foundlings lived under inexcusable conditions. As late as 1934, four years after the initial agreement, Dr. Gesteira and Provedor Arthur Newton de Lemos had a heated exchange concerning conditions at the Home, which Lemos vehemently defended. Gesteira charged that both he and the state governor had personally witnessed underfed and nude children in the Home due to a deficient kitchen and an "absolute lack of clothing."[41] Once the two institutions settled on a modernization plan, the improvements introduced in medical care, hygiene, isolation, and feeding caused mortality rates to fall rapidly and sharply. By 1940, the mortality coefficient for children under two years of age had fallen to 9.72 percent.[42]

To focus on the needs of the youngest foundlings, the Liga added the Juracy Magalhães Pupileira to the complex in 1935, named in honor of the state's *interventor* (appointed governor) and benefiting from the largess of Bahia's public budget. The Pupileira, a Portuguese adaptation of the French *"pouponnière,"* was a specialized institution, dedicated exclusively to foundlings under the age of two. Babies spent a short time in the newborn shelter of the Martagão Gesteira Pavilion before being transferred to the Pupileira. Separate facilities for children of this tender age allowed the staff to concentrate on the developmental stage that *puericultores* considered most critical. It was this age range that presented the highest incidence of mortality and in which deprivation was most likely to cause irreparable damage. Structurally, the Pupileira had space for eighty children, separated into glassed-in units that could hold six cribs each, a bathroom, and a scale for daily weigh-ins. It had special facilities for medical examinations and a large playroom, or *sala de brinquedos*—a rare addition for institutionalized babies. Inaugurated on Christmas Day, the new Pupileira opened its doors to *senhoras* of high society who participated in the tradition of distributing clothes and toys to poor children, typifying what Donna Guy has called women's "performance of charity" within the modern welfare state as a channel to social status and community recognition.[43]

The Pupileira staff attempted to function as a sort of surrogate family for foundling children. Organization leaders expected head nurses and attendants to provide "motherly care" to their charges, tending to the physical and moral aspects of their upbringing. For Liga physician Dr. Eliezer Audíface, it was the female attendants' responsibility to inspire a "joy of life" in children deprived of a home and of motherly attention. In his words, "The attendants do not work on a circuit so that their dedication and work for the children under their care would be like that of a family . . . seeking to awaken that sentiment that lies latent in every woman—the maternal sentiment."[44] Unlike the traditional mission of the Misericórdia, the Liga apparently sought to substitute the role of matriarch rather than patriarch. They assumed that the absence of a maternal figure most endangered foundlings' lives and futures more than the lack of a father. This was one manifestation of transforming from a child-centered approach to the foundling problem to a mother-centered one. For reformists, an affectionate caregiver in the Pupileira was the best chance these motherless children had of growing up without developmental delays caused by institutionalization. Children who stayed within the foundling system beyond the age of two mainstreamed into the general population.

Naming the Pupileira in honor of Juracy Magalhães was also shrewd and reflected at least the media's consensus that the modern Foundling Home represented the appointed governor's personal commitment to the needs of the Bahian populace. In media reports, the Pupileira stood as testimony to the "honesty," "intelligence," and "vigor" of their leader. One journalist present at the inauguration lauded the facility as "the best Christmas present that Juracy Magalhães's government could have offered to the people."[45] Bahia was grateful for a leader who took their concerns seriously and worked for the collective social and economic advancement of the state with a government "of the people, governing with the people, and for the people."[46] By the 1930s, foundling care surprisingly had come to represent governmental commitment to the welfare of *all* Bahians. The investment in modernizing the Home and the attribution to the governor's individual initiative seemed to mark both a new chapter in public expectations of state responsibilities and an old story of personalistic benevolence. But the value placed on foundling care was a radical departure from an earlier era when foundlings lived tragically short, deprived lives and the general public seemed not to notice.

Between the closing of the foundling wheel and the construction of the

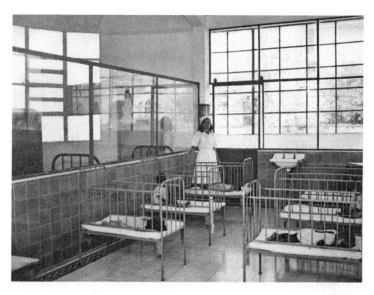

Assistant and foundling children, Pupileira Juracy Magalhães, Santa Casa de Misericórdia da Bahia. (Archives of the Liga Álvaro Bahia contra a Mortalidade Infantil)

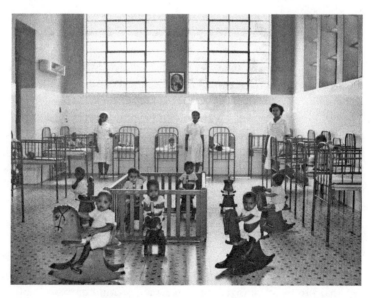

Assistants and foundling children, Pavilhão Martagão Gesteira, Santa Casa de Misericórdia da Bahia. (Archives of the Liga Álvaro Bahia contra a Mortalidade Infantil)

Maternal Shelter, Arnaldo Baptista Marques Polyclinic, Julia de Carvalho Milk Dispensary, and Juracy Magalhães Pupileira, the colonial Santa Casa de Misericórdia had definitively entered the maternalist movement of the twentieth century. In Dr. Bahia's words, the old institution had become a modern partner in the fight against infant mortality—"no longer simply a Holy House of Mercy."[47] Like the "unnatural mother," through science, the Foundling Home was redeemed. Without discounting the vastly improved circumstances for children living in the Home, the Santa Casa de Misericórdia, the Liga, and the state continued to explicitly support the idea that separating mothers and children (at least temporarily) was an acceptable, scientific, and modern approach to dealing with poverty. Barring the case of illness for which treatment options were expanded, separation and institutionalization continued to be the remedies for poverty. The modern Home took in many more infants than were aided by the much smaller breast-feeding stipend program that helped keep children at home with their mothers. And families took advantage of this alternative as long-term childhood institutionalization became a survival strategy for the poor. Even so, institutionalization was an impractical solution, given the weight of poverty in Bahia, and the Liga commenced a new campaign in the 1940s to establish a foster care system to assist this same population of impoverished children.

Even "model institutions" have their limitations. The most ardent champions had to admit that the best science could not compensate for the reality of small children left bereft of a family—in some cases for the entirety of their childhoods. And even the most updated medical ideas could only be implemented to the extent that finances and infrastructural capacity allowed. Despite expertly designed facilities and the expertise of Bahia's top *puericultores*, the Pavilion and Pupileira could never keep up with the needs of local families. They lacked the financial resources to truly embody the ideals of their architects. There were too many women and children in need and an insufficient, undertrained, and underpaid staff. The Liga's second president, Dr. Bahia, for example, repeatedly complained about the staff at the Pavilion whose daily responsibilities exceeded any reasonable expectations and certainly prevented them from providing a high level of care. The small staff of six assistants was responsible for forty children under the age of one, which translated into "taking 40 temperatures, giving 60–80 baths, feeding 200 meals, and changing an average of 300 diapers per day."[48] Under these conditions, it is hard to imagine that these female aides could provide "motherly care" or instill a "joy of life" in forty babies simultaneously. Bahia was also disappointed with the quality of the staff; he attributed the constant turnover to the practice of hiring poor women with little education who, he charged, had no concept of modern hygiene. Of course, the Misericórdia could not expect to attract well-trained nurses due to poor wages and the extreme work-load. Lacking a proper maintenance staff, the residents at the Maternal Shelter were left to clean their living spaces as well as the larger facility while also making time to care for their newborns.

Ultimately, the anti-*roda* movement and the modernization sought to re-define the foundling problem as one originating in Brazilian poverty and not exclusively in Brazilian culture. These ideas reflected a turning tide in the politics of 1930s maternalism. For Dr. Bahia, mothers at risk of relinquishing custody of their children were not failures but rather mothers besieged by cir-cumstances that left few alternatives. Far from "*desnaturadas*," Bahia referred to these mothers as "*desamparadas*": loving, devoted, hard-working moth-ers left "abandoned" by society, the law, and their children's fathers. "Indif-ference," "collective injustice," and "the injustices of men" undermined their natural maternal instincts.[49] Despite their best efforts and long hours spent in low-paying domestic service, their children suffered malnutrition, poor health, and the inadequate supervision of "caretakers" and "ignorant neigh-bors" during the workday.[50] Dr. Bahia repeatedly described single mothers as women "lacking a home and bread" who, in a paradox of the natural order, discovered that their children's needs threatened their own survival.

By the mid-1930s, the Bahian League against Infant Mortality had more than a decade of direct experience in working with local families. That ex-perience combined with the collective knowledge accumulated by older in-stitutions like the IPAI must have provided a more realistic view of mother-hood and child rearing than that inscribed in nineteenth-century medical journals. But that on-the-ground experience did not necessarily preclude twentieth-century reformists from retaining or creating certain biases; for example, fathers and male partners were almost completely written out by the "single motherhood" narrative. Despite those distortions, the interaction between health advocates and poor mothers influenced the development of policies. These mothers presumably helped craft the welfare policies of the midcentury by educating reformers on the economic realities of raising chil-dren in working poor families. Through their daily contact in the public clin-ics and at the Foundling Home, physicians must have learned that Bahian mothers were not "unnatural women" who simply failed to prioritize their children's well-being. These mothers must have explained the challenges they faced with long workdays, low wages, unsympathetic employers, and, in some instances, absent partners. The maternalist movement came closer than ever before to recognizing that the circumstances of average families were complex and difficult, and that their children were part of a larger con-text of family dynamics in which access to resources was often the para-mount obstacle.

Rhetorically, the 1930s discourse on single motherhood reinforced the "abandonment prevention" approach at the Misericórdia. For maternal advocates, keeping children at home rather than at the Misericórdia prevented severance of the "mother-child binary" and enabled and encouraged maternal nursing. The desire for poor women to breast-feed their infants was never separated from the foundling problem. For Dr. Bahia, maternal nursing was an issue of social justice. In his words, "No measure is more humanitarian or more honest than to ensure the poor mother at the very least the right to breast-feed her own child."[51] So breast-feeding, welfare and assistance, and "preventative abandonment" became wrapped together in 1934 into one policy, once again uniting the Liga, the state, and the Santa Casa de Misericórdia.

MOTHERS' MILK AND SOCIAL WELFARE

With the new installations on the campus of the Misericórdia, maternal advocates hoped to provide families with alternatives to the Foundling Home: medical treatment for sick children, temporary housing for new mothers, and sterilized milk for infants in need. Around the city, poor families could access state-subsidized free daycares and specialized maternal cantinas where pregnant and nursing women were served meals free of charge. Reformists instigated this multiangle system of support to keep children at home and supplemented it with the revolving-door policy at the Foundling Home as a fail-safe measure. While clinical and housing options expanded, state-funded welfare assistance sought to reduce the need for families to access them. To bring the system full circle, the Liga and the state devised a small direct funding program to provide the financial means for poor mothers to keep their infants out of institutions altogether.

Support for mothers in need came in the form of cash payments through a welfare program called the *prêmio de amamentação*, or breast-feeding stipend. The program was the first of its kind in Brazil and had as its aim to help impoverished mothers stay home and breast-feed rather than work outside the home and thus nourish their children with potentially dangerous animal milk. Maternal advocates understood that the need to earn a living was often at the root of separations and made exclusive breast-feeding all but impossible. The creation of the Maternal Shelter was the first step toward establishing the *prêmio de amamentação* because mothers and newborns were invited to live there temporarily. During their residency, participants devoted themselves exclusively to their infants, or at least that was the expectation, while receiving a $30-cruzeiro monthly breast-feeding stipend as already mentioned. Thirty cruzeiros was a low wage but certainly not an insignificant amount of money. To contextualize the value of this amount of money, laundresses who worked for the Liga earned a monthly wage of $50 cruzeiros. Servants working for the Pupileira Juracy Magalhães earned $40 cruzeiros per month, and aides in the children's hygiene clinic earned $30 cruzeiros.[52]

The breast-feeding stipend program has a fascinating and complicated genealogy based on both international precedents and local conditions. The Bahian version was modeled after similar programs in France. There were a number of French precedents for financial assistance programs aimed at pregnant women and nursing mothers, dating back to the eighteenth century. The more contemporary attempts at this type of assistance arose in the late nineteenth century, however, and were at times publicly funded and at times the result of collaborations between private charities and local governments. Beginning in 1856, Public Assistance of Paris offered poor mothers stipends equal to one month's payment to a wet nurse. This program was largely ineffectual because many women could not afford to continue paying the wet nurse after the first month, so the stipend only afforded a brief delay to their employment and child-care crisis. Later programs were more comprehensive, providing travel fees to send Parisian infants to their wet nurses' homes in the countryside and up to ten months of wages to pay her. By 1894, Public Assistance was providing up to one year of monthly stipends, though the stipends were insufficient to relieve the need to seek employment, and only a minority of those mothers requesting assistance were able to actually obtain it.[53]

In Bahia, the Liga literally intended to turn Bahian women into the "paid wet nurses of their children," a phrase Dr. Gesteira borrowed from the nineteenth-century French pronatalist movement.[54] In July 1937, the Liga expanded the breast-feeding stipend program beyond the Misericórdia grounds to benefit women and infants who did not reside at the Maternal Shelter. Outside of the shelter, the program required mothers receiving support to register their infants in the local clinic, bring them in for weekly well-baby appointments, and receive the visiting nurse for home inspections. Thus, the welfare assistance program also reinforced reformists' larger mission of medicalizing the habits, routines, and dynamics of poor families. The Liga received regular requests from partner organizations like the Bahian chapter of the Brazilian Assistance Legion (LBA), for example, with recommendations of mothers who were in desperate need of help. Many were wives of Bahian soldiers away on duty. Providing wartime assistance to soldiers and their families was the founding mission of the LBA, so supporting the Liga's welfare outreach efforts served that objective. In 1943, Maria de Nazaré Portela and her infant son, Maria do Carmo and her daughter Ruth,

Maria José de Sousa and her daughter Maria Emilia, and Guiomar Damiana Santos and her son Carlos Alberto were all beneficiaries of the breast-feeding stipend via the personal advocacy of Ruth Aleixo, local LBA president and First Lady of the state of Bahia.[55]

The welfare program could not accommodate all women in need, not even all those who came through the Maternity Center. Most enrolled mothers were referred through the Maternity Hospital, the public clinics, or at the registration desk at the Foundling Home. Between open registration and the breast-feeding stipend, the infamous turning wheel gained a completely new narrative. Rather than an uncaring and morally corrupt mother depositing an unwanted child, the new system of public aid freed desperate, grieving mothers from the tragedy of passing through the Misericórdia's gates and resigning themselves to their final and irrevocable option. In Dr. Bahia's words, mothers arrived in tears at the Foundling Home but left "grateful to the state for providing the assistance that would allow them to retain and breast-feed their beloved children."[56] This new narrative "redeemed" *mães desnaturadas*, appealing to the notion that there was nothing more natural than a loving mother with an infant child at her breast. The generosity of the state had the ability to cure distortions caused by poverty and bring the instinctive relationship between even poor mothers and their children back into equilibrium.

Unsurprisingly, the overwhelming majority of mothers in the program worked as domestic servants. Most were unmarried mothers, but not exclusively so. In general, Brazilian physicians avoided the debate that raged among French physicians and politicians over whether marriage should be a prerequisite for public assistance. Bahian physicians saw the short residency in the shelter as a time for mother-child bonding. Coupled with the subsequent stipend, that emotional attachment could help keep families intact even if mothers and fathers were unmarried. As mentioned, fathers were sidelined in the breast-feeding stipend program. Enrollment documents did not record any information on the children's fathers, not even registering their names. The paradigm of impoverished single motherhood either presumed fathers were absent from the lives of their children or relegated fatherhood to a nonessential and even irrelevant aspect of the campaign to improve child health and reduce mortality. Erasing fathers erased the dynamics of fatherhood, patriarchy, and partnership from the lives and experiences of these families as they accessed welfare aid.

The one characteristic that the participants in the program seemed to share was that they were all mothers of more than one child. In fact, organizers made a particular attempt to support women with twin infants. In any given month, mothers with twins accounted for approximately half of all participants. Many participants in the *prêmio de amamentação* program had several children, and their brief profiles reflect how challenging motherhood was for Bahian women in the early twentieth century, given the uneven medical knowledge about difficult pregnancies, high infant mortality, and few options for birth control. Adding to these difficulties was the struggle to raise families on the paltry wages earned in domestic service. Apolinaria Bispo, who worked as a laundress and began receiving stipend payments in December of 1942, had given birth to twins Jurandir and Yaci in October. At thirty-one years of age, she had experienced seven pregnancies, three of which ended in miscarriage. In 1942, Bispo had three living children, including the twin babies; her older three children had died in infancy. At the very least, Bispo had a husband to help support her, and the evidence suggests that married Brazilian women, whether impoverished or not, experienced multiple pregnancies throughout their reproductive lives. For unmarried women, such as Fernanda Lopes, who entered the program after the birth of her twins Cleonice and Carlos in December 1941, the economics of family life could also be precarious. The records do not reveal, however, whether unmarried women like Lopes had long-term partners, so it is difficult to accurately reconstruct her family life. Both Apolinaria Bispo and Fernanda Lopes found themselves in the same situation of need after the birth of their twins, demonstrating that poverty was often acute for Bahian families whether parents were legally married or not.[57]

Approximately twenty women could live at the Maternal Shelter and participate in the program at one time. But funding was the only limitation to the number of nonresidential participants. By 1941, the *prêmio* program had already benefited 500 Bahian children and their mothers. By the close of 1945, that number had climbed to 1,173, so the program had a significant impact on the lives of hundreds of families.[58] Mortality rates were also well below average among children in the program. Physicians attributed this success to medical supervision, maternal education, and of course the health benefits of breast-feeding over bottle-feeding.

For years, the Liga counted on the support of the local Rotary Club, one of many partner organizations. Consequently, the Liga enlisted their aid to advocate on behalf of the breast-feeding stipend. In 1940, the prominent jurist and club member Carlos Ribeiro declared to the local paper *O Imparcial* that "mothers' milk is the property of children."[59] It is unclear whether Ribeiro meant to suggest that children had a right to their own mothers' breasts or that all infants had a right to breast milk, because the *prêmio de amamentação* program ultimately incorporated both of these ideas. In a fascinating twist on the long-standing poverty and wet-nursing debate, participants in the *prêmio* program could augment their stipends by contributing breast milk to the Julia de Carvalho Milk Dispensary. During their residency at the shelter, mothers earned an additional $1.50 per liter for any excess breast milk donated to the dispensary. The entire sum was turned over upon departure. The offer also extended to *prêmio* participants after they left and to poor new mothers in the larger community.

Bahia claimed the distinction of being the first state in the nation to open a breast milk distribution center. On the occasion of its inauguration in 1937, Appointed Governor Magalhães even donated funds to purchase an apparatus called a Bettinoti Polyextractor that allowed eight women to pump breast milk simultaneously. Breast milk collected at Julia de Carvalho was destined for a number of distribution points, including the Pavilion, the Puericulture School, and the two Infant Hygiene Posts in the neighborhoods of Liberdade and Rio Vermelho. These institutions jointly distributed an impressive quantity of breast milk for needy infants. Within a few years, the Bahian League against Infant Mortality facilitated the provision of more than 1,000 liters annually, and by 1941 a total of 10,738 liters.[60] This was all possible thanks to women like Lidia Santos who contributed $877.30 cruzeiros' worth of her breast milk in 1943, Lourença dos Santos who contributed $754.80 worth, and Dionisia Pereira who contributed $408.80 worth in 1943.[61] Their milk, and that of other poor women like them, sustained hundreds of infirm or needy infants and saved the lives of children who otherwise had no option for safe and healthy nourishment. The breast milk expressed by Bahia's desperate poor also aided financially privileged children whose health or family situations required milk from a woman other than their own mother. In Dr. Bahia's words, the breast milk collected helped nourish "the children of physicians, including those of some of the professors of our [medical school], as well as [the children of] eminent families of high society."[62] "*Nutriz*," "wet nurse," became the common terminology for women who donated to the milk bank and the participants of the *prêmio de amamentação* program in general.

Among those *nutrizes* of 1950 was Bernadete Rodrigues, a twenty-five-year-old Afro-Bahian single mother of two who worked in domestic service.[63] Like all of the mothers who donated milk between 1950 and 1953, Rodrigues's entry listed her as living in "precarious social and moral conditions," and similar to a few others, her "legal conditions" were recorded as equally so. The fact that Rodrigues had given birth twelve days before seeking to donate milk for remuneration evidences just how "precarious" her financial situation must have been. In 1952, the Liga's partner organization Pro-Matre referred twenty-one-year-old Maria de Lourdes Conceição Santos. Santos was another domestic who had given birth to her first child just ten days before seeking out the milk bank.[64] Rodrigues's and Santos's ex-

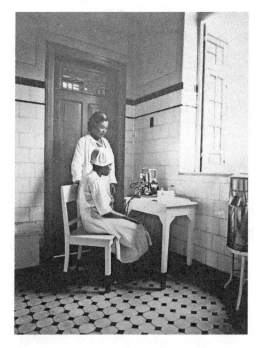

Nutriz *Pumping Room, Maternal Shelter at the Santa Casa de Misericórdia da Bahia. (Archives of the Liga Álvaro Bahia contra a Mortalidade Infantil)*

periences and the experiences of dozens of working women like them demonstrate the crises of poverty underlying many families' struggle to provide sustenance for their children. Small stipends may literally have made the difference between having the resources to feed themselves and their children or not.

Proponents of the *prêmio* program obviously did not regard the breast milk of the city's poor as dangerous, contaminated, and uncivilized as had a prior generation. Rather, they argued that breast milk was essential to the lives of impoverished children and conveniently available as a public service to the larger society. Despite the decades of medical condemnation of wet nursing, the *prêmio de amamentação* apparently made wet nursing acceptable by sanitizing the process through scientific monitoring and public oversight. Breast-feeding for remuneration had been thrust into the twentieth century. At the Lactário, staff separated mothers donating breast milk to a designated sterile room where they utilized the latest mechanical technologies. While clinical and rationalized, the image of a poor mother pumping breast milk in the facility appears cold and dehumanizing; these methods totally distanced nursing mothers from any living child—their own or another's.

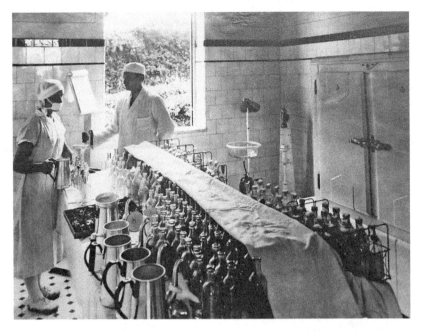

Julia de Carvalho Lactário, Santa Casa de Misericórdia da Bahia. (Archives of the Liga Álvaro Bahia contra a Mortalidade Infantil)

The ironies of the Bahian breast-feeding stipend are irresistible. First, it evidences an obvious racialization of discourses of motherhood, in this case further intertwined with real experiences of poverty and servitude. That impoverished women seeking public aid were sought out as sources of breast milk does not necessarily mean women of color were exclusively and irrevocably bound to a "mammy" narrative. It does imply that for poor Afro-Brazilian mothers, the "social justice" of nursing their own children of which Dr. Bahia spoke came with the continued assumption that their bodies were convenient and available for service to the community at large. And the institutional labeling of these women as *"nutrizes"* and *"amas"* donating milk for the children of Bahia's wealthiest families only makes this more problematic. That poor women could best serve the state as "paid wet nurses to their own children" was an idea inherited from French pronatalism, but Brazilian traditions were different from French ones. The Brazilian wet nurse was a cultural icon representing slavery and miscegenation. Labeling poor women as wet nurses was racially loaded and reflected a continuing association of skin color with servitude.[65] The language certainly evoked that of the nineteenth century more than that of a modern welfare state in construction.

Taking these complications a step further, insiders and outsiders commonly depicted the state of Bahia and its capital of Salvador via maternal and mammy metaphors, as explained in the introduction. The "Old Black Mammy," the "City of Women," the "Wet-Nurse City" all culturally placed Bahia within Brazil. And *baianas* of color typified that traditionalist trope of Bahian regional identity. This association begs the question of to what extent the long-held imaginary of *baianas* as natural mothers and mother-substitutes in the form of wet nurses provided a sort of implicit subtext in the politics of aid to single and "abandoned" motherhood. These mothers on assistance, however, were both "junior" partners in Bahia's most lauded and emblematic modernization effort (public health) and *nutrizes* to their own and unknown children, tradition at its most unequivocal and iconic expression. At the very least, Bahia was a place where race, maternity, and region intertwined, and this was as true in something concrete like the institutionalization of family welfare as it was in contemporary artistic representations and intellectual analyses.

THE BREAST-FEEDING STIPEND PROGRAM EVIDENCED A troublesome slippage between the old and the new. The so-called archaic continued to creep into modern terminology and reformists' assumptions. While reducing the foundling population and keeping more mothers and children united seemed to promise the opportunity for practicing "Motherhood" with a capital *M* as Dr. Gouveia conceived, the participants in the breast-feeding stipend program never became "*Mães.*" They were still *nutrizes.* To be fair, the rhetoric of "wet nursing their own children" may not have been of utmost importance to these mothers when keeping their newborns and feeding themselves and their other children hung in the balance. Moreover, they may have understood the exchange of breast milk for small stipends as a minor complication if it meant acquiring sorely needed financial resources. And for the children who circulated through the Foundling Home, the improvement in conditions there were undeniable and life saving. But these programs demonstrate that family welfare policies, while absolutely necessary and beneficial, responded to a cultural logic where racial ideologies, gendered assumptions, and class prejudices met. That logic was coded into both the language and the practice of the burgeoning welfare state with identifiable consequences for the development of institutions and maternal aid programs.

One of the contradictions of the developing welfare state was that state and private organizations theoretically provided an impressive number of services as a right of citizenship, but social and economic inequality remained extreme and largely accepted as the natural order of society. In Bahia, maternalist advocates intended health and welfare programs to impact all aspects of poor families' lives. In this way, the movement's leaders were quite idealistic in thinking the best way to address extreme inequality was for a poor state to attempt to continually expand to mitigate the consequences of that inequality. The continued investment in using the Foundling Home as a temporary escape hatch for impoverished families was an example of that. For the mothers of foundlings, once considered "unnatural women," the lived reality of inequality, structural racism, and poverty posed the greatest constraint on their ability to constitute and maintain stable families. With the emergence of family welfare programs, these women confronted a reformism that defended but narrowly defined their "natural" state of motherhood and the "natural" order of things for their families and for their role in the larger society.

CHAPTER FOUR

Motherhood as Science

THE *CURIOSA*

*D*URING THE YEAR OF 1940, MIDWIFE MARIA MA-dalena Figueiredo of Salvador delivered ninety-five babies.[1] This was not unusual, as Brazil's traditional midwives assisted mothers from all social classes in the vast majority of deliveries and had done so for generations. Throughout the colonial and imperial periods, practitioners like Figueiredo provided advice and support to women as they gave birth and raised their children with little interference from beyond the immediate family circle. Midwives enjoyed a great deal of mobility and autonomy; parish registries recorded births and deaths without the intrusion of government. Moreover, midwives typically infused their practice with a popular Catholicism that further reinforced the connection between Church and family life cycles. Birthing and child rearing were community-oriented activities, not clinical ones, and generations of knowledge passed informally between female practitioners and clients and mothers and daughters. This sharing of expertise among women marked a significant feature of the social and family histories of Brazil, but it should not be painted as overly romantic. Women shared resources on a small scale because public health institutions were nonexistent, and battling illness and poverty on the family level added an additional burden on the most marginalized sectors of society. The lack of medical facilities and formal means of assistance meant families struggled to stay healthy, and poor families were most vulnerable to disease and need. In that context, midwives like Maria Madalena Figueiredo were vital resources for local families, but raising healthy babies still posed a formidable challenge.

While her position was rather typical even into the 1900s, Figueiredo was among a select group of midwives who had a relationship with the state of Bahia via a program headquartered at the Third Health Post. She and several contemporaries enrolled in the program that involved an exchange of benefits and responsibilities on both sides. The partnership was one mani-festation of the increasing medicalization of birthing. By the early twenti-eth century, the medical community and the state prioritized family health in general and infant mortality rates in particular to a greater extent than in any prior period. This initiative was one of a few developments in the state-family connection, linking medical agencies and female practitioners or so-cial advocates.

The role of the midwife, disparagingly called a *"curiosa,"* was a critical el-ement of this process of uniting medicine, bureaucracy, and Bahian women. Considering midwifery as a practice, change was quite modest in the first half of the century. Most women continued to call for a traditional midwife to aid them during childbirth, and those living outside the state capital really had no possibility of making an alternative decision. Programs like the one in which Figueiredo participated were barely viable compared to the lofty ex-pectations of their organizers. Midwives largely continued their work with-out hindrance, despite their medical rivals' best efforts to slander them. The period did witness the beginnings of a slow transition to institutionalized clinical practice as the dominant pattern in birthing, but this took several decades. In addition to the actual transformations under way, the midwife-mother relationship held a symbolic cultural importance in that it served as a type of cautionary tale for women in making "proper" decisions. For medi-cal reformers, midwifery was a common target utilized to define and distin-guish between what they considered legitimate practitioners, safe spaces, and trustworthy counsel.

On this more discursive level, censuring midwifery also reinforced bio-medicine's take on the practice or exercise of womanhood and motherhood. To privileged women, the experts' message was consistent: trade supersti-tious, overly sentimental, backseat mothering for an active, scientifically in-formed maternity, the "other maternity" to use historian Maria Martha de Luna Freire's words.[2] Independent, "empirical," and spiritual, the folk mid-wife ushered local women into a tradition-laden performance of their mater-nal duties, according to critics, a far cry from the "other maternity" physicians championed. Moreover, their deep-rooted community authority served as a reminder that most mothers depended on local midwives, disregarding what physicians considered the intrinsic risks of nonbiomedical birthing and heal-ing methods. Physicians charged privileged mothers with failing to prioritize their children's well-being, opting instead for convenience, vanity, or ease. They assumed that the common employment of female household help rep-resented wealthy mothers' attempts to distance themselves from child rear-ing. Regarding the employ of midwives, physicians expected to supplant them as the primary advisors on questions of healthy child rearing. The anticipated transition would entrench biomedical practitioners as both health-care providers and sources of knowledge about treating the body and preventing illness.

Biomedicine's conquest of birthing entailed a gendering of knowledge and expertise. Within it, midwives and midwifery were both source and symbol of female knowledge. Biomedical champions of both sexes sought the formalization and professionalization of childbirth, reinscribing childbirth with knowledge legitimized by men. Furthermore, midwives customarily attended to various health issues, so biomedical specialists endeavored to replace them with a general scientific approach to mothering—not limited to childbirth. Childbirth was one entry point for a more ample medicalization. In the 1930s and 1940s, men and women of science worked to equip local women with the tools to adopt and promote biomedical mothering. As the example of Maria Madalena Figueiredo demonstrates, one method involved negotiating with folk midwives to alter their practices and influence the recommendations they shared with their clients. Simultaneously, biomedical experts attempted to displace that generational knowledge dominated by networks of women (including midwives) through organized outreach programs in scientific mothering. Mothering outreach to the city's poor mothers occurred in the clinics and programs described in chapters 2 and 3. Yet incorporating women of means required particular efforts in Bahia and in cities like Rio de Janeiro and São Paulo.[3] The maternalist movement gained allies among Salvador's well-to-do women, many of whom gained specialized puericulture instruction through innovative educational programs.

Physicians of the 1930s and 1940s urged privileged women to replace their reliance on "uneducated" women like midwives with intimacy between mother and child as well as self-acquired and professional scientific expertise. The modern bourgeois housewife organized her life and her professional, educational, and charitable pursuits around caring for children. Ironically, this rhetoric was contradictory, as it simultaneously emphasized affective intimacy and a secularization of women's sentiment. Reformists expected mothers to act with reason, to refuse to heed midwives and nannies out of feelings of affinity, intuition, or custom. Yet maternalist advocates also expected mothers to draw upon their "natural" intense emotions and insist on closeness with their children while stopping short of overindulging them. Thus, progressive mothers were expected to measure and rationalize their affect.

Hence, this "other maternity" reflected a compromise between two contradictory notions—the benevolence, even divinity, of the maternal instinct on the one hand, and the supposed irrationality of women on the other. The "modernized" maternal expectations fit well with the medical community's assertion of sole legitimacy in the world of health. Biomedicine—universal, secular, and disinterested—could balance women's instincts, whereas midwifery only exacerbated women's tendencies toward emotionality and superstition. According to this logic, only biomedical practitioners could guide and instruct mothers in the successful fulfillment of their "sacred duty" both within the home and outside in the community. Delivering newborns was only one aspect. Thus, reformists encouraged women of all classes to eschew their local midwife and the body of knowledge she wielded in favor of the male obstetrician, the nurse-midwife, and the children's health specialist. In addition to introducing biomedical practitioners into family life, experts also advanced a stricter differentiation between sources of knowledge about birthing and mothering and a reconfigured (and gendered) hierarchy of specialists.

"SAD AND PERNICIOUS" TRADITIONS

Midwifery as a practice and midwives themselves were, of course, more than an abstraction of medical discourse. For twentieth-century physicians worldwide, taking on midwives as their principal rivals was a logical progression. Midwives were specialists in childbirth, reproductive issues, abortion, and women's and children's general health. In Bahia, physicians had made quite a bit of headway in establishing biomedical expertise in treatment, but few inroads into the world of birthing. As in many places, local midwives customarily built long-term relationships with the families they attended. Brazilian families generally used the term *"comadres"* to refer to midwives, a word that dates back to medieval Europe, signifying the close relationship between mothers and the midwives who helped bring their children into the world. Bahian midwives tended to be unmarried black and brown women of limited resources who typically learned the practice through apprenticeship with more experienced relatives. Similar to other large Brazilian cities, such as Rio de Janeiro and São Paulo, Salvador had a small community of biomedically trained midwives (*parteiras*) with degrees from the School of Medicine. Unlike their *parteira* counterparts, *comadres* were women who learned the practice on the ground. Despite licensing requirements and other regulations on the books, midwives' work was largely unencumbered by legal interference.[4]

This was a situation that Bahian physicians had railed against since the mid-nineteenth century. Members of Bahia's Tropicalista School, for example, could make few local references when they decried the perils of midwifery in the 1860s. Local case studies were in short supply in the attempt to contrast midwifery with obstetrics. At that point, neither the medical school of Bahia nor of Rio de Janeiro maintained separate facilities for birthing or for training students in delivery. Most medical students completed their course without ever witnessing childbirth. Yet members of both faculties denounced the threat posed by Brazil's "ignorant midwives."[5] The Tropicalistas relied heavily on rhetoric, examples reproduced from foreign literature, and the limited experience of the physicians within their own small cohort to sound this alarm.[6] Decades later, their counterparts of the 1930s and 1940s did not occupy the prominent position in the world of obstetrics that they desired either, but these later physicians had the opportunity to work with many more thousands of mothers and children since the advent of the public clinics. They had more credibility and influence due to their greater interaction and status within the urban community. This did not mean these physicians had the power to sideline midwifery unopposed, but they had more ammunition to defame the practice than did their predecessors. The institutionalization of prenatal and children's health services provided medical critics a more informed basis from which to characterize the local practice of midwifery, though it was still a biased one.

It is impossible to accurately document the number of births attended by Bahian midwives, but they likely delivered at least two-thirds of the infants born annually in the state. Lacking comprehensive data, physicians estimated the prevalence of midwifery by extrapolating from the medical histories of the prenatal and well-baby population at the free clinics. Small samples from the 1920s suggest that 75–80 percent of enrolled infants had been delivered by a traditional midwife. In 1932, Dr. Álvaro da Franca Rocha estimated that 85 percent of Bahian babies were delivered by midwives.[7] Nearly ten years later, Drs. José Adeodato Filho and Domingos Machado gave an estimate of 75 percent.[8] Thus, not much had changed by midcentury. Folk midwives still delivered most newborns, greatly outnumbering institutional or outpatient birthing options.[9] Samples from other Brazilian cities bore out this exact pattern as well. The journal *Revista de Ginecologia e d'Obstetrícia* estimated that traditional midwives delivered 85.2 percent of babies born in Rio de Janeiro in 1922.[10] For São Paulo, the Serviço de Pre-Natal da Inspetoria de Higiene e Assistência à Infância determined that an average of 85 percent of mothers gave birth with the assistance of folk midwives between 1930 and 1940.[11] As in Bahia, local physicians developed these estimates based on the families who passed through the public clinics.

Whether "*curiosa*," "*comadre*," or the generic "*aparadeira*," the midwife spelled trouble to Brazil's medical community. In this, neither Bahia nor Brazil was unique. The replacement of folk midwives by nurse-midwives and male physicians was a worldwide trend. The global conquest over traditional forms of healing and birthing evidenced a gradual acceptance of biomedicine as the most legitimate source of knowledge and most efficacious method for curing the human body. Similar to their European and American counterparts, Brazilian physicians argued that midwives' nonscientific and "superstitious" methods were responsible for the high instance of neonatal disease and injury, maternal fatality, and stillbirth.[12] In Bahia, these statistics were difficult to determine, and attributing them exclusively or even tangentially to midwifery involved more than a little conjecture. For the decade of 1929–1939, the Prenatal and Infant Hygiene Inspectorate recorded an annual average of 669 stillborn infants in Bahia out of an average of 5,707 live births, a total of 12 percent. This statistic is more tragic, considering that another 30 percent of the successful births ended in death before the infants' second birthdays. The data on maternal fatalities told another disturbing story; 543 women died in childbirth, an annual average of about 11 per 1,000 births.[13] Thus, while Bahian physicians relied on inference, speculation, and unsubstantiated circumstance to denigrate midwifery, the patterns they decried were appallingly real.

The medical argument against midwifery generally fell into three categories that reflected a certain interpretation of Brazil's quest for "order and progress"; the emerging specialization of women's and children's medicine; and a deep-rooted, gendered cultural politics. Often all three of these criticisms blended together. First, physicians argued that a widespread faith in superstition, loosely defined, compromised the precarious state of Brazilian civilization. As the medical community acquired more familiarity with prenatal patients, they gained a basis of experience from which to draw, usually disapproving, interpretations of their patients' decisions. Dr. Domingos Machado, for example, recorded the following case study in 1941. Like many of his contemporaries, Machado juxtaposed the rational, scientific methods employed by physicians with the supposed rash and dangerous practices of the "untrained" midwife.

> E.C.P., record no. 12.894, *parda*, residence: 22 Roça da Julinha. Thirty-two years of age, a domestic from Bahia.
> She came to the Service nine months pregnant (!), having experienced a large hemorrhage without apparent cause . . .
> The advice of the prenatal specialist was in vain, as some days later we learned of the death of the patient due to repeated hemorrhages during labor.
>
> This would not have happened if the patient had listened to the advice given and come to the Maternity Center where she would have received the perfect technical assistance for her case . . . They could also have used medications that she could not have had access to in her home.[14]

In his summary of the events that caused E.C.P.'s death, Dr. Machado emphasized the specialized nature of biomedical birthing, the rigorous scientific method of excluding all possible factors and only thus determining the unique needs of the individual. His patient chose not to seek medical advice during her pregnancy and only turned up at the health clinic as a last resort. Safe pregnancies and deliveries required intervention long before the final weeks of gestation. The patient sought clinical treatment when prenatal experts could have offered prevention, her physician argued. Only through medical assistance in the controlled space of the Maternity Center could a pregnant woman have access to modern medications and procedures. For Machado, the patient was ultimately culpable for her own demise because she trusted in the methods of the *aparadeira* rather than the rational physician and structured institution. Her "ignorance" caused death in a case where biomedicine could surely have saved her. In Dr. Machado's words, "This was a case that ended in maternal fatality by the woman's own fault exclusively and that of an '*aparadeira*.'"[15]

For Machado and his colleagues, the ascendancy of science meant that practitioners did not have to cede to the erratic nature of childbirth. Childbirth, reproduction, and many other functions of the body could be harnessed, controlled, and directed, rather than merely witnessed or guided. As in Machado's reflections, the interventions of a physician could presumably *determine* the outcome of a difficult pregnancy. This stood in opposition to traditional midwifery, wherein the assumption was that expectant mothers could determine the outcome of their pregnancies through their *own* everyday activities—such as consuming specific foods and avoiding certain behaviors. The midwife, therefore, observed spiritual and natural signs and guided or instructed the expectant woman. For champions of biomedicine, the determinative structuring and ordering of seemingly chaotic circumstances was the great contribution that many expected science to make to an overall transformation in Brazilian society.

Looking comparatively, physicians beyond Bahia produced similar discourse about the relationship between systematizing childbirth and stabilizing society. In Rio de Janeiro, the influential pediatrician Fernandes Magalhães and the obstetrician Clovis Corrêa da Costa spent much of the 1930s and 1940s promoting the development of clinical networks that could be used for childbirth or to supervise in-home birthing programs.[16] Though the doctors' proposals differed, they equally cited the disorganized nature of childbirth and the prominence of folk midwives as cause, outcome, and signal of larger social problems. For Costa, the sorry state of childbirth assistance in Rio served as a reminder that the *sertão* (underdeveloped backlands) existed right in the heart of the nation's capital—the "center of culture, progress, and civilization."[17] As illustration, in the "*curiosas*" section of his major text on puericulture, Costa described a horrific childbirth crisis that occurred in the favela of Morro da Saúde. In this case, a laboring mother needed immediate medical attention because her baby had become stuck at the neck in the birth canal. The ambulance dispatched could not reach her home due to the condition of the roads. As a result, the mother descended the hill of the favela, physically supported by family members—in the rain and via dangerous, steep, and likely unpaved roads—with the fetus partially lodged, "dangling between her legs."[18] Rather than point to the extreme danger and distress experienced by mother and child and the obvious failures of public health infrastructure even in the heart of civilization, Costa closed the anecdote by describing it as truly a *"cena sertaneja,"* a scene typifying the *sertão*.[19] He reduced the plight of impoverished mother and child to a disturbing and demeaning attempt at satire. Though couched in the specific language of littoral versus interior, the familiar theme of midwifery as confirmation of national backwardness repeated and recurred. Like many others, Clovis contended that Brazilian underdevelopment showed no rural-urban distinctions but rather marked the frontier between medicalized and "traditional" spaces within the city.[20]

Within the second category of critique, physicians interpreted the cultural position of midwives as a reflection of the lack of professionalization within the medical community itself. As physicians argued that safe birthing exceeded the capacity of the folk midwife, they also maintained that specialization was essential to the proper development of the Brazilian medical academy. And that academy experienced great growth in the opening decades of the century with new medical schools opening in Rio Grande do Sul, Minas Gerais, São Paulo, Paraná, Para, Recife, and a second faculty in Rio de Janeiro.[21] Conceptions of pregnancy and childbirth as intrinsically life-threatening bolstered the push for specialization in obstetrics. Experts argued that these were pathological processes rather than natural ones and therefore required specific expertise and differentiated preparation. The obstetricians criticized their own colleagues along with the families who employed midwives by contending that neither group fully understood the dangers of childbirth. Critics argued that few medical students elected obstetrics, failing to recognize it as a skilled practice. Similar to community members, these physicians interpreted the long history of midwifery to mean that birthing was not a viable and challenging use of their training—or at least their critics accused them of making that assumption. Dr. Diogenes Vinhaes summarized this succinctly in 1935:

> In our current society, which is still backward, even some physicians
> consent to . . . the sad and pernicious tradition of allowing midwives

to assist in delivery . . . Obstetrics cannot be left to the midwife. It is an intelligent and technical exercise. There is no such thing as a natural birth . . . There is no comparison with the other natural functions of the body. Birthing bleeds, bruises, deforms, impairs, shocks, and kills.[22]

The hazards of birthing implied that obstetrics entailed serious, respectable work for the ambitious physician. In this way, the midwife-obstetrician contrast paralleled the history of the Brazilian barber-surgeon.[23] As they did for "cutting," physicians argued that birthing assistance was not an unskilled, mechanical occupation but a professional, scientific career pursuit. All civilized nations embraced this modern perspective, according to its champions; the specialized practice of the learned obstetrician was replacing the outmoded vocation of the *curiosa*.

Finally, many physicians' criticisms of midwifery bore a not-so-subtle resemblance to the old gendered notion of unruly, dishonorable, public women operating beyond their sanctioned "place." Midwives were autonomous and not regularly attached to "decent" households; thus, they maintained an unstable relation to patriarchal authority. Critics often played upon the metaphor of midwives being women in or of the streets, working on a circuit and profiting from unrestrained freedom of movement and unsupervised liberty of action. From Rio de Janeiro, Dr. Costa similarly argued that *carioca* midwives moved freely about the city and "in all levels of society, from the shacks of the 'favelas' to the stately colonial homes on the elegant beaches."[24] From Bahia, Dr. António Simões asserted, "Many are the mothers who have paid with their lives and those of their children for the imprudence and ignorance of these sad figures of the death circuit."[25] If a male obstetrician was unavailable, physicians argued, an expectant mother needed a *parteira*, a female nurse-midwife. She needed "a woman with education and a diploma at the head of the bed as she prepared to fulfill the most noble of her missions, not the ignorant and reckless mercenary woman from the streets."[26] "Mercenary woman" is a label that was also commonly used to refer to wet nurses. This language certainly suggests that physicians believed midwives and wet nurses belonged to the same cohort whose incompetent methods of caring for those entrusted to them resulted in deaths that would have been preventable. The class implications are striking as well. For many, midwifery was dangerous because the women who practiced it were unregulated and unbound in addition to being "uneducated." Physicians assumed these mercenaries delivered babies strictly for monetary reward rather than out of a commitment to health and welfare. This depiction of midwives as uncontrolled women evoked contemporary arguments in the press that poor women's unconventional behavior threatened the modernization efforts under way in Salvador. "Mercenary women" like midwives and wet nurses came from the streets, moving in and out of familial households for personal gain, whereas competent women with proper education were confined within the intellectual and physical boundaries of modern medicine.

Some outside the medical community also took up the crusade against midwives. In July of 1931, Oscar Oliveira sent a passionate letter to the Bahian director of public health, denouncing two midwives working in his community. Oliveira claimed two foreign women were abusing "our good faith" by exercising their profession without licenses and even practicing abortions. One purported to be a physician, according to Oliveira. He urged an official investigation into this case of "charlatanism" that would license the two midwives locally if in fact they were formally educated. If not, Oliveira implored the department to penalize them in the name of "legal morality."[27] The notion that private citizens could look to the state to arbitrate and enforce moral conduct was also a marker of the times in which Oliveira lived.[28] In his letter, Oliveira characterized the problem of midwifery in much the same way as Bahian physicians did. Though he expressed concern about abortions, the larger offense for Oliveira was that his neighbors operated without official authorization or supervision.

Concerned citizens like Oscar Oliveira had legal support for meddling in the affairs of their neighbors. Oliveira was incorrect in his assumption that the state had any serious intention to prosecute midwives but not that the supervision of midwifery fell within its purview. In January of 1932, the federal government issued new legislation to strictly delineate the functions midwives were permitted to exercise, part of a larger regulation of the medical professions. According to the statute, Brazilian law only authorized folk midwives to assist healthy pregnant women and newborns in the clients' own homes and without prescribing medications unless mother or child's life was at risk. The state separated health care from midwifery, as the law prohibited midwives from exercising their customary role as healers. The statute also spatially confined the practice to clients' homes; midwives could not attend women in their own homes nor in any type of facility. As physicians themselves insisted, the law required midwives to contact physicians at the first sign of difficulties and then suspend their treatment "until the arrival of the professional."[29] This statute achieved various ends. It gave the state a concrete basis in modern law by which to supervise midwives and other nonmedical specialists, drawing a line in the sand between the sanctioned and the improper practice of their expertise.[30] By recognizing the work of midwives as appropriate only to routine deliveries, it reinforced the superiority of medicine over midwifery for complex conditions or risky pregnancies. Moreover, exaggerating the spatial distinction presumed biomedicine as the more formal and technical exercise. Theoretically, this contrast would help potential clients distinguish between competing practitioners if, in fact, community members needed help making the distinction.

Obstetricians encountered difficulties in attracting business for several reasons. First, local women were well aware that physicians had comparatively little experience and thus entrusted childbirth to midwives, who represented generations of knowledge. The folk midwife also remained a powerful figure in Brazilian society due to the degree of discretion required for success in this field. Midwives guarded vital family secrets and intimacies related to abortion, sexuality, and clandestine births, for example. This entailed a deep relationship of mutual trust that physicians would need decades to build. Second, Brazilian women were largely unaware of medical advances that could make birthing more comfortable and safer, so they did not organize around these issues as their counterparts had in the United States in the late 1800s. Furthermore, gender mores insisted that women not display their bodies before men, and this tradition would take time to soften.[31] On the practical level, the community of physicians with interest in delivering babies was small in Bahia, as was the population of nurse-midwives. Although Bahia was a pioneer in the institutionalization of maternal care, the state lacked infrastructure for birthing until the first decade of the twentieth century. And throughout the first half of that century, obstetrics was not widely practiced in Bahia beyond the city of Salvador.

THE CLINICAL OPTION

Regardless of physicians' preferences, the reality was that there were few alternatives to midwifery in Bahia and elsewhere in Brazil. Bahia was home to one of the nation's first women's health hospitals, the Climério de Oliveira Maternity Center (Maternidade Climério de Oliveira), jointly founded by the state and the Santa Casa de Misericórdia two decades prior.[32] Dr. Climério de Oliveira of the School of Medicine spearheaded the long campaign that eventually resulted in Bahia's Maternity Center, which was the physical realization of a commitment the medical school had made in their 1854 educational reform.[33] Salvador's society ladies, organized as the Comitê de Senhoras da Sociedade Bahiana, greatly assisted in initially financing the Maternity Center through fund-raising.[34] As was the general pattern in Bahia, local benefactors were absolutely essential to the creation of public health infrastructure. Given the paltry attempts at obstetrics, the opening of the Maternity Center was quite literally the birth of a clinic. Previously, only the Santa Izabel Hospital offered an underutilized and unsanitary birthing room with a poor reputation. The Climério de Oliveira Maternity Center was an important marker in the history of obstetrics and gynecology as respected, desirable medical specializations. Importantly, it served as a training center for physicians and nurse-midwives as well.

In small numbers, Bahian woman began to elect clinical birthing over at-home midwife-assisted delivery. The Maternity Center's client base consisted almost exclusively of poor women, though the facility was open to expectant mothers of all backgrounds. The Maternity Center initially had space for sixty patients, and expectant mothers could admit themselves as early as thirty-four weeks into their pregnancies. By the end of their first decade, physicians and nurse-midwives at Climério de Oliveira were delivering hundreds of babies annually. By 1927, over five thousand women had elected to labor there.[35] This represented only a fraction of the total number of infants born in Bahia, however, and the Maternity Center continued to be the only institutional birthing option in the state. The vast majority of patients were single, impoverished women of color who were overwhelmingly employed in domestic service (more than 80%).[36] They were the same clientele who frequented all of the family health centers in Salvador.

Among the mothers who chose to deliver at the Maternity Center was Bernadette Menezes Teixeira, who gave birth to a son, Antonio Alberto, on September 13, 1935. On February 3, 1936, Maria Xavier dos Santos delivered her daughter Elza there as well. Either nurse-midwives or physicians would have assisted at the births of these children. Bernadette Menezes Teixeira, along with Maria Xavier dos Santos and her husband Alfredo dos Santos, found themselves lacking resources to provide for their infants shortly after their births and subsequently admitted the children to the Foundling Home.[37] These stories suggest that an initial experience in the public health system via the maternity ward perhaps encouraged families to see public welfare as a more realistic option for subsequent periods of need. Staff members in the clinics and aid programs certainly referred patients back and forth between their agencies, reinforcing the system as a whole. Climério de Oliveira was more successful in attracting patients than the birthing room at the Misericórdia had been. Although for many poor women, it must have been impossible to leave their families for two or more weeks while awaiting childbirth. Remaining at home was one of the great advantages of midwifery. To reach mothers in their homes, the Maternity Center maintained an ambulatory service that offered consultations and transport to the clinic. In emergency situations, the ambulance at times doubled as a delivery room.[38]

The popular press lauded the modern facilities of Bahia's Maternity Center. The *Diário de Notícias*, in particular, ran a series of favorable reports.

Modern installations, however, were only the first element necessary to convince women to turn away from midwives and consent to giving birth in a clinic. Brazilian women depended on their midwives, and for the wealthy, internment in an institution was dishonorable. In that effort, the *Diário de Notícias* became a key ally, providing contrasting stories on unruly street women with ones about disciplined, progressive ladies who donated to philanthropic causes like the Maternity Center and delivered their children there. As the historian Mark Overmyer-Velazquez argued for a different modernizing urban context, the role of the popular press was fundamental in crafting cultural and political differentiations, "orienting [their readers] in relationship to one another and to the city spaces in which they lived and worked."[39] To reinforce the message, the *Diário* published thank-you notes from grateful husbands to the Maternity Center staff, acknowledging the professional, attentive service their wives received there. The newspaper presented the Maternity Center as a locale capable of not only "civilizing" birthing and taming the chaos of unregulated women, but also providing a respectable experience for decent families as authorized by male heads of household. Even pictorial exposés on the Maternity Center represented their patients as well-dressed white women, serenely nursing their newborns.[40] In truth, these images characterized the minority of patients. Despite the media campaign, women of means rarely chose to give birth at Climério de Oliveira. For those women and their families, the household was a space of privilege and safety; only women without resources gave birth outside the sanctity of the domestic sphere.

Looking comparatively, the 1934 census counted only eighteen public gynecological and obstetric facilities in all of Brazil. Six were located in the Federal District and surrounding state of Rio de Janeiro. As a group, those eighteen institutions delivered 24,612 babies that year. However, more than twice that number were born in Bahia alone in 1934, part of a total of 963,541 Brazilian babies overall.[41] And the size of these institutions remained small. In bustling industrial São Paulo, there were 323 beds for childbirth in 1936—a year that saw 29,859 babies born in the city. By 1940, the Climério de Oliveira Maternity Center in Salvador had increased capacity to eighty beds.[42] It is clear, therefore, that only a small minority of women delivered their children in a medical clinic, whether in Bahia or elsewhere, and this was due to both preference and limited access.

The creation of Bahia's Maternity Center and the difficulties its leadership faced signified a number of transitions at play in Brazil and in the practice of medicine. It evidenced public and private benefactors' interest in safe, healthy births for the well-being of the community at large, even if facilities were only equipped for minimal capacity. Moreover, it demonstrated the ways in which biomedicine, gender, race, and class would factor into who could legitimately claim expertise in birthing in the twentieth century. With the establishment of clinics like Climério de Oliveira and physicians' insistence that birth was a medical event to be directed by a specialized professional, male expertise in obstetrics was firmly recognized. In one scholar's words, "Birthing came to be considered a man's business."[43] This was true in medical rhetoric and increasingly in popular opinion. Yet male physicians did not attain a monopoly over the *practice* of birthing assistance even as their assertions of methodological superiority were increasingly trumpeted by various voices. As the example of the Climério de Oliveira Maternity Center demonstrates, medical authority and a gendered definition of "competence" did not mean the complete displacement of female practitioners. Through the mid-twentieth century, women continued to deliver the vast majority of Brazilian babies, either as independent practitioners or as nurse-midwives attached to private or state institutions.[44]

THE "OFFICIAL" CURIOSAS

Despite the growing patient population at Climério de Oliveira, one birthing hospital could only aspire to attend to a small segment of Bahian mothers. Even for those fortunate enough to gain one of the few open spaces, many women could not leave their families unattended for a long stay. Many preferred to give birth at home where they could continue to manage their households. Given institutional constraints and women's preference for midwives, the state attempted an in-home birthing program in 1938 as mandated by the recently created yet newly defunct Children's Department. In the private sector, Dr. José Adeodato Filho inaugurated a similar effort that same year with the Bahian branch of Pro-Matre, modeled after the *carioca* institution of the same name.[45] Beyond Bahia, in-home birthing programs appeared in Rio de Janeiro and São Paulo in the 1930s and 1940s, some headed by state agencies and some by philanthropic organizations. A common thread, however, was that these programs relied heavily on the expertise of female visiting nurses to aid patients and nurse-midwives to deliver infants. The field of nursing—and obstetric nursing in particular—entered a significant period of formalization and professionalization during the 1930s and 1940s as well.[46] This provided increased educational and occupational opportunities for Brazilian women and proved a vital resource for in-home birthing programs. In addition to their corps of nurse-midwives, many agencies incorporated the work of folk midwives into ambulatory birthing services. This was the case for Bahia's Inspectorate of Prenatal and Infant Hygiene as they inaugurated in-home birthing assistance in 1938.

Salvador's Third Health Post served as headquarters for the in-home birthing program, and it provides a concrete example of the successes and failures of the state's attempts to offer domiciliary obstetric services.[47] Because of its relatively large prenatal program (initiated in 1932), the post employed more visiting nurses than did most other similar facilities in the city. The comparatively ample staff of thirteen visiting nurses made thousands of home visits to pregnant women that took them into patient's households with regularity. But having sufficient staff to attend to the unpredictable nature of home delivery was another matter altogether.

Dr. Álvaro Bahia, as inspector of Prenatal and Infant Hygiene, envisioned expanding the post's model into a citywide effort. Perhaps the doctor hoped to capitalize on new legislation that promised federal funding for in-home birthing programs.[48] Officially, the new birthing program was to utilize visiting nurses to attend to and supervise expectant mothers through the seventh month of pregnancy, and nurse-midwives for months eight and nine. Nurse-midwives would then direct the patient to the Maternity Center if a space were available.[49] Otherwise, expectant mothers would presumably call upon a traditional midwife. With a small cadre of nurse-midwives attached to the health posts, the odds that one was available to actually assist during labor and delivery must have been remote. Clinical prenatal programs sought to divide the services of traditional midwives into distinct roles among a defined hierarchy of nursing and obstetric professionals. Puericulture theory's emphasis on preventative medicine called for a total approach, requiring experts to provide counseling on prenatal care, birthing assistance, and infant and child "hygiene," but via practitioners with differentiated levels of training. Traditional midwives, on the other hand, fulfilled all of these functions as part of their routine services.

For Dr. Bahia, it quickly became obvious that the insufficiency in personnel made the in-home birthing program all but impossible. And the deficiency was dramatic; the state employed a total of three nurse-midwives in 1938 and five in 1939: Maria Emilia da Silva and Maria José de Barros of the First Health Post, Judith Mainetto de Moraes and Edithe Vieira de Carvalho of the Second, and Marietta do Prado Quaresma of the Third.[50] The staffing problem did not result from the state losing nurse-midwives to private practice; rather, there was simply a very small community of licensed midwives with medical school training in Bahia.[51] Although the School of Medicine had offered a midwifery course since the mid-nineteenth century, it did not confer degrees in that field in any significant numbers until the 1930s. Between 1930 and 1950, the medical school graduated 214 *parteiras* and 5 *parteiros*.[52] Placing Bahia in a comparative context, there were 242 licensed midwives practicing in clinics in all of Brazil according to the 1934 census, 45 percent of whom practiced in the Federal District and the states of Rio de Janeiro and São Paulo.[53] A comprehensive home-delivery assistance program staffed by nurse-midwives was not going to happen in Bahia given the personnel constraints.

Consequently, the initial attempt to expand into in-home birthing largely failed. The visiting nurses' and nurse-midwives' hard work and dedication was admirable, as were physicians' intentions to serve Bahian women in new ways, even if a bit naive under the circumstances. As the third decade of the century came to an end, state physicians weighed a number of strategies to overcome the limitations impeding a further medicalization of birthing. Dr. Bahia felt that one potential solution lay in bolstering the esteem of obstetrics within the profession, an idea partially inspired by Clovis Corrêa da Costa's work in Rio de Janeiro.[54] He appealed to professors at the School of Medicine to encourage their students of midwifery and medicine to observe home births and even participate in home deliveries as part of their training. Thus, the Maternity Center would be reserved for difficult cases, and a larger total number of expectant mothers would deliver with biomedical assistance. His argument ran contrary to the one made five years earlier by Dr. Virgilio de Carvalho, the director of the Third Health Post's prenatal program.[55] Carvalho had recommended intensifying advertising in the popular press with the goal of persuading *more* women to seek admittance to the maternity ward. Given the size of the Maternity Center, this proposal was even less realistic than Dr. Bahia's hope that local physicians would enthusiastically make home visits to the city's poor. These strategies could not effect the change physicians sought; the only possible intervention into home birthing would have to be in alliance with Bahia's traditional midwives.

Recognizing their limited reach, clinical staff attempted to reconcile biomedical birthing with traditional midwifery. Lacking the personnel and infrastructural resources to replace midwifery, public health authorities turned their attention to incorporating popular midwives into their sphere of influence. Working *with* rather than *against* traditional midwifery was a telling resolution, given the generally derogatory view that physicians held of these practitioners.[56] Encouraging folk midwives to continue their practice with so-called regular births also undermined physicians' insistence that childbirth was inherently risky, thrusting the human body into an abnormal state. Nevertheless, Salvador's Third Health Post and similar health posts in Rio de Janeiro initiated free educational programs in scientific and hygienic methods for folk midwives in the 1930s.[57] After training, these midwives did the labor of the health posts' in-home birthing programs while the state monitored their activities. Both components of the partnership were oriented around the assumption that midwifery was dangerous, but as a practice, amendable with proper instruction. This conception of redemption-through-science underscored *puericultores'* standpoint on mothering practices among the poor in general.

According to Dr. Bahia, the clinics sought to receive midwives kindly and use the training as an opportunity to emphasize what *not* to do during delivery. For the doctor, the goal was to teach midwives "to commit fewer errors and be less culpable for the problems they unintentionally cause."[58] Upon enrollment, the state provided an "obstetric kit" that served two purposes, from the perspective of the clinic's doctors: attracting midwives with the promise of free materials and providing sterilized equipment for use during home deliveries. The kit included alcohol, medicinal soaps, cotton, iodine, talc, quinine capsules, and silver nitrate drops among other items. It was a slightly reduced version of nurse-midwives' supply kit and a bit more robust than a similar delivery kit visiting nurses often left with pregnant women as they made their neighborhood rounds. As the kits demonstrate, hygiene was the major component of training. Physicians like Álvaro Bahia were particularly concerned about midwives' immediate postnatal procedures with newborns, and issuing that warning was a common element of the campaign against midwifery.

Midwives in the state's program undoubtedly learned about tetanus prevention via postpartum treatments of the umbilical cord as well as the administration of silver nitrate drops as a precaution against neonatal blindness. For the medical community, these serious but preventable conditions typified the gap between biomedicine and empiricism, between modernity and backwardness. For Dr. Bahia, umbilical tetanus, for example, was "a discredit to the progress of the people and should be eradicated in cities that claim to have modern sanitary organization—because the illness results exclusively from . . . the ignorance of *'aparadeiras'* or *'curiosas.'*"[59] Hygienic birthing methods and sanitized instruments certainly provided a critical benefit to Bahian women and their newborns, but that would have been the case for either home or clinical delivery. Confronting the very real problems of infant morbidity and mortality was paramount to the well-being of poor families. Thus, doctors and midwives at the Third Health Post engaged in vital work through their endeavor to successfully assist women in safely delivering their children. Yet the diffusion of novel methods also entailed creating new meanings around the birthing experience and new expectations for practitioner-patient interaction.

The midwifery program also sought to track registered practitioners as they completed their work in the community. Other than these small-scale efforts, neither the state nor the Bahian League against Infant Mortality had any reliable means of determining who made up the population of local midwives or gathering anything other than generalized, anecdotal information about their methods. The program allowed for a connection between the state and traditional midwives, although the numbers were quite modest. State officials understood that their program attracted few midwives and that the overwhelming majority continued to work independently. Considering the work of the participants themselves provides a better gauge of the impact of this partnership than the meager numbers might suggest. Many Bahian midwives delivered dozens of infants per year. Therefore, those attached to the Third Health Post likely applied biomedical methods as they attended to hundreds of births collectively, to the extent that these midwives accepted the procedures the clinic encouraged.

The objective of tracking was to determine the demographics of midwifery, the number of infants delivered and the number of fatalities, and the state measured its success in "reeducating" midwives by these statistics. Clinical staff asked the *curiosas* to report each birth they attended within eight days. The post even offered monetary awards to the participant presenting the lowest number of stillbirths and maternal deaths.[60] In 1940, that award should have gone to Amancia Pereira da Conceição, who delivered 126 newborns and 7 stillborn children. Conceição must have been one of the most sought-after and experienced midwives in her region, considering she delivered many more babies than the participant average. The remaining women delivered an average of 20 infants that year. Taking the surviving 1940 records as an example, it is clear that midwives remained the dominant providers of birthing assistance right through midcentury. Those participants alone delivered nearly 700 infants (and 41 stillborn children) that year, which must represent only a fraction of the total births that occurred in homes with midwife assistance, given that the program was only mildly successful in attracting, registering, and tracking them.[61] Yet even this small cohort could potentially reach more women than could a maternity center with only eighty beds. These "official *curiosas*," along with visiting nurses and nurse-midwives, were critical in taking biomedical birthing procedures out into the community. In fact, by 1946, the federal Serviço Especial de Saúde Pública (Special Public Health Service) created folk midwife training programs in several rural and forest areas of Brazil—in Goiás, Minas Gerais, Espírito Santo, and parts of Bahia.[62]

On the one hand, it is accurate to understand the midwifery training program as an attempt at co-optation and control. Physicians continued to view traditional midwives and their practices as "sad and pernicious," so there was no pretension of equality. They sought to rein in the freedom of occupational and physical movement that these "women of the streets" typically enjoyed, and the physicians who led these initiatives were quite explicit in that intention. They endeavored to undermine folk midwives' popularity and to eliminate their body of knowledge as well as the familial practices stemming from it. On the other hand, the program grew out of the state and medical community's recognition of their own limitations. This was a pragmatic decision, an effort to reconcile abstract medical and social theories with the widely accepted esteem of midwives, the paucity of state resources allocated to public health staffing, and local women's prerogative to make their own choices.

During these same years of the 1930s and 1940s, more and more women became champions of medicalization in their own right and elected biomedical birth over midwifery. Many even took on maternal medicalization as a profession, educational pursuit, or avocation. These women were on the opposite end of the spectrum from the *curiosa* in terms of their social standing as well as their relationship to scientific technique and medical opinion. And unlike folk midwives (at least stereotypically), they employed biomedical mothering techniques with expertise, thereby meeting the medical community on their own terms. On the cultural side, the privileged "professional mothers" embodied a modern femininity that met biomedical experts' approval and embraced a more appropriate and sanctioned usage of the maternal instinct than did the imprudent, mercenary women whom they challenged.

HYGIENIC EDUCATION FOR WOMEN

The medical community found important "civilian" allies in middle- and upper-class women whom they connected to as mothers and as advocates. From the biomedical perspective, the ideal for this sector of mothers involved abolishing the reliance on midwives altogether. Rather than entrust their well-being to midwives, physicians expected these mothers to seek obstetrical assistance and to become experts themselves in healthy child rearing in accordance with the latest scientific precepts. At least, this was the ideal. And their social role was twofold as well; that is, proponents expected these mothers' personal decisions to contribute to widespread societal change. First, prosperous women fulfilled a crucial function in the generation of an "improved" Brazilian nationality through their familiarity with science and application of hygienic principles to their families' daily lives. Within their households, privileged women could mentor their servants in hygiene and model biomedical mothering procedures. Second, as allies and social reformists, they could instruct poor mothers in medically approved child rearing either by example or by direct intervention. This advocacy opened new opportunities for middle-class women's employment outside the home, often a necessity in an increasingly competitive consumer society. As advocates, medical professionals, and philanthropists, scientific mothers proved a vital link between the growing disciplines of obstetrics and pediatrics and the larger community of Brazilian women and families.[63]

Women of means, therefore, played an essential role in spreading the message of medicalized motherhood. Puericulture experts considered middle- and upper-class women most "permeable" to their concepts of optimizing children's physical, moral, and psychological health. These notions appealed not only to these women's "bourgeois sensibilities" but also to their pretensions of class and racial differentiation.[64] Of course, a similar statement could be made about the physicians who espoused these ideas and organized scientific education programs for women. They were also helping define a bourgeois conception of parenting in which the physician arbitrated family matters rather than the priest, the patriarch, or the midwife. In this conception, good middle-class mothers were well versed in puericulture, understanding and implementing the latest medical techniques and tips for the hygienic education of the child.

To medical reformists, even women of means needed to alter their child-rearing behaviors and to renounce the generational women's knowledge they shared. The most common criticism leveled at middle- and upper-class women was that they favored their own convenience over the welfare of their children, especially if this entailed handing over their maternal duties to substitutes. They hired folk midwives for childbirth and regularly solicited their advice for familial health issues. They trusted wet nurses and nannies to feed and supervise their children even though these servants were not up to date with new theories of hygiene. Medical professionals considered all of these female assistants unprepared for their tasks. Because mothers employed female assistants and put their faith in that generational knowledge, physicians argued, the children of wealthy families were in no better position than those of poor ones. Consequently, the realization of their privilege was compromised. Addressing students in his opening lecture on pediatrics at the School of Medicine, Dr. Pinto de Carvalho, for example, reminded his class of the importance of maternal education to their future practice. He warned that women of all backgrounds were prone to heed the counsel of other women to the detriment of their children's health. "Women with low education are not the only ones who obediently turn their ears to the disoriented advice of midwives, neighbors, and girlfriends who know everything," the professor cautioned.[65] By criticizing the child-rearing practices of women of means, physicians contended that their own influence was imperative to the health and rational organization of the modern home. They sought to discredit the possibility that even women of this social standing would make the healthiest decisions for their children without medical supervision. They struggled to overturn the power over knowledge and practice that poor women held—domestics within the home and midwives as independent counselors. Domestics surely did not enjoy the local esteem that midwives held, but their child-rearing labor was essential. Physicians associated these two types of power, over knowledge and over practice, as parallel threats to scientific mothering.

Despite the surge of discourse, biomedicine's crusade in favor of new knowledge and transformed practice proved incomplete. There was a conspicuous tension between medical principles and local realities as seen in the incorporation of the treacherous folk midwife into the state's birthing program. Reformists implored Bahian mothers to demote their servants, but only as far as conceivable. No one expected families to give up household help altogether; rather, mothers could rigidly divide the child-care responsibilities appropriate to female domestics from those of the modern *dona da casa*, the lady of the house. Similarly, physicians vacillated between seemingly contradictory notions of womanhood and motherhood. They worried that women's emotional, irrational, and traditional nature caused them to trust in "midwives, neighbors, and girlfriends who know everything" instead of the secular science of biomedicine. But that same emotionality, nostalgia, and religiosity could be invoked to return the intimacy and spirituality between mother and child. The subject of maternal nursing among women of means demonstrates well this murkiness in Brazilian medical discourse and was typical of global trends in the period. Around the world, reformists attributed the failure to nurse to a vague notion of the seductions of modern life that turned women toward social and professional pursuits and away from familial obligations.[66]

Bahian physicians described maternal breast-feeding as a "sacred duty" or "holy mission"; women who willfully chose not to nurse were not true mothers. In depriving the newborn of the maternal breast, women failed God's purpose for the female sex. If a woman chose vanity or pleasure over nursing, she endangered her child's life and failed in her obligations as a mother and a wife. Bahian physicians wanted local women to know that infant deaths due to a lack of maternal breast-feeding were the mother's own fault, as Dr. Machado wrote of his deceased patient's decision to consult her midwife. They condemned the supposed selfishness of middle- and upper-class women who preferred "anti-hygienic" activities such as the theater, dances, and social outings to staying home with their infants.

Dr. Calcida Vieira dos Reis made this point quite clearly in 1927 by arguing that the modern young woman knew "the sounds and rhythms of music, the latest news in the social and political world, but often lacked knowledge of the best rules for nourishing her baby."[67] For Reis, this problem was generational and familial; parents forgot to educate daughters in domestic duties and in how to be a wife and "true" mother. Reis criticized women whose pride prevented them from nursing. She painted a picturesque, romantic scene of the experience of nursing and challenged any woman who would choose personal interest over intimacy with her child.

> If nursing distorts the figure, what does it matter? It should be much more . . . delightful for a woman to have the little being of her womb at her bosom . . . little mouth sucking slowly, sweetly, daintily . . . Satisfied of hunger, the little head slowly leans lightly, the eyes close, the little hand loosens from the source of life . . . This scene is much more beautiful than even the most beautiful figure that any mother could possess.[68]

Dr. Reis and her colleagues who admonished affluent women to be their children's primary caregivers acknowledged a tension between modern life and maternal duties. Yet that tension did not necessarily mean that modern life and maternity were incompatible. Reis herself was an atypical Bahian woman, completing medical school in 1927 and working at the Liga. If Reis was a mother herself, she undoubtedly employed household help in her own home. She was one of a small but growing number of female physicians with degrees from the Bahia School of Medicine, numbering approximately sixty-one by 1950.[69] Rather than eschew modernity, physicians urged middle- and upper-class women to take on motherhood itself as a profession.

A professional mother would be her children's primary educator, intelligent and knowledgeable in modern scientific methods. Modern motherhood required the time-honored, orthodox notions of intimacy and self-sacrifice, but it also necessitated a degree of technical preparation that was supposedly a defining characteristic of the age. *"One must learn to be a Mother,"* wrote Dr. Almeida Gouveia in 1940; "being a Mother is a social process."[70] Professional, scientific mothers would have no need to turn to the guidance of midwives. They would not be at the mercy of their unqualified household servants and neither would their children. Certainly, Dr. Reis, Dr. Gouveia, and others wrote for an audience of their peers. However, well-to-do families had access to these prevailing medical ideas through popular newspapers. Press coverage of both "unruly" women and charitable society ladies helped cultivate the notion of "maternity as modernization and civilization."[71] Of course, this was the "other maternity" practiced under the auspices of medical authority, but it appealed to women seeking to align themselves with the progressive transformations under way in Bahia.

Naturally, bourgeois women needed the theoretical tools to fulfill these new domestic and societal roles. They needed new sources of knowledge on children's healthy development, an alternative basis of information that did not derive from midwives and from the established family and community networks. Before moving to Rio de Janeiro in 1936, Dr. Martagão Gesteira of the Bahian League against Infant Mortality laid the foundations for a comprehensive educational institute for training in scientific motherhood. The Escola de Puericultura Raymundo Pereira de Magalhães opened in 1937 thanks to a large donation made by the sons of a well-known sugar baron and commercialist and named in their father's honor. The Raymundo Pereira de Magalhães Puericulture School was the first institution of its kind in Brazil, established to provide "teaching and propaganda on infant hygiene with special emphasis on preparing future mothers."[72] It occupied a spacious and elegant building in the centrally located neighborhood of Campo Grande, right on the border with Vitória, which was home to some of Salvador's most affluent families. The school was the culmination of years of small-scale efforts at institutionalizing women's and girls' education in scientific motherhood.

Puericulture education was not a new idea; it had roots in nineteenth-century France and maintained a lifelong advocate in Dr. Adolphe Pinard, father of puericulture. Bahia's Puericulture School owed its creation to a long-running discussion among the first generation of *puericultores*, like Pinard, on the subject of maternal instruction. Pinard and his contemporaries agreed that puericulture education was the key to solving France's depopulation and infant mortality problems. For Pinard, education for girls and aspiring schoolteachers was not complete without scientific training in child care. "We must imbue the young girl with this idea, namely: that if she has breasts, it is for feeding. We must ceaselessly prepare her for that function which is so natural, so great and so beautiful, *motherhood of the breast*."[73] To achieve this, he advocated for puericulture education as a part of primary schooling and personally taught schoolgirls throughout his career. As in Brazil, the French approach reflected physicians' suspicion that maternal and caretaker errors were responsible for childhood fatalities. Therefore, puericulture education in the schools focused primarily on educating girls for their future roles as wives and mothers.

In Bahia, puericulture education in the schools was greatly discussed and little realized. Noteworthy efforts were attempted, but there is not sufficient evidence to suggest that puericulture education was ever institutionalized within the public school system. Instruction in puericulture did find its way very early in the century into the Normal School of Bahia, a teacher-training institution. The first physician to organize and teach puericulture to aspiring Bahian teachers was Dr. Alfredo de Magalhães, the president and founder of the IPAI, a private agency. By 1935, Bahian law theoretically mandated puericulture education for all aspiring schoolteachers in the state's Normal Schools. For the younger set, the IPAI provided a homemaking school for girls. Similarly, the Liga maintained a child-care education program for school-aged girls annexed to the Fernandes Figueira daycare beginning in the late 1920s.[74] Years later, in 1934, the staff also organized a training program for puericulture nurse-assistants. These were the initial but limited approaches to women's child-rearing education, generally prioritizing teacher training.[75] Establishing an entire institute was a much grander and more ambitious effort. Investment in a full Puericulture School in 1937 further reflects the institutional gains women's and children's health made during the interwar years.

The most comprehensive effort to date, the Raymundo Pereira de Magalhães Puericulture School was inaugurated by the Liga to great fanfare on October 17, 1937, during Children's Week. The timing was strategic. Federal Minister of Education and Health Gustavo Capanema was on an official visit to Bahia that week. The minister was an honored guest at the inauguration, along with Martagão Gesteira on a special return trip from his new federal post in Rio de Janeiro, as well as the Bahian appointed governor Juracy Magalhães, whose government contributed 60 *contos* for the institution and authorized a recurring annual grant. The mayor of Salvador and other officials were also on hand to publicly affiliate themselves with a popular good cause. As expected, the ceremony garnered a great deal of press coverage owing to the illustrious state representatives in attendance. Minister Capanema even participated in the day's events by conferring the prize to the winner of the annual Better Baby Contest. The press interpreted his attendance as an unequivocal confirmation that the state of Bahia was on the cutting edge of social reform. In Capanema's words, the school represented "one more beautiful affirmation" of Bahia's commitment to social welfare.[76]

In terms of curriculum, the educational program of the school divided into three academic tracks based on three distinct profiles of students. The primary course, called the "elementary" track, worked with young girls and poor mothers receiving health services at the Puericulture School's hygiene clinic. An intermediate course was for *senhoras* and *senhorinhas* who wanted specialized puericulture training for their own roles as mothers and proper supervisors of their household help, as well as advanced preparation for community work. The final track was an advanced course, called the "superior course," for students from the medical school to gain specialization in infant hygiene.[77]

The elementary program for young girls, named the School for Little Mothers—Escola de Mãesinhas—was an idea imported from the United States. The child advocate Dr. S. Josephine Baker conceived of and founded

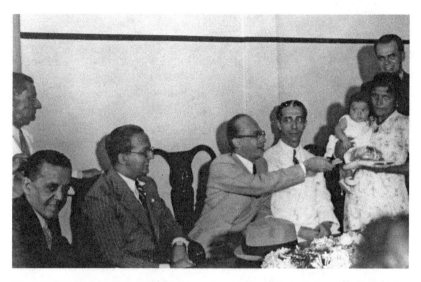

Minister of Health and Education Gustavo Capanema presents the Better Baby award to Walter Tapuz Ramos, held in the arms of his mother, Lindaura, on October 17, 1937. Behind Ramos stands Dr. Álvaro Bahia; seated to the left of Capanema are Juracy Magalhães, governor of Bahia, and Dr. Martagão Gesteira. (Archives of the Liga Álvaro Bahia contra a Mortalidade Infantil)

the first Little Mothers' League in New York City in 1910.[78] At the time, Baker was director of the New York Child Hygiene Bureau and would become one of the most influential child advocates in the history of the United States. Alarmed by the high infant mortality rates among immigrant tenement residents, Baker had specific goals for the Little Mothers' Leagues. She understood that preteen and teenage girls often had vital child-care responsibilities at home, supervising younger siblings while their parents worked long hours in factories. Instructing these young girls through small leagues and in-school puericulture classes was a strategy aimed to reduce infant mortality. Baker also saw immigrant girls as an important assimilation aid for parents who often did not speak English and perhaps were unfamiliar with American child-rearing conventions. Therefore, the Little Mothers' Leagues offered civic education as well as child-care skills. Proponents hoped that young girls could then exert influence over their own mothers' behaviors. By 1915, there were dozens of Little Mothers' Leagues across the United States working with nearly 50,000 girls.[79] Unlike French precedents, Little Mothers' Leagues encouraged young girls to become community advocates for better children's health. The architects of the Bahian Puericulture School found a middle ground between the US and French models, embracing both motherhood preparation and local activism as facets of their educational mission but for different segments of their student body.

In the Escola de Mãesinhas, young girls learned the basics of caring for infants and small children. It certainly shared many of the same goals as the Little Mothers' Leagues, though it is difficult to determine whether the Bahian program served primarily poor girls as did its predecessors. Certainly, Bahia never had an immigrant population comparable to New York's, and unfortunately, data on the background of Escola de Mãesinhas' participants were either never collected or no longer exist. Some clues suggest the socioeconomic status of the families to which these children belonged, however. School attendance is one factor. It is unclear whether participating girls also attended regular school or whether school attendance and literacy were requirements for participation. Little Mothers' Leagues in the United States drew their participants from local public schools, but in Bahia this seems unlikely. In 1937, Dr. Álvaro Bahia wrote that the Liga could not reach an agreement with the state Department of Education on how often girls would attend puericulture classes and, therefore, kept matriculation in the Escola de Mãesinhas independent from the public education system.[80] Considering that poor adult women who used the school's health services were also theoretically on the "elementary" track, it is likely that literacy was not a requirement, as most of these women would not have been literate.

Comparing enrollment rates in the Escola de Mãesinhas with that of the older students at the Puericulture School, the dropout rate was much higher for the elementary than for the intermediate course. Like their American counterparts, poor young girls in Bahia would have had family responsibilities that may have prevented their participation in a four-month course. This would be less likely for children of well-to-do families who employed servants to perform household tasks and care for young children. Looking at the first six years of courses, on average 73 percent of students who began the intermediate course graduated with a diploma after the program concluded. By comparison, only 31 percent of the girls in the Escola de Mãesinhas remained in the course until its conclusion.[81] The most telling evidence comes from contemporary photos of the graduates of each track. Even accounting for the difference in ages, the students of the elementary course were noticeably darker skinned and more plainly dressed than their seniors. All of this evidence taken together suggests that the student base of the Escola de Mãesinhas was similar to that of the Little Mothers' Leagues, and the program certainly reached a poorer sector of society than did the school's intermediate course.

Sanitary nurses taught elementary classes, educating young girls about child care using dolls in the *apartamento de boneca*, the doll's apartment.

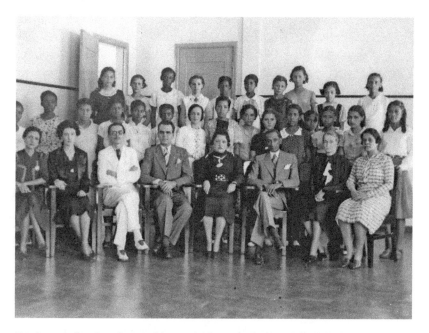

Teaching staff and graduates of the Escola de Mãesinhas in 1938, Escola de Puericultura Raymundo Pereira de Magalhães. (Archives of the Liga Álvaro Bahia contra a Mortalidade Infantil)

Their students were typically between ten and fourteen years of age and learned basic principles of infant hygiene, diet, and sewing. Girls also practiced feeding and bathing with the real children enrolled in the school's free daycare. In addition to the obvious gendered nature of female domestic education, the girls' program revealed a great deal about contemporary attitudes and models of hygienic family organization. Each space in the doll's apartment had a definitive purpose, and children were to sleep in bedrooms separated from adults, which was a major complaint that hygienists had with the living situation of many poor families. "Future mothers" also learned the importance of order. The apartment's wall clock served as a reminder to rigorously observe structured mealtimes and bedtimes. Within its first eight years, the Puericulture School graduated ninety-one Little Mothers.[82] Similar to Pinard's model program in France, at the Puericulture School little Brazilian girls were prepared for their future roles as mothers and, perhaps for many, their future roles as domestic servants. They were not necessarily groomed to become community child advocates; social advocacy was a major objective of the intermediate course.

The heart of the Escola de Puericultura was the intermediate course for young women from the "best" Bahian families. It was a rigorous introduction to the scientific principles of puericulture taught by the president and other Liga physicians: Dr. Álvaro Bahia, Dr. José Adeodato, Dr. Ruy Santos, and Dr. Álvaro da Franca Rocha. These instructors were also teaching faculty at Bahia's School of Medicine. The intermediate program truly embodied the goal of training women in the latest puericulture principles; obviously it was geared to nonspecialists but without completely diluting the scientific theory. Coursework included topics such as infant hygiene, pathology, psychology, children's physiology and anatomy, diet, and sewing. As expected, women taught the dietary and sewing courses, Professors Amelia Rocha and Lourdes Oliveira. But the school was academic and scientific in its orientation; it was not a finishing school. Because of this, the Puericulture School met some initial resistance from the very community it was constructed to serve. Rumors circulated among the *famílias baianas* that the content of the courses was inappropriate for the virginal sensibilities of young society ladies. According to Dr. Álvaro Bahia, the first course offering nearly failed because community members accused the Liga of teaching biological facts that young women did not need to know, facts that their parents hoped to prevent them from learning.[83]

Those who suspected that classes at the Puericulture School went beyond simple homemaking and etiquette were absolutely correct. In Dr. Bahia's infant hygiene class, for example, students studied eugenic theory, prenatal and infant care, as well as societal issues such as family legislation and foster care. The course of instruction was completely in line with expectations for middle- and upper-class women. Graduates would have the scientific background to supervise domestic responsibilities within their homes and to perform certain child-care duties themselves. Although students did not train in obstetric nursing, they did learn medically recommended postnatal procedures. In his detailed lesson on "The First 24 Hours, Hygienic and Educational Care," Dr. Bahia taught prevailing medical attitudes on bathing, feeding, and expected physiological changes in newborns as well as treatments for the umbilical cord.[84] He taught about the common hygienic errors committed by folk midwives. The inclusion of this section on what to do immediately after delivery is suggestive. If Bahia and his colleagues expected their students to someday give birth in maternity hospitals, this lesson on delivery and the first hours afterward would prove unnecessary. If the physicians expected or conceded that most of their students would eventually give birth in their homes, however, this knowledge could easily be put into practice. These principles could even help in "supervising" the work of a folk midwife. Outside of the classroom, puericulture students gained hands-on training by practicing their new principles on the infants enrolled in the school's free daycare and the foundlings at the Santa Casa de Misericórdia.

The school maintained high enrollment, graduating 222 *puericultoras* in its first eight years.[85]

The most salient feature of the course was its focus on privileged women as reformists and children's health advocates in their own right. The curriculum and even the design of the building incorporated practical experience and activism. In order to guarantee that puericulture education would never become divorced from the larger mission of advocating for poor mothers and children, the school's second floor housed well-baby and prenatal clinics, a maternal cantina, a children's hygiene museum, and both breast milk and sterilized milk dispensaries in addition to the daycare already mentioned. Like all of the Liga's programs, these were free services directed at poor women in the community. Given the school's location, the daycare was a convenient option for domestics working for families in the neighboring affluent areas.

Students had ample opportunity to witness "the spectacle of the poor single mother" up close, to borrow a phrase from Dr. Bahia.[86] As with the other clinics around the city, those at the Puericulture School maintained a steady clientele. In 1940 and 1941, for example, physicians there attended to 7,681 well-baby visits. Meanwhile, dozens of expectant mothers also sought examinations at the school as evidenced by the seventy-four prenatal consultations performed during that same period.[87] Between the mothers and children, there were hundreds of patients who visited the clinic for the first time during those years, demonstrating that the clinic consistently grew in popularity. Additionally, local mothers could also come to the school to obtain milk and infant formulas. This program was extraordinarily popular and literally distributed tens of thousands of nutrient "doses" annually to children in need. In this way, the marriage of theory and practice at the Puericulture School represented its founders' commitment to instructing wealthy Bahian women in advocacy. Perhaps puericulture students had limited interaction with the women who utilized these services, though they "practiced" their new skills on these women's children, but the integration of education with public clinics meant that the school set its sights beyond simply educating affluent women to be hygienic mothers at home.

Liga president Álvaro Bahia (1936–1964) continually reminded his students that they were not simply learning to be better "future mothers," but that their certificate of completion came with specific obligations to their society and their nation. Upon graduation, they became *puericultoras*—champions of the health and welfare of defenseless children and advocates for abandoned and single mothers. These larger ramifications were not lost on the program's students either; they wholeheartedly embraced their mission as one that would change the nature of Brazilian society. As one student observed in 1939, "When all the young women out there learn of the necessity of puericulture education, the problem of childhood will be reduced to a minimum and the average type of Brazilian man will be different."[88] Her reference to average types in universal terms evoked the eugenic notion of the perfection of the Brazilian race over successive generations. Students also expressed the specific responsibilities that women of their class yielded in modern times, advocating for child health issues among the poor. Leticia Trigueiros best expressed this mission in 1941 when she addressed her classmates on the occasion of their graduation as *puericultoras*:

> The objective of the modern woman [should] be the conquest of the professions for which she is most apt . . . [The] ideal that should be the ideal of all women . . . [is] the elevation of the cultural level of our poor classes. Infant hygiene, prenatal clinics, hospitals, dispensaries are not worth anything if we do not have a population capable of utilizing and enjoying their benefits. It is this work that is required of women in our days.[89]

As Trigueiros explained in her eloquent address, educated women could perform the vital role of convincing the popular classes to take advantage of modern health facilities. Her words resonated with the common charge of "ignorance" and "misery" leveled against poor mothers, as she highlighted the distinction between the incapacities of the "poor classes" and the professional aptitude of well-to-do female health advocates. Moreover, according to the speaker, modern women need not become the competitors of men. Rather, educated women could fulfill a public, professional occupation through social work, which was more suited to women's specific talents and energies than to men's.[90] With this, Trigueiros echoed many middle-class women's professionalization movements in Europe and the United States.

But, for Brazil, the practice of scientific motherhood held particular significance for the continuing process of national modernization. Educated women of this class performed a patriotic duty by nursing and rearing the next generation of great *men*, giving Brazil "strong sons, for her increased greatness."[91] The conservative daily *O Imparcial* lauded the achievements of the school's 1941 graduates in doing their part to empower Brazil through raising "vigorous, virile sons."[92] This gendered notion of national progress had been embedded in the maternalist movement since its inception. In 1933, for example, future Puericulture School director Dr. Álvaro da Franca Rocha wrote that Brazil's imminent prosperity rested on a "politics of *puericultura*," since prosperity was "intimately linked to the health, heartiness, and education of the people. Today's child, tomorrow's man, represents a type of capital that accumulates during the years of his minority. [That capital] will

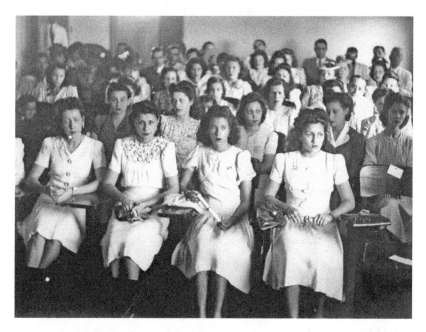

Puericultoras *at their graduation ceremony in 1943, Escola de Puericultura Raymundo Pereira de Magalhães. (Archives of the Liga Álvaro Bahia contra a Mortalidade Infantil)*

pay abundant interest when he reaches the age of virile activity, according to his degree of health and level of education and intelligence."[93] Similarly, at the Puericulture School, participants and visitors argued that ultimately men would produce Brazilian modernization and that women must have the intellectual tools to properly raise these men from their infancy. Women's roles were no less important than men's, but their social and national contributions in modern times were inseparably linked to child rearing and to nurturing men's activities. Brazilian progress was gendered male, because progress implied productivity, capacity building, and industrial output.

When the second-semester graduating class of 1941 invited Maria Esolina Pinheiro to be a guest speaker, she expressed this gendered perspective quite clearly. Pinheiro served as technical assistant of the Children's Biology Laboratory of the Federal District's Secretariat of Health and Assistance and was former director of the Rio de Janeiro Social Services School. She was in Bahia in 1941 to conduct an advanced course in social work on behalf of the Red Cross. Pinheiro's fascinating address warrants an extended excerpt here:

> The child represents the man of tomorrow. And what doesn't the world expect of this Man? It requires him to be healthy and balanced, beautiful as an expression of his race, strong as an expression of his power . . .

it requires the personality to adjust to his social function. And who fulfills the educational role—woman! . . .

Brazil has not yet begun to show the world the force of its destiny, the heights of its greatness. The more we protect [our] human capital, the sooner this hour will strike . . . preparing the foundation that will place Brazil among the Best Nations of the World. It is woman on a par with man who is preparing this foundation, every time she breast-feeds her son, protects her husband, educates the youth, and beautifies her life.[94]

Pinheiro's speech should also be read in the context of a nation preoccupied with war, though Brazil did not enter the conflict until the following year. Pinheiro became a vocal advocate of women's mobilization to serve the war effort as professional nurses, social workers, teachers, and volunteers. For her, the home front contributions of men and women were as significant to national defense as were the efforts of Brazilian soldiers. When she spoke of the modern requirements of men and the educational role of women, therefore, she made reference to Brazil's pending involvement in the war and argued that the patriotism of both men and women was critical to seeing the nation through the difficulties of the current age. According to one graduating *puericultora* at that ceremony, their certificate should be the ideal of all women just as the reservists' certificate should be the standard for all men.[95] Women's advocacy both inside the home and within the community set the stage for men to maximize their potential and thereby propel Brazil's progress, revealing the "greatness of the *patria*."[96] This did not make women's activities peripheral, but rather narrowly delineated and with singular purpose. Pinheiro was a perfect choice of speaker because her own career demonstrated that middle-class women could translate scientific training into a serious, prestigious, and nationalistic professional pursuit.

Graduation at the Puericulture School was mainly an event for participants and their families, but on occasion the ceremonies attracted influential citizens, whose participation added legitimacy and strategically reminded everyone in attendance of the government's interest in family issues. The Liga's president also took advantage of the opportunity to urge the graduates and their guests to contribute financially to the institute or the larger movement in some way. When the media baron Assis Chateaubriand addressed the graduating class of 1944, he congratulated the state of Bahia for having identified and worked on the problem of childhood for years. The connections between Bahia's Puericulture School and maternalist politics on the national level are significant. Chateaubriand's influence proved decisive in encouraging President Getúlio Vargas to relocate Dr. Gesteira, the Liga founder, to Rio de Janeiro to lead the construction of a National Puericulture Institute similar in organization to its Bahian progenitor. But it incorporated a few new services, expanding on the Bahian model to include prenuptial eugenic counseling, a pediatric treatment facility, a birthing center, and a research branch.[97]

The establishment of the Puericulture School evidences the overlap of various tensions of Brazilian political and social change. It opened its doors at a time when women's education, familial roles, and access to professional employment were intensely debated topics, particularly among activists. At the school, organizers and participants reinforced the notion that the purpose of women's education was to create better mothers for the next generation of Brazilian men and to support mobilization around issues that were gender and class appropriate. They sought to create an entirely new sector of female child-rearing experts and entrust to them the mothering tutelage of the less fortunate. Scientific motherhood served the twin goals of forming coalitions with middle- and upper-class women and counteracting the wisdom vested in the long-recognized authority of lower-class black and brown midwives that women had shared for generations.

The design of the Puericulture School, the course of instruction, the expectations for the various classes of participants—all revealed the contradictory nature of the discourse of national progress. Organizers differentiated their approach according to the socioeconomic class of the target female population, and these distinctions had racial implications. The divergent methods demonstrate the expectation that women's participation and contribution to Brazilian "progress" would be differentiated hierarchically by class and race as well. For example, while the images and words of puericulture graduates on the intermediate track often graced feature articles in local newspapers, Little Mothers and poor mothers did not receive media attention. Local papers depicted the young girls and the poor mothers as merely a nameless, homogenous collective rather than specific individual participants or clients with their own perspectives on mothering and family health. Their choices, their actions, and their achievements appeared only as school organizers' and supporters' accomplishments.

THROUGH THE SCIENTIFIC MOTHERHOOD CAMPAIGNS of the early twentieth century, Brazilian women became "simultaneously subjects and objects" for modern social medicine, according to Maria Martha de Luna Freire.[98] This was certainly the case. But, of course, "woman" was not an undistinguished, uniform category. Many women participated in the study and the objectification as the case of Bahia's *puericultoras* demonstrates. Women figured as both the actors and the acted upon. Women could and did participate extensively in the medicalization of childbirth and child rearing and not only in the obvious way. Medicine was changing as were the priorities of the state and even the city of Salvador itself, but neither the medical nor the bureaucratic communities enjoyed the power or prestige to dictate family dynamics unchallenged. Biomedicine tackled competing knowledge as a treacherous curiosity, and as women, as poor citizens of color, and as respected alternative practitioners, Bahian *curiosas* embodied the problem. Yet the process that transformed childbirth from a familial event to a medical one was lengthy, and it relied on the tools of both public discourse and clinical practice. Physicians, nurses, popular midwives, professional advocates, and women of all classes worked in tandem at times as well as in opposition. Ultimately, the association with backwardness and danger irreparably damaged the social esteem of the *curiosa* as did the concrete gains that biomedical resources and improved hygiene contributed to the wellbeing of Brazilian families over time. Moreover, the expansion of the public health system offered badly needed assistance to families, including birthing, among other services. But the growth of the system as a whole helped solidify and legitimize biomedicine through greater accessibility to the community at large and eventually encouraged more families to view obstetrics as the superior option.

While scientific motherhood and other eugenics-inspired programs called for national revolution, they reinforced more fixed notions of social place that were both gendered and racialized. As in other places, Brazilian obstetrics built from an assumption of differential authority and expertise between male and female practitioners, but the notion of differentiated competence existed among women as well. The perception of disparate capacity also extended to a delineation and hierarchy of female roles by class and race in pursuit of Brazil's much anticipated "progress," yet *all* women had a part to play theoretically if they mothered children. In the rhetoric of maternalism, motherhood united women through a shared purpose and gave national significance and political relevance to all—though none of this challenged the deeply engrained culture of gender and racial privilege. And it only bolstered the idea that proper womanhood and proper motherhood were the same. Moreover, scientific motherhood, while differentiated, allowed women's household and public roles to "modernize" and medicalize without being fundamentally redefined.

CHAPTER FIVE

Bahia's Estado Novo

THE *PAI DOS POBRES*

Veja só . . .
A minha vida como está mudada
Não sou mais aquele
que entrava em casa alta madrugada
Faça o que eu fiz
porque a vida é do trabalhador
Tenho um doce lar
e sou feliz com meu amor
. . .
É negócio casar

See here
how much my life has changed
I'm no longer the guy
who came home in the early hours of the morning
Do what I've done
because life is for the worker
I have a sweet home
and I'm happy with my love
. . .
Marriage is good business[1]

I N 1941, THE *SAMBISTA* ATAULFO ALVES SANG IN
praise of President Getúlio Vargas's New State, the four-year-
old Estado Novo. With the tune "É negócio casar," Alves thanked the Estado
Novo for taming his wayward masculinity and turning unproductive *malan-*
dros into successful fathers and husbands committed to hard work and un-

wavering in their dedication to Brazil. In the final stanza, the *sambista* sang, "The Estado Novo came to orient us / In Brazil, nothing is lacking but you have to work / [Brazil] has coffee, petroleum, and gold / And for he who fathers four children, the president sends an award . . . *É negócio casar.*" Thus, the words Alves composed with cowriter Felisberto Martins proved a veritable hymn to the themes of the Estado Novo as they pertained to working men and their families. Within the New State's social policy, the nation's productivity correlated directly to patriarchal duties and the fecundity of working-class men. Success in fathering was the larger success of Brazil, and the president personally wanted to encourage and reward fathers for their role in shaping it.

Alves and Martins's words echoed a widely shared vision of President Vargas, affectionately called the "Father of the Poor," "Pai dos Pobres."[2] For working family men, Vargas's Estado Novo (1937–1945) did provide resources, stability, and a legislative apparatus to support their roles as heads of household, so the song lyrics were correct in labeling marriage "good business." Family and fatherhood were integral to a larger inclusive national project. But, of course, there was a debt to be paid for Vargas's concessions to working-class patriarchy. In return for helping working men create and maintain their families, the state expected loyalty, labor pacification, military service, and acceptance of a certain interpretation of Brazilian national identity, especially during the tumultuous period of World War II.

In Bahia, in the same year that "É negócio casar" played on the radio, Joaquim Amancio Pita and Manoel Simplicio dos Santos found navigating fatherhood in the Estado Novo more complex than the lyrics would suggest. Both Pita and Santos had their infant children interned at the Foundling Home, Pita after his wife, Maria Ignacia, fell ill within days of giving birth to their daughter Deusuita, and Santos upon the death of his partner, Bernandina, two months before their son Nelson's first birthday.[3] Though Bahia's welfare infrastructure had expanded greatly since the beginning of the century, fathers facing tragedies could not access those services easily if at all. Clearly, these men and men like them were in the minority of those Bahians seeking assistance. Many more mothers than fathers found themselves in extreme financial vulnerability, lacking sufficient resources to sustain their children. Furthermore, men could more easily elect not to parent their children, even in a patriarchal society, without risking the moral condemnation that fell upon women. But Bahia's family health and welfare system revolved around a local politics of motherhood. Health and welfare advocates assumed that mothers needing aid were partnerless, and lacking a male partner became a crucial element of the rhetoric of social assistance. Most of these mothers worked as domestics, as was typical for working women of color, and thus family advocates assumed them to be alone in the effort to care for their children. If anything, "the problem of single motherhood" was a rallying cry for the movement in favor of better public health and increased options for social welfare. While Alves accurately sang of the Estado Novo's interest in fatherhood, Bahians like Joaquim and Manoel were not really reflected therein. In an era when the figure of the Father of the Poor dominated social policy, family assistance in Bahia seemed to marginalize *os pais dos pobres* (the fathers of the poor).

In this chapter, I argue that there was a significant disconnect between the paternalism of the Estado Novo and the maternalism of Bahian health and assistance policy. Both versions of family policy were a means to an end, either for the immediate purpose of class conciliation/increased production or for the longer-term goal of stimulating generational "improvement" in the Brazilian population—especially within the poor. Bahian family reformism remained mother-focused even within a father-focused national discourse and the policies emanating from a state-supported vision of patriotic patriarchy. While Vargas's social policy built from an expectation of working-class female domesticity and male productivity, Bahian health-care advocates recognized the reality that there were many families in which mothers were critical wage earners or even the sole providers for their children. "Protecting" mothers and children meant keeping them together, healthy, and in decent conditions, not necessarily out of the workforce. Given the essential nature of household service in Bahia and the fact that domestics composed the vast majority of enrollees in social welfare programs, this must have seemed implausible. While the Vargas administration worked toward the consolidation of a welfare state offering benefits to industrial working men, Bahian maternalism continued a long-standing trajectory of orienting social assistance around the actual and perceived needs of working women. In this way, female domestics, their children, and their alternately problematic and cooperative interaction with social reformists sat at the center of the state-building process that linked Bahian assistance to the developing Brazilian welfare state.

Moreover, I argue here that being female, poor, and alone was a rhetorical orientation of Bahian assistance. Bahian maternalism did not present an explicit challenge to national paternalism. If anything, Bahian physicians and family advocates cast their work as local expressions of federal directives. Under the Vargas administration, the idea of a national, comprehensive welfare state was new, but social policies aimed at family well-being and reform were quite old and local.[4] The divergence between Bahian approaches and the national ones elucidates the ways regional projects enjoyed a boost from national attention while maintaining the distinct character inspired by local interests and local actors.

The eight-year dictatorship of President Getúlio Vargas (the second stage in a consecutive fifteen-year term) initiated unprecedented state consolidation, making the Father of the Poor the most influential political figure of the twentieth century in Brazil. Committed to national progress and economic development, the Vargas administration created an enduring model for the extensive role of the state in labor relations and social policy. These interrelated functions were the main thrust of pro-labor, or *trabalhista*, politics. *Trabalhismo* sought the "valorization of the working man" and the "improvement of the race in order to give the nation strong and healthy people."[5] Unfortunately, labor legislation and even social assistance policy designed in Rio de Janeiro failed to outline how such measures were to be implemented or enforced locally. For example, protective laws benefiting female and child factory workers were often ignored in practice. Moreover, new legislation did not even concede the reality that most wage-earning Brazilians were not employed in urban industry. The Vargas administration was, nevertheless, the first to implement welfare state policies of a national scope, however inadequate and slanted toward Brazil's industrial minority.[6]

Finally, another type of gap existed between aspirations and reality within the growing welfare state because the federal government never succeeded in funding their family assistance projects without levying the resources of private organizations and local elites. Rather, the state worked in tandem with influential institutions and their benefactors. The need for cooperation required modern institutions to integrate into a much older tradition of local patronage, blurring the lines between state-directed citizen's welfare and elite charity. Philanthropic Bahian individuals and families gave liberally to support aid programs, but they were never called upon to consider their own privilege in utilizing the labor of the poor mothers who worked as their household servants. The expansion of social assistance credited to the benevolence of the Father of the Poor represented, in fact, networks of interests and organizations (in the Federal District and far beyond) that championed the centrality of mothering, fathering, and raising children to a successful twentieth century for Brazil.

VARGAS-ERA FAMILY POLICY

On December 24, 1932, President Vargas sent a telegram to his personally appointed state governors. In the brief lines of this "Christmas Message," the president strongly argued that no issue more closely connected the perfection of "the race" and the progress of the nation than maternal and child welfare. Repeating claims that advocates had made for decades, Vargas insisted that Brazil's future was compromised by a lack of attention to its children. He pointed out that infant mortality rates in the capital city of Rio de Janeiro were comparable only to those of "tropical" Africa and Asia, implying that efforts to elevate Brazil to the level of "European civilization" had been unsuccessful. Vargas urged his appointed governors, the *interventores*, to afford greater attention to maternal assistance, prenatal care, and child development because these issues were a matter of national salvation. For years, maternalist reformists and child advocates held up Vargas's famous "Mensagem de Natal" as evidence of the president's personal commitment to social welfare and proof that disadvantaged women, children, and families were an indisputable priority of his administration.[7]

When Vargas issued this call to battle against infant mortality, his provisional administration was only two years old. The president came to power on the back of a military coup, the Revolution of 1930, orchestrated by a group of military and allied conspirators who felt disenfranchised by the closed *café com leite* politics of the First Republic and dissatisfied by the Liberal Alliance Party's defeat in the presidential elections. The initial years were rocky to say the least; Vargas faced challenges from military dissidents and a major one from residents of the state of São Paulo, who threatened secession if the president continued to stall on his promise to implement a constitution. Despite this tumult, the *paulista* confrontation helped force a Constituent Assembly that officially confirmed the president and set about crafting a constitution. It quickly became clear that regional integration, centralization, cultural nationalism, and economic growth were firmly on the president's agenda.[8] Beyond that, social reformism found its way onto the Vargas platform even prior to the better-known Estado Novo years (1937–1945), as the new constitution confirmed.

The 1934 Constitution was the first in Brazil's history to define and pledge special protection to the family as the bedrock of the nation. According to this new supreme document, those families that warranted the state's promise of security were first and foremost based on "indissoluble marriages," and men and women occupied distinct and complementary roles within them.[9] Adult men should ideally be the breadwinners; the constitution forbade the labor of all minors under fourteen years of age, the nighttime labor of all minors under sixteen, and the labor of women and all minors under eighteen in "unhealthy industries."[10] Some of these directives appeared in an earlier statute on the protection of working women during pregnancy.[11] In all Vargas-era legislation, the expectation that women give birth and care for children always trumped wage earning. These visions of family were atypical, since most Brazilian families were not united by unbreakable, formalized marriages. And few enjoyed the luxury of conveniently selecting their working hours and workplaces or neatly dividing their generational and gender roles.

Familial health and maternal and child well-being secured a few references in the 1934 Constitution, affirming their perceived relevance to both Brazilian society and nation building. The union, the states, and the municipalities pledged responsibility

> to promote eugenic education; to support maternity and childhood; to assist large families; to protect youth against all manner of exploitation—including physical, moral, and intellectual abandonment; to adopt legislative and administrative measures to reduce infant mortality and morbidity and social hygiene measures that impede the transmission of communicable disease . . .[12]

With these far-reaching parameters, the state promised proactive measures and defensive ones in favor of Brazilian families and, in particular, their youngest members. And interestingly, these articles equated familial health with size and morality. Codifying these duties was primarily symbolic because Brazil did not have any nationwide family assistance institutions in 1934. But these articles did provide a language and framework for the later Estado Novo family policies that endeavored to concretize, at least partially, the federal mandates defined by the constitution.

Between the "Christmas Message" and the constitution, Bahian maternalist advocates won an ally in President Vargas, who played the role of symbolic patron of the maternalist movement throughout his years in power. The president's explicit request that maternal and children's issues be a priority of public initiatives gave credibility to a movement that was already in full force in Bahia and dated back to the first years of the century. Before Vargas came to power, maternal and child welfare had never received federal, much less presidential, attention of that magnitude. But the Vargas administration pledged to make a clean break with the failures of the past and with everything that was not in the best interests of the Brazilian people. The Bahian people had myriad opportunities to experience the discursive side of that promise through the president's many radio broadcasts. As a number of scholars have confirmed, a successful public relations machine was a critical part of governance, especially when the regime moved from the Senate-confirmed presidency of 1930–1937 to the closed politics of the Estado Novo.[13]

President Vargas proclaimed his New State on November 10, 1937, by addressing the Brazilian people via radio, informing them that upcoming elections were cancelled and that he would remain in office "serving the nation."[14] Influenced by fascist constitutions such as those of Italy, Poland, and Portugal, the New State, or Estado Novo, was a regime designed to meet the challenges of an industrializing and modernizing society unencumbered by the burdens of party politics and representative democracy. In justifying his *auto-golpe* (self-coup), the president argued that Brazil had entered a period of crisis caused by subversive elements—some real Communist challenges and some manufactured—and the failures of political parties. Such extraordinary circumstances called for a courageous head of state to make exceptional decisions. To avoid chaos, restore the legitimacy of institutions, provide for growth and security, "to readjust the political organism to Brazil's economic necessities . . . no other alternative [was] possible other than the one taken, instituting a strong regime of peace, justice and work."[15]

And Vargas's Estado Novo was strong indeed. November of 1937 ushered in an authoritarian regime characterized by the centralization of federal authority, intervention into the economy and industry (including the creation of state-owned firms), and social legislation aimed at improving conditions for the average Brazilian worker. The administration promoted a shared sense of nationalism over regional identities and interests, the strengthening of the military, and, importantly, the repression and censorship of dissent. From Brazilian workers, Vargas asked for conciliation and compliance instead of independent labor organizing. He asked for workers to trust in the government to ensure safety in the workplace, stability, and fair wages and working hours. The president often referred to those guarantees as "justice" or "dignity" for Brazilian workers, and of course, his forces of repression were present and available to enforce *conciliação* between labor and management if workers expressed dissatisfaction with their side of the bargain. This was the underpinning of *trabalhista* politics. In return for cooperation, pacification, and productivity, the regime pledged to help working men provide for, protect, and exert authority over their families.[16] As Ataulfo Alves sang, "the Estado Novo came to orient" working men and reward compliant fathers for their hard work on behalf of the nation and their steadfast responsibility within the domestic sphere.

More than any administration that preceded his, Getúlio Vargas's presidency prioritized consolidating Brazil's national identity and using that uniformity of people and purpose to stimulate economic development. The "March to the West" most dramatically enacted this integrated approach; in that campaign, the state attempted to settle Brazil's vast backlands while incorporating rural and indigenous residents and exploiting the interior and the forest for agricultural production.[17] Brazil's domestic civilizing mission built on the assumption that homogeneity and integration were essential to national security and fiscal prosperity.[18] During the Vargas era, politicians and intellectuals referred to the process of creating homogeneity as the consolidation of the race. A bounded and identifiable Brazilian race reified the ideal of a racial democracy, a discrimination-free, conflict-free, raceless national unity. Repeating the notion of *the* race/*a raça* meant rhetorically creating it, adding an official voice to the chorus insisting that Brazilian race relations were inherently harmonious despite wide disparities in income, education, and political power.

Racial consolidation found its scientific justification in eugenics. Brazil maintained a vibrant, influential eugenics movement in the first half of the century. The language of eugenic regeneration was fundamental to the Vargas regime, serving as a guiding principle for organizing youth, education, and health and welfare programs. As contemporary propaganda boosted, the Vargas government served Brazilians by "working toward the eugenic perfection of the race."[19] Several leading eugenicists carried the race-improvement banner into institutions by holding prominent positions in the federal bureaucracy. Unified nationalism, racial consolidation, and eugenics all underscored the import of engineering, and then reproducing, a committed and cooperative labor force. A strong and healthy population would demonstrate love of country *and* love of work. Vargas articulated this connection during his public speeches and broadcasts. His administration made an explicit correlation between mothering, child rearing, and economic development. Working *men* were vital human capital, but those men had to survive to adulthood, and here was the link to progressive mothers and healthy babies. This was an old idea, but one that gained a federal seal of approval during this period. As the Estado Novo's new institutions surveyed the population, they found undernourished and weak children, "an unpleasant reflection of the typical Brazilian man."[20] Therefore, for Minister of Education and Health Gustavo Capanema, state support of mothers and children proved imperative to "the quantitative and qualitative formation of our race."[21]

Vargas consciously used puericulture as a means of incorporating the popular sectors and stimulating patriotism, as Nancy Stepan has shown.[22] The Vargas administration placed a high priority on inculcating a patriotic spirit in Brazil's children to solidify and perpetuate the race. National symbolism was central, as was a positivist emphasis on civic culture in which all citizens could participate, including those who elected Brazilianness over their immigrant roots. The commitment to symbolic inclusion and healthy child rearing for all further buttressed the perception of racial harmony, of a compliant people undivided by origins, skin color, and phenotype. The annual Semana da Pátria, Week of the Fatherland, for example, provided an ideal opportunity to showcase the critical strides the Vargas government was making toward racial improvement. Youth groups were organized in a militaristic style, particularly on the Dia da Raça/Day of the Race, when parading schoolchildren marched in a celebratory display of national pride and the

cordial blending of racial, regional, and socioeconomic diversity that signified *brasilidade*.[23]

World War II provided greater urgency to the gendered rhetoric on familial stability and the significance of robust working men for the nation.
Brazil needed healthy men and boys for its military capacity, especially after eschewing neutrality and joining the Allied cause in August of 1942. The
connection between strong children and strong nations was not a Brazilian
invention. And these ideas certainly preceded the Second World War, but
the context of this war reinvigorated the call to protect mothers and children (i.e., reproduction and puericulture) and to ensure that sons be combat-
hearty should future conflict arise.

Internationally, the Pan American Child Congresses of the 1930s and
1940s provided an ideal occasion to probe the connection between maternalism, pronatalism, and warfare.[24] Brazilian professionals contributed frequently to those meetings and engaged in regional dialogues about puericulture. The theme of war dominated the 1942 meeting, for example, held in
Washington, DC, just over a month before Brazil joined the Allied effort. In
an unequivocal statement of final recommendations, the delegates agreed
that international cooperation during wartime was essential to ensure "the
American republics may utilize to the fullest extent the resources of all in behalf of American childhood, upon which the future of the free nations of the
Western World depends."[25] Within this conception, maternalism and child
protection preserved Pan-American peace. In the end, warfare was good for
babies, as the renowned activist S. Josephine Baker provocatively surmised,
and it certainly was for the expansion of welfare services.[26] Brazil, therefore,
was fully in accord with broader dialogues on leveraging the attention paid
to the citizenry during wartime into resources for working families with
children.

As President Vargas repeated on several occasions, Brazil's economic
prosperity, defense, and the "securing of the race" depended on work: on the
production, energy, and labor of individual citizens. Vargas often described
those workers in masculine terms, and this is unsurprising, given the emphasis on action and output as well as the context of military mobilization. In his
words, a strong nation required a type of "virile willpower."[27] The government's deep investment in providing justice and dignity for the "*homens de
trabalho*" made an authoritarian state into a "true democracy," according to
Vargas at least.[28] While ensuring decent working and living conditions supposedly fulfilled the state's promises to men, the language around women's
employment was always one of "protection," as it was for children.[29] Vargas
sometimes spoke of protecting male labor but not nearly as often and not exclusively within the protection framework. But for women, the state pledged

to guard them against what was inherently conceived of as an adult male space: the industrial factory, which was to be occupied by women and children only out of economic necessity. The Estado Novo sought to safeguard women and their roles as mothers from the dangers and demands of factory work. Women factory workers were operating beyond the safety of the home, removed from the oversight of male family members who could defend their interests, and exposed to the potential abuses of employers. In law and rhetoric, working women appeared as unguarded laborers or as struggling single mothers in need of welfare aid. Either way, working Brazilian women were typically cast as vulnerable or defenseless, reliant on the patriarchal protection of an altruistic state.

Taken as a whole, promoting fatherhood was more characteristic of Vargas-era family policy than was the promotion of motherhood, certainly during the Estado Novo years.[30] Ideally, family patriarchy would reflect the order, stability, and hierarchy that the Estado Novo sought to develop in all arenas. The family could be a space of discipline like the shop floor, the school, and the barracks; and hard-working male heads of household would be the agents of discipline, just as the Father of the Poor ensured the well-being of the collective Brazilian family while requiring their obedience and due deference.[31] Thus, the state wagered that content fathers made productive workers and acquiescent citizens. Prior to the Estado Novo, the 1934 Constitution had already guaranteed a nationwide minimum wage, an eight-hour workday and six-day work week, medical assistance and disability protections, education for the illiterate, and paid annual leaves. These provisions applied regardless of sex, but Estado Novo family policy introduced specifically gendered privileges.

The New State instituted special concessions for working fathers to assist them in establishing traditional families and in providing for their legitimate and natural children. Even the legislation designed to "protect" children and women actually advanced a conception of fatherhood.[32] Between 1940 and 1943, Vargas signed various new laws on family, amplifying a small but significant body of twentieth-century family legislation.[33] Prior to this, the Civil Code of 1916 and the Juvenile Code of 1927 had also addressed fatherhood. While establishing some limits, the Civil Code absolutely codified the patriarchal mandate, or *patrio poder*. The code decreed men's authority over wives and children, as the "head," "legal representative," "provider," and "administrator" of the family.[34] By law, married women were "relatively incapable" and precluded from accepting work or residence outside the home, executing contracts, or managing property and inheritance without the consent of their husbands.[35] And the Código dos Menores, or Juvenile Code, with its focus on abandonment and delinquency, set punitive measures for parental failures. This meant that the state could step in and suspend the patriarchal rights of criminal, immoral, abusive, or absent parents as well as those of parents unable to control the behavior of their habitually delinquent children.[36] But Vargas's family policies were the only ones to codify *benefits* and *incentives* to fathers beyond merely guaranteeing and enforcing their authority over wives and children.

New legislation promised federal loans to engaged couples for the purchase of a first home. These loans were also available to married couples who did not yet own their home, though couples with children received preference over those with none, and those with the most children were pushed to the top of the list of potential grantees. In all cases, the Federal Bank reduced interest rates on these home loans as couples grew their family size. Moreover, the law created a new official category of Brazilian family, the "numerous family," composed of parents and eight or more children under the age of eighteen. The fathers of numerous families were entitled to a number of benefits and preferences, including family wages. Exactly as the lyrics of "É negócio casar" recorded, to prolific fathers, the president sent an award. They paid lower taxes than single and widowed men and women without children. Fathers of numerous families received preference over fathers with fewer children and single men for civil servant jobs and for promotion. They would also see their sons favored in admission to recreational and sports societies.[37]

The preferential treatment of prolific fathers had more than just population increase as its aim; the state championed a particular model of stable, hard-working, and disciplined fatherhood. Unlike the protected mothers in earlier legislation, fathers had to demonstrate paternal responsibility in order to access their legal benefits and entitlements. Fathers had to prove annually that they attended to the "physical, intellectual, and religious" upbringing of their children.[38] More than husband, the state endeavored to reinforce men's roles as heads of families and responsible fathers to multiple children. Familial support, moreover, was not merely a top-down concession; it was also a response to pressure from below demanding compensation for dangerous working conditions and the contribution of labor to national growth. These demands were clear, for example, when Brazilian women petitioned for and won rights on behalf of injured and deceased partners, even in cases where couples were not legally married.[39] Family policies formed part of a pact with the working classes, a bargaining chip in the negotiations between state and society.[40]

As argued above, the Estado Novo's patriarchy benefits were not exclusively or even primarily about marriage, and this was a point of contention between the pragmatic Vargas and his more conservative minister Gustavo Capanema along with Capanema's allies in the Catholic Church.[41] Despite

Capanema's preferences, the state's patriarchy benefits rewarded stability and order over even the sacrament of marriage. Therefore, the Estado Novo encouraged fathers to recognize their children born out of wedlock, making the process free of fees and eliminating legal distinctions between "natural" and "legitimate" children. The law made no differentiation in benefits and family wages for fathers of "legitimate," "legitimated," or "recognized/natural" children.[42] "Numerous" households with parents bonded through consensual unions were eligible for all benefits, thus offering a further incentive to recognize children. On the other end of the spectrum, the law punished irresponsible parenting, establishing the mandate to institutionalize children whose fathers were too poor to provide for them.

As Vargas and Capanema envisioned working-class families, they had mainly dual-parent, father-headed households in mind. Protection of female and child laborers could demonstrate to the restive worker that the government sought to protect his wife and children from abuses. Yet Vargas-era reforms made little impact in Bahia, where industrial labor was not a possibility for the majority of working mothers or fathers. For Bahians, the series of decrees related to family and labor may have symbolized the president's commitment to these issues, but they would not be enough to provide better working conditions for most parents.

Census data confirm that Bahian men did not fit the industrial labor mold so typical of Estado Novo rhetoric. This did not make Bahia out of sync with most of the rest of Brazil, since industrial work was rare in nearly all corners of the nation. The growing metropolises of the South were the great exception to this pattern.[43] Bahia was among the most populous states in the nation with 3,918,112 residents in 1940; however, it did not fall among the most industrial.[44] Salvador was home to around 300,000 *baianos* but only 87 industrial firms in 1944.[45] Several hundred more industrial establishments were located outside of the city, and Bahia, similar to many other states, had more than tripled the number of industrial firms between the censuses of 1920 and 1940.[46] Yet Salvador's industrial production fell behind the other large capital cities—such as Recife with 253 firms, Belo Horizonte with 192, and the outliers of Rio de Janeiro and São Paulo with 2,150 and 3,549 firms respectively.[47]

All this meant that factory work was not typical for Bahian men. Men and women of African descent made up the majority of Bahia's working population, 71 percent in 1940, given that the state was home to the largest population of people of color.[48] Bahian men worked in agriculture, fishing, forestry, and service, but not primarily in industry. Of males over nine years of age, fewer than 4 percent worked in industry. Looking comparatively, São Paulo State's population of male industrial employees (8%) was more than double that of Bahia. Similarly, Rio de Janeiro state (7%) and the Federal

District (11%) also far outpaced Bahia in the percentage of men employed in industry.[49] Ten years later, in 1950, male industrial workers had doubled to 6 percent of the total male Bahian population; this meant 101,152 men working in what were called "transformative industries."[50] But the southern states had seen their numbers grow even more rapidly—São Paulo State to 18 percent, Rio de Janeiro State to 17 percent, and the Federal District to 22 percent.[51] Since the majority of Bahian men did not work in industry, their state-guaranteed patriarchal rights (based on the idealized factory employee-father) were ambiguous at best.

If those men and fathers were missing in national labor discourse, Bahian working women were even further afield. Thousands of women worked in the textile factories of São Paulo and Rio de Janeiro. As late as 1950, only 20,427 Bahian women—barely 1 percent—found employment in industrial firms. Most women worked in domestic service, and a significant number also found employment in the informal sector as street vendors or artisans.[52] Brazil's new labor codes did not apply to domestics and informal workers. In fact, domestic service was specifically disqualified in the century's preeminent labor legislation, the Consolidação das Leis do Trabalho signed by the president on May Day of 1943.[53] Families of means were not bound to any federal guidelines in their employment of household servants. Therefore, most working Bahian mothers would find little to no protection in the Vargas-era labor codes designed for factory employees. The Vargas call for social justice, the valorization of the "*homen de trabalho*," and the protection of (working) wives and children presumed a wage-labor model that was not the reality for the majority of Brazilians, and certainly not for the majority of Bahians.

Balancing motherhood with the insecurity of domestic labor placed working women and their children in a precarious situation. Anecdotal accounts from Bahian physicians suggest that employers were often unsympathetic to their maids' maternal responsibilities. The constitutional right to paid maternity leave, periodic breaks to breast-feed infants, and protection from firing due to pregnancy could not be enforced in informal arrangements. In reality, they were often ignored even in the factories. But domestics who became pregnant often feared they would lose their jobs, and nursing an infant while working in household service was nearly impossible.[54] The lack of set working hours was also hostile to raising children. "Sleeping in" service meant separation from children and leaving the youngest ones to trusted friends, relatives, and caregivers. Physicians attributed a large portion of the infant mortality rate among poor children to this practice. Separated from their mothers during the workday, domestics' children consumed animal milk and other supplements because of the inability of their mothers to nurse, opening the possibility of gastroenteritis related to bacterial contamination.[55] Thus, Bahian women found little advocacy either as workers or as mothers; the common combination of motherhood with household service had no place in Estado Novo *trabalhista* politics. Bahia, however, maintained its own politics of who the needy were and what needy families looked like.

Despite the disparities between federal policies and local realities, Bahian advocates received Vargas-era family policy with great enthusiasm. They lauded the Father of the Poor as an ally in the campaign to improve the health and welfare of mothers and their children. What was in the interest of mothers and children was close to the president's own heart and the key to Brazilian prosperity.[56] Vargas's own words and those of Capanema gave the movement a boost. The first Christmas Message was followed by another one on Christmas Eve 1939, in which the president issued another veritable call to arms, imploring men of "noble sentiments," "heroic and generous women," and "conscientious" physicians to aid the cause.[57] He further warned Brazil's fortunate to perform their philanthropic duty lest they be branded selfish and superficial. In this way Vargas, like Bahian advocates, explicitly divided Brazilian families into two tiers: those who needed assistance and instruction in the healthy rearing of their children, and those who provided the expertise and resources to fund those efforts.

The annual radio broadcasts during Children's Week, which the Vargas government made an official civic event, further promoted his vision of a unified nation where Brazilians joined together in a common mission to aid mothers and children. Naturally, Children's Week provided the perfect platform for patriotic speeches to honor the accomplishments of the Estado Novo in addressing social concerns, advancing the wartime effort, and highlighting Brazil's bright future. In 1942, Bahians listened to Minister Capanema remind Brazilians that their national identity was not based on racial prejudice and domination; therefore, any social distinction resulted from differences in health and morality.[58] And to date, Capanema went on to argue, Brazil did not demonstrate the desired levels of health, which could only be remedied through strengthening families and aiding them in raising healthier children. By 1945, Capanema declared the Estado Novo government victorious in its endeavor to definitively mobilize the entire population in favor of children's health and to coordinate a network of protective services across the nation.[59]

In Bahia, maternalist advocates asserted that by bettering the lives of mothers and children, they were doing the good work of the Estado Novo. Many argued that Bahia's maternalist movement substantiated the state's claim to national relevance and modern social modalities. One of the most explicit debates over the meaning of the Estado Novo for Bahian maternal and child programs occurred in 1938 with the closure of the state Children's Department. Appointed Governor Landulpho Alves caused a public uproar that year by closing down the agency as part of a restructuring of the Health Department. Alves subsumed the activities of the Children's Department (formally an autonomous institution) under the authority of the Health Department and created a new branch called the Prenatal and Children's Hygiene Inspectorate.[60] Structurally, both institutions fell under the authority of the appointed governor's brother, Isaías Alves, Bahian Secretary of Education and Health. Opponents claimed that the closure put Bahia out of line with the goals of the Estado Novo and was a personal affront to the wishes of the president. Had not Vargas himself outlined the government's commitment to maternal and child welfare in the famous Mensagem do Natal six years earlier? And did President Vargas not "govern all of Brazil?"[61] An unsigned editorial in *A Nota* condemned the restructuring and suggested that Alves's failure demonstrated a lack of comprehension of Vargas's program for national regeneration. "In the Estado Novo," argued the author, "we cannot allow that the delegates of personal confidence of the president of the republic are the saboteurs of *his* programs."[62] Thus, the argument ran, the president instilled his personal confidence in Alves as his local representative in the state of Bahia to advance the objectives of the Estado Novo. And Vargas himself insisted that children's programs be a fundamental aspect of his plans for a reformed Brazil.

In this back-and-forth quarrel in Salvador's leading papers, the Children's Department, founded in 1935, became the direct accomplishment of the Estado Novo. Even Dr. Martagão Gesteira, who founded the Children's Department as well as the Bahian League against Infant Mortality, commented from his new home and federal position in Rio de Janeiro. Gesteira expressed disbelief that such a meritorious and successful organization could be abolished when the policies of children's welfare were the "most impressive directions of the Estado Novo," connected to President Vargas's plan to "restore the vital energies of the nationality."[63] Gesteira stated his protest before the National Academy of Medicine and organized an official letter of objection sent from the Academy to Vargas. For his part, Secretary Alves defended the decision to close the Children's Department by issuing a heated response to Gesteira's accusations that had been relayed nationally in the press.[64] Alves suggested that Gesteira's shock over the closure was personal, not professional. Adding to the complication, the Children's Department of old was only nominally a public service; the building where the organization and its staff operated was the property of the Liga. It had never functioned as a self-sustaining governmental institution, fully funded with public resources, as was typical.

As far as the state government was concerned, children's welfare remained a top priority in Bahia, and services were only being restructured for increased efficacy. In fact, the appointed governor and the secretary likely sought to better align Bahian social services with Vargas policy, since the president himself had dismantled the old Children's Hygiene Inspectorate (Inspetoria de Higiene Infantil) and replaced it with the Maternal and Childhood Protection Directorate (Diretoria de Proteção à Maternidade e à Infância) just four years earlier.[65] For Secretary Alves, the Bahian Children's Department had made the mistake of attempting to treat the problems of childhood in isolation, and the new organizational structure would link social and health concerns. Clearly angered by the accusation of failing to heed the Mensagem do Natal, Alves argued, "The Government of Bahia does not need lessons in how to execute the call of President Vargas, fulfilling the patriotic duty to support the cause of the child."[66] The State Children's Department was quietly reestablished under Appointed Governor Renato Pinto Aleixo six years later when Minister Capanema required that all states have one.[67]

Though Alves, Gesteira, and others bickered in the press, Bahia's powerful brothers were correct that Estado Novo policies privileged efficiency, institutional restructuring, and vertical integration. Their attempt to reorganize public services to increase rationalization and productivity followed the general federal pattern in health, education, and cultural institutions, among others.[68] As in various arenas, the Father of the Poor centralized all maternal and child health and welfare services under the direction of the federal Ministry of Education and Health, headed by Capanema. In 1940, Vargas signed the decree that created the National Children's Department, which he, Capanema, and Director Dr. Olinto de Oliveira envisioned as a headquarters that would coordinate and oversee the activities of an entire network of state-level Children's Departments and municipal juntas.[69] Creating the National Children's Department (Departamento Nacional da Criança; DNC) meant the extinction of the Maternal and Childhood Protection Directorate established six years earlier. Thus, the administrative shuffle on maternal and child issues continued. The ministry charged the DNC with supervising all public and private institutions and research centers that dealt with issues related to maternity, childhood, and adolescence as well as promoting the creation of new facilities—ambitious and far-reaching goals that presumed recognized central authority, adequate resources, and effective long-distance communication. In Capanema's words, the DNC would be "a system of complete and efficient services designed to assure *all* mothers of the most favorable conditions for conception, pregnancy, birth, puerperium, and rearing and to give *all* children a guarantee that their physical, moral, and intellectual development would be normal and happy from birth through adolescence."[70] The popular appeal of the minister's inclusive words was clear, discursively eliminating any distinctions of class, race, or region.

On the financial side, the statute that created the National Children's Department did not include any specific details about the organization's budget other than to decree federal funding and invite donations from private individuals wishing to collaborate in the mission of a state agency. According to Title IV, Article 141 of the Constitution, 1 percent of the federal, state, and municipal budgets had to be allocated "in support of maternity and childhood." With the opening of the DNC, a portion of these funds passed to private institutions in the form of subsidies, via the Conselho Nacional de Serviço Social and its local affiliates.[71] In Bahia, this amounted to a grant of 250 *contos* in 1940, out of 4,000 *contos* awarded nationwide.[72] The federal government allocated more to Bahia than to any other state, with the exception of Mato Grosso (300 *contos*). In 1944, Bahian organizations received $540,000.00 cruzeiros in federal funding. By this year, Bahia's awards were far outstripped by those granted to organizations in Rio Grande do Sul (Cr$706,000.00), Minas Gerais (Cr$1,413,000.00), São Paulo (Cr$2,633,000.00), and the Federal District (Cr$2,162,000.00).[73]

Every year, Bahia's Santa Casa de Misericórdia received the largest award. Of the thirty-six Bahian organizations that received subsidies under the Vargas administration, nearly half of them were local chapters of the Misericórdia—the capital site and its smaller sister institutions in the interior. And this was typical of federal investment in the brotherhood across Brazil. In one scholar's words, the large subsidies such as those awarded in Bahia turned the Misericórdia into "essentially a state charity."[74] Among the other organizations (orphanages, shelters, hospitals, parochial schools, and puericulture and health services), the League against Infant Mortality and the IPAI claimed approximately 70 percent of the remaining Bahian allocation. The Liga fared very well, receiving a subsidy that was among the largest awarded in Brazil to any institution other than the various sites of the Misericórdia.[75] The examples of the Liga, IPAI, and Misericórdia demonstrate that child and maternal causes enjoyed a funding priority over the other types of charitable work being done in the state of Bahia.[76] And it certainly did not hurt that Dr. Álvaro Bahia, president of the Liga; Dr. Alfredo Ferreira de Magalhães, president of the IPAI; and Dr. Christovam Colombo Moreira Spinola, relation of the *provedor* Clovis Moreira Spinola of the Misericórdia, all served on the Bahian board of the Consêlho de Assistência Social that consulted on the awarding of local grants.[77]

Furthermore, Bahian maternalist organizations enjoyed personal connections to Brazil's top leadership, dating back before the establishment of the Estado Novo. The Liga, for example, had a standing relationship with Vargas and Capanema, who both made official visits to Bahia's child and maternal facilities in the 1930s. President Vargas even toured the Climério de Oliveira Maternity Center and the Juracy Magalhães Pupileira during a November 1936 visit to attend the inauguration of Bahia's Cacau Institute.[78] Ironically, during his welcome speech at the Cacau Institute, Appointed Governor Magalhães sealed his break with the Vargas regime (exactly one year to the day later) by promising that Bahia would only back the most capable presidential candidate in 1937 to succeed the eminent Vargas.[79] Those elections would never come. For his part, Minister Capanema became "visibly excited" and spoke with enthusiasm in praise of the work being done for mothers and children during the opening of the Puericulture Institute in 1937.[80] The Bahian League against Infant Mortality capitalized on these visits and connections by referencing them in appeals for subsidies throughout the Estado Novo years. Those links could only have helped in the quest to receive federal subsidies and meant that Bahia's welfare infrastructure, which already surpassed that of many other states in the nation, would find its distinction even further advanced in the 1940s.

Though directly subordinated to the Ministry of Education and Health, the DNC structure involved a complicated and extensive bureaucracy. While the 1940 decree called for the establishment of state Children's Departments, more specific details on how these institutions should be organized were slow to emerge. Four years later, in October 1944, Capanema issued a statement setting general guidelines on the types of assistance that state Children's Departments could provide but without setting definite expectations. Keeping to this vertical organization, he instructed state Children's Departments to execute the orders emanating from the DNC, which intended to supervise all local activities. He authorized four general categories of service: medical maternity assistance, social maternity assistance, medical-hygienic protection of children, and social protection of children.[81] Clearly, the sheer number of projects that potentially fell within these broad boundaries meant that state authorities were largely left to their own discretion to design maternal and children's programs, if any were offered at all. In Bahia, Interventor Alves and Secretary Alves did not heed the requirement to (re)establish a Children's Department. After the debacle of the 1938 closure, it must have seemed politically imprudent to reverse policy and dismantle the bureaucracy supposedly created to improve services. Rather, Appointed Governor Alves kept his brother's structure intact and left the issue for his successor to resolve.

The Bahian example reveals that despite encouraging maternal and children's welfare as a governmental priority, the Ministry of Education and

Health could not control how states interpreted this mandate nor determine their fiscal decisions. The weakness of many institutions undermined centralization efforts, as did the unintentional flexibility that this situation afforded for local politicians to set their own agendas. In the case of the DNC, these limitations were apparent from the beginning and exemplified by the inability of its director and of Minister Capanema to designate specific procedures, timelines, or evaluation methods—much less to ensure that guidelines created in Rio de Janeiro were faithfully implemented across the country. New statutes bureaucratically solidified the vertical integration of maternal and child health and welfare, but on the ground, local circumstances and politics continued to prove most influential on social policy.

In Bahia, the public fervor over the closure of the Children's Department clearly demonstrated that local issues of maternal and child welfare had been decisively linked to the philosophies of the Estado Novo. Social advocates understood these programs as Bahia's contribution to larger issues of national regeneration and insisted upon the importance of aligning Bahian politics with the priorities of Vargas's reforms. In this way, Bahian advocates and national leaders were definitely speaking the same language, and powerful and productive ideas propelled the institutionalization of family health. Despite those shared idioms, Bahian maternalist advocates and the Vargas administration were not operating under the same set of assumptions. Whereas Vargas and Capanema sought to protect and aid wives, partners, and children in order to secure the loyalty and cooperation of working-class patriarchs, Bahia's welfare aid remained resolutely mother-focused without even the implicit presumption of mothers' relationship to men.

WORKING WOMEN AND ABSENT MEN

Despite the patriarchal politics of the Estado Novo, Bahian welfare policy retained its focus on healthy mothers and babies during the 1930s and 1940s. Progressive mothers and prolific fathers are not mutually exclusive, of course, but this difference between local and national approaches further brings the ideas and politics behind Bahian maternalism into relief. In 1938, for example, while Vargas associate Assis Chauteaubriand affirmed that "healthy men are [Brazil's] best capital," philanthropic organizations in Bahia held a prolific mother contest, awarding society ladies for the quantity and eugenic quality of their large families.[82] The first prize of 5 *contos* went to Antoinetta Souza Miranda, who at age thirty-six had thirteen healthy children.[83] In 1941, while the federal government issued new decrees to assist working fathers, the state of Bahia and the Liga supported fifty-eight impoverished mothers and their infant children with monthly stipends through the *prêmio de amamentação*. In 1943, Olinto de Oliveira, Vargas's personally selected director of the DNC, reminded all local women's, children's, and youth organizations that they needed to undergo inspection to qualify for federal grants.[84] At the same time, the state physicians António Simões and Hosannah de Oliveira reinvigorated discussion of their colleague Virgilio de Carvalho's proposal that Bahia build a Casa da Mãe Pobre, a Poor Mother's Home, to assist "*mães desamparadas*."[85]

Within Bahian maternalism, there was really no conception of working poor families; deprived children came from fatherless homes led by struggling, abandoned mothers. Fathers and male partners were almost completely written out by the "single-motherhood" narrative. Assistance programs sidelined fathers, typically enrolling mothers and children without recording any information on the children's fathers, not even registering their names. In the Prenatal and Infant Hygiene Posts as well as the Liga's clinics, staff members did not consistently collect information on the partners or fathers of their patients. The closest data recorded women's marital status and the legitimacy or illegitimacy of their children, leaving fatherhood, male-headed families, or even nuclear families tangential in these records. In general, the Bahian paradigm of impoverished single motherhood either presumed that fathers were absent from the lives of their children, or it relegated fatherhood to a nonessential and even irrelevant aspect of the campaign to improve child health and reduce mortality. Maternalist advocates encouraged a holistic approach to social welfare—but one predicated on the assumption that the state needed to protect working women and their children from hapless men and absent fathers. In this way, Bahia's justification for health and welfare assistance to mothers inverted the popular Estado Novo narrative.

One interpretation for this discrepancy would be that Bahians were pragmatic; motherhood was simply more relevant than fatherhood to the local context. Bahia did not have to, did not want to, or did not need to appeal to fathers in the labor market as did the Vargas administration whose policies were chiefly aimed at the industrial South. Alternatively, one may consider the Bahian approach old-fashioned rather than "modernized," holding on to the moral notion of a sacred bond between long-suffering mothers and their unfortunate children. Or, perhaps some mix of both of these possibilities accounts for Bahia's maternalism in the face of the Estado Novo's paternalism. A more intriguing and complex interpretation would be to consider the single-motherhood narrative in Bahia's aid model as absolutely central to the conception of welfare and assistance that guided program development there. The silences and unasked questions on fatherhood and partnership left the impression that mothers seeking health care and assistance raised their children on their own and beyond the parameters of the traditional, patriarchal family model. This vision of families-in-need that presumed unprotected mothers of illegitimate children was intimately linked to constructs of both gender and race and to the realities of Bahian inequality.

Bahian ideologies of social welfare arose within different circumstances and dialogues about mothering, servitude, and child rearing than did the Estado Novo version. Servitude is fundamental here due to the population of women served by assistance programs. From the 1880s, Bahian maternalists were well aware that domestic servants performed most of the "mothering" in society. Initially, their concern was with the supposed failures of nannies, wet nurses, and maids, both enslaved and free. But by the Vargas era, Bahian programs had shifted focus from domestics in service to domestics raising their own children. The official invisibility of their partners suggests that advocates conceived of domestics as outside of the familial model, as women broken from conventional family bonds and permanently appended to the homes in which they served. In the very recent past, household labor had been a form of bondage, so the assumption that domestics had no personal lives beyond service, that they were "members" of their patrons' families, pulled the cultural baggage of slavery's social and labor relations. And wealthy families tended to presume that poor people, even the free, maintained looser and less formalized ties in general.[86]

Thinking in terms of gender, working "unprotected" in the homes of strangers, surrounded by nonkin men and with the potential of sexual abuse, was a position to which only certain women were subjected. Women working in those situations culturally suggested that they had either no male to protect them or a male who failed to adequately provide—hence a condemnation of men of the popular classes and of men of color in particular. All of this reinforced the assumption that domestics fell under the authority of the head of household in which they labored, rather than that of a husband or a senior male relation. This was explicitly clear in the exclusion of domestic service from the labor protections and regulations in the Consolidação das Leis. Seen through this lens, patriarchal authority and domestics' own family obligations and intimacies were incongruous in that they did not allow for rival patriarchs and rival households. Thus, within a certain racialized cultural logic, it proved easier for maternal advocates to conceive of female servants as abandoned mothers rather than as wives or companions.

At the Bahian League against Infant Mortality, the figure of the desperate single mother had been around since the beginning of the institution. During the 1923 opening ceremony for their first clinic, Dr. Martagão Gesteira spoke on behalf of the organization's efforts to aid poor but deserving

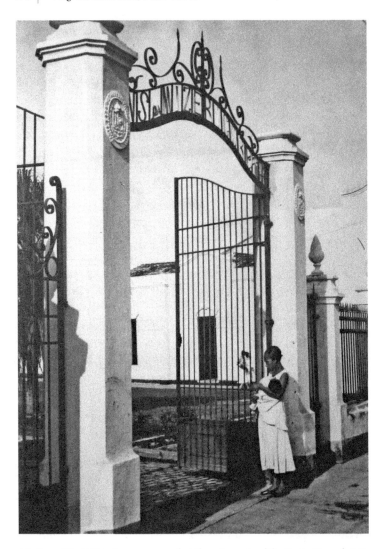

Mother with child in her arms posed at the entry gate of the Santa Casa de Misericórdia, en route to the registration desk at the Foundling Home. (Archives of the Liga Álvaro Bahia contra a Mortalidade Infantil)

mothers.[87] Ten years later when the Liga inaugurated services at the Foundling Home, Gesteira lamented the fate of women abandoned and ignored by their "seducers" and kin, who never learn to love their "fatherless" children.[88] But it was the Liga's second president, Álvaro Bahia, who articulated this point fervently and often, referring to maternal advocacy work as providing a form of justice for impoverished single mothers.[89] For Dr. Bahia, single motherhood was a social ill that left women overburdened by the attempt to sustain their children all on their own. One way that poor mothers would exercise their "rights," according to the doctor, was through the ability to breast-feed their own children. This was a new formulation. Bahia's use of the word "rights" had specific aims; it was much more common for maternal nursing to be expressed as a right of the *child*.[90] Dr. Bahia was certainly not the first to draw attention to the complications poverty and women's wage labor wrought for maternal nursing. At the medical school there had been a small contingent of physicians since the late nineteenth century who argued that the children of wet nurses were at an especially high risk of infant mortality. Soon this line of reasoning extended to all female household servants who had to be separated from their babies in order to earn a living. By 1927, the Juvenile Code even made it mandatory for wet nurses to officially register, which included demonstrating that their own children were healthy and had reached a minimum age of four months.[91] Thus, it was in this vein that Dr. Bahia connected "single motherhood," household service, and the "right" to breast-feed.

These ideas also had a global political dimension. Brazilian child advocates frequently quoted the Geneva Convention's "Declaration of the Rights of the Child," adopted by the League of Nations in 1924,[92] which defined children as a distinct group deserving of specialized protections and guarantees. In January of 1940, the federal Maternal and Childhood Assistance Division ratified a document called the Rights of the Brazilian Child, modeled after a similar and pioneering code adopted by Uruguay's Inter-American Child Protection Institute in 1927. The Rights of the Brazilian Child consisted of twelve articles that guaranteed the right to health; education; safety from violence and exploitation; family; nutrition; maternal love; and freedom from judgment based on family background, illegitimacy, poverty, race, religion, or mental or physical deformity. This framework of rights elaborated children and mothers as discrete categories within families entitled to particular claims on state and society.[93]

Labor law did not extend into private homes, so the right to nurse children, of which Dr. Bahia spoke, required the cooperation of servants' employers. Dr. Bahia never spoke explicitly about the tension between wealthy families' demands and the child-care responsibilities of their female servants. The Bahian League against Infant Mortality and other private organizations needed the support and financial patronage of these families, so any direct condemnation would have been foolish. Nevertheless, the Bahian *"mãe pobre"* or *"mãe desamparada"* became a recognizable type, a symbol of the campaign to aid abandoned women and children. Appealing to the plight of these symbolic mothers proved very useful in marshaling resources from sponsors.

Thus, the "social forces," to use Dr. Bahia's vague language, preventing impoverished women from breast-feeding remained largely ambiguous. Highlighting the need to work outside the home over inflexible patrons and domestics' low wages distanced employers from culpability in the plight of that "poor mother." By remaining elusive on the causes of working mothers' alienation from the right to nurse their infants, Dr. Bahia and other maternalist advocates avoided problematic accusations by placing the blame squarely on the shoulders of irresponsible, absent (poor black and brown) men.[94] However, one can read the single-motherhood rhetoric as a backhanded critique of domestic service. Mammies, maids, and nannies may have been treasured fictive kin, but those fictions did not erase the real relationship of employer and employee. Well-to-do households were not protected spaces for domestics, but in fact perilous ones for servants' bonds with their own children and for those children's physical well-being.

All of this represented perhaps a surprising degree of conversation around rights for a country with a self-confirmed president who was ruling by decree and had appointed his allies to govern the states.[95] But rights and enfranchisement were a silenced irony for the Vargas administration in general. Brazilian women finally attained suffrage in 1932, for example, after years of struggle, but that achievement rang somewhat hollow when elections were suspended. Similarly, the 1930s were a landmark decade for Afro-Brazilian politics due to the successful mobilization efforts of the Frente Negra Brasileira, the Black Brazilian Front, but the Frente and all other political parties became casualties of the Estado Novo.[96] The labor movement had been effectively subdued through co-optation and the menace of state violence. Guarantees for mother and child proved a safe conception of "rights" in an era of closed political participation for Bahia and across Brazil. Brazilians had rights as recipients of state benevolence but not rights as actors.

Mothers' and children's rights could conceivably be the inverse of fathers' responsibilities. Rather than enforcing responsibility, the federal government relied mainly on incentives as the surest and least polemic means of encouraging fathers to recognize their children and sustain their households. Even so, there were some punitive federal laws to oblige support of children that predated Vargas. But the law fell short of complete protection for those born out of wedlock, since it did not require parents to declare themselves for a child's civil registration. The Penal Code, for example, made it a crime to fail to support a child under eighteen years of age, but fathers and mothers could always elect not to recognize their children born out of wedlock in the first place. And the law made it difficult for children, their mothers, or those representing their interests to sue for paternal recognition.[97]

For his part, the Liga's president shared some controversial opinions about holding fathers accountable even if it meant pushing aside traditional views of privileging the peace of legitimate homes.[98] This certainly made sense within the abandoned single-motherhood paradigm. Álvaro Bahia's stance on paternal obligations was even stronger than that written into the state of Bahia's "General Regulation on Childhood Assistance." The authors of that document interpreted Article 125 of the 1937 Constitution as a mandate to states to replace the notion of *patrio poder* with *patrio dever.*[99] Article 125 defined ensuring their children's upbringing as parents' "primary duty" and "natural right."[100] Hence, in the codes of the state of Bahia, this article meant that parental obligations trumped patriarchal rights, but bold wording on paper did not always mean much in practice.

While the federal government tried to court men into responsible fatherhood, the Bahian welfare state took much less interest in working men than working women. Regional conceptions help explain the cultural or symbolic side of motherhood and mothering in Bahia's welfare paradigm. Metaphors of race and motherhood are inescapable for the study of public health and social welfare and conflated in deep and intriguing ways with Bahia's own cultural narrative and its imagined place in a "progressive" nation. Salvador was a "City of Women" and a city of *baianas* in particular, populated and served by poor women of color and their children. By the 1930s, the *baiana* as a black woman/street vendor was already a recognizable character representing the supposed traditionalism of the state.[101] These narratives melded well with the vision of women of the popular classes as independent, unattached, and struggling to sustain their children without the help of a male partner. Bahia's prototypical laborers were of a different kind than those lauded by the Estado Novo. Their work seemed to bear little relation to the industrial development Brazil was pinning its hopes for "modernity" on; nevertheless, local advocates lauded poor mothers' integration into the welfare state as proof of Bahia's successful modernization.

CHARITY, BENEVOLENCE, OR RIGHTS (AND WHOSE?)

Despite the contrast between Estado Novo paternalism and Bahian maternalism, there was one significant arena of overlap—the national and local expressions of wealthy women's philanthropy and activism. "Heroic and generous" women of influence, to use Vargas's words, were certainly prepared to heed his call to support the cause.[102] This was particularly true after Brazil declared its entry into World War II and promised troops in aid of the Allied cause in August 1942. The greatest mobilization of women on behalf of social aid came with the establishment of the wartime assistance league, the

Legião Brasileira de Assistência (LBA; Brazilian Assistance Legion), spear-headed by First Lady Darcy Vargas. The LBA attended to Brazilian mothers in need, primarily in this case as wives of deployed soldiers. Supporting them in the absence of their husbands proved to be an extension of the larger project of validating working-class patriarchy.

Within days of Brazil's entering the war, First Lady Vargas founded the Brazilian Assistance Legion in cooperation with the Federation of Commercial Associations. As was the custom in the Estado Novo, the LBA organized from the top, with Darcy Vargas immediately calling upon the First Ladies of the states of Brazil. In her August 28 telegram to the wives of the appointed governors, Darcy Vargas affirmed that "the Brazilian woman must fulfill her mission to protect the families of brave soldiers" during a time when the nation faced the gravest challenges.[103] Her telegram invited the First Ladies to each establish a local chapter of the LBA; they would model women's civic engagement from the highest echelons of power and prestige. Once established, the LBA maintained a brigade of visiting assistants, provisioned food and milk, advocated for women and children with health and welfare agencies where needed, helped families file civil registration, and opened daycares and maternity centers.[104] For the men abroad, LBA volunteers served as *madrinhas*, or godmothers, "tendering moral and affective comfort to those in combat."[105]

It is accurate to consider the LBA an organization devoted to serving Brazilian families and the home-front war effort, but it was also explicitly linked to the immediate domestic goals and politics of the Estado Novo. In fact, it was the Minister of Justice and Internal Affairs Alexandre Marcondes Filho who officially authorized the statutes of the LBA, under the regulations of Decreto-lei no. 4.684.[106] That presidential decree required all organizations whose objectives related to "national defense" to secure the ministry's prior authorization before beginning operation. In the name of national security, Vargas signed Decree-law 4.684 to impede "dangerous elements" from using popular mobilization during the war against the interests of the state.[107] Thus, the LBA was formally recognized as an element of Brazil's national defense. Moreover, the LBA was the first assistance organization with national scope; it grew to boast a volunteer corps of more than one million Brazilian women, who offered their time, labor, and expertise in what amounted to a gendered and politicized mass mobilization of wartime activity. Darcy Vargas's leadership signified gendered but nonthreatening politics and a particular vision of self-sacrificing elite motherhood that channeled the activist energies of influential women into their traditional roles as champions of family and the downtrodden.

The LBA's orientation fit squarely within the political and economic logic of the Estado Novo, which saw Brazilian workers as a corporate body. During the war, the state expressed *trabalhista* politics in militarized language and associated order and productivity with national defense and success on the battlefield. For the LBA, this meant that soldiers' families and workers' families were the same. The organization's programs, therefore, prioritized deployed soldiers' families but sought to aid working families in general. Darcy Vargas would later reflect with appreciation on "our humble soldiers of peace, the industrial and commercial workers" who supported Brazil's brave soldiers overseas.[108] The LBA's conflation of soldiers with workers and the Estado Novo's *trabalhista* politics were clearly evident in the association's funding scheme, demonstrating the overlap between Brazil's military response and the state's industrial orientation. On October 15, 1942, President Vargas signed a monthly allocation for the LBA into law to be funded from three sources, all by means of the Ministry of Labor, Industry, and Commerce. First, he promised the LBA a subsidy directly from the federal budget. From the Pension and Retirement Funds, the ministry was required to pull one-half percent from the payments made to all retirees and pensioners. Additionally, current employees contributed a mandatory one-half percent of their salaries to the LBA, and their employers were required to match that total.[109] This sum equaled Cr$10,200,000.00 for the coffers of the Legion in 1942 and Cr$40,800,000.00 in 1943.[110] Of course, the LBA also relied on private benefactors to support their efforts, but the rationale here was apparent. The LBA aided workers and their families during wartime, and thus the resources to fund their activities should come primarily from the industrial sector via the ministry that regulated all labor guidelines and worker-industrialist relations. As the LBA helped father-headed households during a time of need, male workers in the factories contributed to assist the wives and children of their deployed comrades. These were the deserving poor.

The LBA's most public national campaign occurred in 1943—an ambitious crusade in support of the Brazilian child, called the Campanha de Redenção da Criança (Campaign for Redemption of the Child), launched by Darcy Vargas and the newspaper/radio tycoon Assis Chateaubriand, who served as one of the organization's vice presidents. The redemption language is telling; it combined the eugenic ideal of regeneration with the moralizing tone of child saving. Darcy Vargas and Chateaubriand envisioned raising funds from Brazil's most affluent families and redirecting those resources to construct and support Puericulture Centers in the abandoned hinterlands. Their charitable but paternalistic vision of reform reflected Chateaubriand's own political leanings. Hailing from the Northeast, he was an influential figure of the Estado Novo who advocated for a highly structured and hierarchical social order. Chateaubriand fell in and out of favor with President Vargas over the years, assisting his candidacy in 1929 and then advocating for the return to democracy that would oust Vargas in 1945. He was a highly significant figure, and his personal support for the cause of infant health helped spark the president's own interest.[111] Though he favored a strong, interventionist federal government, Chateaubriand also argued that the wealthy held a special responsibility to allocate a share of their resources to the cause of national development.

Writing to Capanema in September of 1944, First Lady Vargas described the Child Redemption Campaign as a mission in "human solidarity," a means of instructing the Brazilian people in their duty to the nation's children.[112] Its organizers also had nationalist eugenic ambitions. Dr. Hermes Bartolomeu of the DNC encapsulated this sentiment best when he stated that the campaign sought "to ensure children's survival as well as a strong and healthy race for the nation."[113] Once the campaign was under way, the DNC provided technical support, and Chateaubriand's newspaper conglomerate, the Diários Associados, took charge of publicity across the country. His *Diário de Notícias da Bahia* reminded its readers that the goals of the Redemption Campaign were neither sentimental nor abstract. Rather, "a stronger and healthy people will always be a hard-working, efficient, and prosperous people destined . . . to exert great influence among nations."[114] His *Estado da Bahia* called the campaign "a grand, national movement"—philanthropy with the "highest social aims."[115] To promote the LBA's movement, Minister Capanema personally chose "Protection of Children in Collaboration with the LBA and the Campaign for the Redemption of the Child" as the national theme for Children's Week of 1945.[116]

In anticipation of the first project, LBA representatives toured some of Brazil's most deprived regions to determine which communities were in greatest need of puericulture centers. The exploratory team consisted of Bartolomeu; Josefina Albano of the LBA; and Rosa Alvarez, a US public health specialist. In Bahia, the team visited several locations and concluded that the small Recôncavo town of São Felix would reap the first fruits of the Campanha de Redenção. Financing came from a Cr$600,000.00 donation made by the wealthy Morganti family of São Paulo.[117] On March 7, 1944, honored guests from the LBA and the DNC presided over a grand ceremony to kick off construction on the São Felix site. Following the raising of the flag and the singing of the national anthem, Mayor Julio Ramos de Almeida delivered a passionate speech about the significance of the day and the choice of his town as the location of the first LBA Center. National pride was on full display on that Tuesday, since the crusade was, in Mayor Almeida's words, "the most patriotic fruit of the campaigns initiated by the Estado Novo."[118] Like Mayor Almeida, even with private funding, many must have understood the Child Redemption Campaign as an extension of official Estado Novo policy.

The selection of São Felix for the first puericulture center provides another opportunity to read the politics and patronage networks of the Estado Novo on a local level. Most of Bahia's traditional rural aristocracy hailed from the Recôncavo, and it had been the site of political infighting among clans that provoked a federal intervention in the 1920s.[119] But it is unclear what impact any of this would have made on a national audience reading about the Campanha in one of Chateaubriand's many newspapers. Certainly São Felix warranted health services, but many other regions of the state and the nation did as well. The choice of São Felix was in no way inevitable. Yet this small town in a tobacco-producing region on the Paraguaçu River must have conjured images of depression and want for wealthy *paulistas* like the Morgantis. São Felix, and the state of Bahia in general, likely summoned visions of backwardness and a region in desperate need of a modernizing influence. Few regions could have symbolized the past in the southern imagination better than the Bahian Recôncavo: agricultural, black, and oligarchic. If health services could improve the population of a traditional town like São Felix, Brazil could still hope to engineer a working populace suitable as a basis for economic progress. The campaign appealed to the sense of duty and patronage of families like the Morgantis, imploring them to part with a small piece of their fortunes on behalf of the "grateful impoverished" masses.[120] By "redeeming" the Brazilian child, the privileged residents of the industrialized urban centers could reach out to the supposed economically and culturally distant areas of the nation. They could help counteract the vestiges of the past—the rural poverty, the blackness, the obsolete aristocracy. In so doing, Brazilians of means could take pride in resuscitating "the child of today, man of tomorrow—the primordial element in the future development of national agriculture and industry."[121]

Chateaubriand was back in Salvador in the inaugural year of the campaign. He was the honored guest speaker for the graduating class at the Puericulture School. In a flowery and enthusiastic speech, Chateaubriand insisted that national progress began with a public commitment to the Brazilian child. He reminded those present at the ceremony that the protection of pregnant wives and of children represented the greatest security the state could provide for the (male) Brazilian worker, whether urban or rural.[122] For Chateaubriand, building these types of institutions was the real work of the Estado Novo, taking control of Brazil's destiny by ensuring the healthy development of its future generations, just as Mussolini had done in Italy. "A strong state," he maintained, "must consider children's welfare and the eugenic defense of the race."[123] In sum, the selection of Bahia as home to the Redemption Campaign's first center illustrates the power of the persistent southern perspective of northeastern (and western) "underdevelopment" and the networks of influential individuals machinating behind the scenes.

Those networks were formidable enough to generate funding from Brazil's wealthiest families and to command the attention of the federal government.

While the Campanha received a great deal of national press, particularly through the Diários Associados, the Bahian LBA remained busy with its own local initiatives. During the war, the Bahian LBA worked collaboratively with maternal and child welfare programs to assist soldiers' families. Chapter president and Bahian First Lady Ruth Vilaboim Aleixo wrote to the Liga on several occasions, for example, requesting that the organization award the *prêmio de amamentação*—the breast-feeding stipend—to poor and desperate wives in need of immediate assistance due to their husbands' deployment. The LBA advocated for women like Raimunda Aurelina dos Santos and her son Edison who needed financial help in 1943. They reached out on behalf of Maria de Nazaré Portela, whose husband Geraldo was away serving in 1944.[124] Furthermore, like many state chapters, the Bahian LBA created independent facilities and, like many maternal and child facilities in Brazil— even to this day, the centers honored Darcy Vargas by carrying her name. In 1943, the Bahian LBA opened the Darcy Vargas Creche—a large, modern free daycare center with space for thirty babies—in the Graça neighborhood of Salvador. The following year, the organization expanded the Darcy Vargas Creche into a full "Casa Maternal" where domestics and factory workers could leave children under age three while they worked. The expanded Casa included a small playground for the children. It also had a cafeteria where "humble domestics" like Martinha Guedes were served a "succulent bowl of soup" after stopping by during the workday to nurse their infants.[125] Though Bahian organizations like the LBA and the Liga depended on local partnerships, their interests diverged over time. After the war, for example, the LBA had to reconceptualize its mission.[126] Bahia's LBA increasingly devoted its resources to aid orphans and other institutionalized children. This conflicted with the Liga, whose affiliated physicians insisted that child advocates should expand options for foster care rather than allocating resources for improving institutions.

The LBA and the Bahian League against Infant Mortality both relied on federal subsidies for their institutional survival, and this was the case for dozens of social welfare organizations across Brazil, even though federal money was perpetually in short supply. The institutional weakness, financial constraints, and limited reach of the DNC meant that the Estado Novo never fulfilled Capanema's goal of uniting *all* maternal and child assistance programs under one strong federal institution. The DNC itself suffered from lack of resources, as a matter of fact. Even the LBA, which carried the full esteem of the Vargas surname, suffered long delays and suspensions of payments from its sponsoring agencies.[127] The prized National Puericulture Institute had more than 80 percent of its initial budgetary allocation reapportioned for other initiatives before the first stone was set.[128] And it continually suffered from lack of funding and autonomy after being incorporated into the University of Brazil's School of Medicine.[129] In financial terms alone, family advocates imagined more comprehensive and far-reaching programs than would ever become reality, and the Estado Novo certainly did not create an adequate health-care infrastructure to meet the health needs of *all* poor mothers and their children. Most women and children outside of state capitals had very limited access to specialized health care throughout this period, but the federal government did provide subsidies across Brazil to private institutions aiding women and children. The Estado Novo did not create new local institutions in general, but rather depended on privately controlled ones to execute its call for "maternal and childhood assistance" under state supervision.

The reliance on private resources was an integral aspect of the paradigm of *assistência social*, social assistance or social welfare. In this approach, the state authorized and often proffered subsidies, but the leadership of assistance organizations and the administration of their services remained in the private sector. Thus, the state worked in cooperation with nongovernmental organizations and their benefactors. This model was typical of emerging welfare states in Latin America, as religious and secular private organizations provided various types of social aid long before the involvement of the state.[130] The Bahian example illustrates this well, and as I argued in chapter 2, local synergies between the public and the private sectors long predated the Vargas era as an assistance model. These were reciprocal arrangements, and this framework of public-private social assistance left room for state aid to slant toward organizations with direct, personal connections to the federal government or those that fit neatly into Estado Novo politics.

The link between private organizations and the federal government was strategic from several perspectives. Clearly, those connections added prestige and legitimacy to local efforts. Uncovering them opens a window into how the Estado Novo functioned outside of Rio de Janeiro through networks of favored private institutions and alliances among influential people, showing a side of Vargas-era politics that seems quite similar to regimes past. The association with social welfare also provided a showcase for the state's regard for average families. Taking this point a step further, the social service work on the local level gave Brazilians beyond the Federal District an opportunity to witness or even benefit from "individual" acts of benevolence and patronage made by Brazil's wealthy and powerful. Outside of the industrial South, where *trabalhista* politics were less impactful, this version of state power and charity was a salient symbol of the Estado Novo. Iraildes Caldas Torres has argued that this paradigm of *assistência social* turned Brazilians into dependents rather than citizens with rights of access to state resources, revealing a "relation of power and dependency between the [actor] who 'gives' and the [object] who 'receives.' Social welfare [was] not presented to its users as a service, but as a kindness accompanied by a spirit of charity and solidarity."[131] For the case of the LBA specifically, Torres argues that its efforts were essential to demobilizing industrial labor and winning the goodwill of working people.

Torres's analysis resonates beyond the LBA; however, some caution is necessary in interpreting Estado Novo social welfare. The federal state certainly strategically employed the image and activities of the president and first lady, but it is inaccurate to consider Getúlio and Darcy Vargas, or even Gustavo Capanema, as master manipulators of a naive and unsuspecting public. And while the LBA served the philosophies of the Estado Novo expertly, one cannot underestimate the enormous mobilization of women's expertise that the organization levied and employed during WWII. Finally, however inadequate, the federal government's investment in social services was not simply propaganda. Through subsidies, the Vargas government did help provide health and welfare services to tens of thousands of women and children in Bahia alone. Bahian organizations faced little interference in putting those stipends to use according to their own missions and within the context of local realities and patronage networks.[132] The most meaningful critique, therefore, is a reassessment of the supposed historical rupture that Vargas proclaimed. The Brazilian government was not wholly reimagined and reborn in the Estado Novo with a novel, contemporary approach to the well-being of its dispossessed citizens. In the nationalization of family health and welfare, "modern" institutions helped secure a tenuous compromise with the popular classes while reinforcing a much older tradition of patronage, patriarchy, and patriarchalism.

The fact that the Vargas government largely left social projects in the hands of philanthropic organizations, particularly those with deep local connections like the Bahian League against Infant Mortality and the Misericórdia, meant that state support combined with local modes of patronage. If anything, the Bahian maternalist movement demonstrated that modern social programs could be completely rooted in patronage networks and traditional notions of charity. The largest personal benefactors of the Liga and the Misericórdia illustrate this convenient union between old sugar money and a newer scientific approach to social problems. Between its foundation and the end of the Estado Novo, the Liga acquired a number of facilities donated in full by illustrious Bahian families. Many of these families represented agricultural elites, and several were the inheritors of the old colonial sugar aristocracy. The names of these benefactors were permanently linked to clinics and graced invitations to fund-raisers and special events. For example, the sons of the sugar baron and commercialist Raymundo Pereira de Magalhães donated the prized Puericulture School in 1937, which was given their father's name. Other important benefactors included Alice and Álvaro Catharino, both descendants of two of Bahia's wealthiest and most influential families: Alice, the granddaughter of Manuel Machado, and Álvaro, the son of Co-mendador Bernardo Martins Catharino. The patriarchs Machado and Cath-arino were both Portuguese immigrants who made their fortunes in Bahia as owners of two of the most successful textile companies: Confecção e Teci-dos Paraguaçu and Companhia Progresso União Fabril. The Catharinos do-nated a building for the Instituto Baptista Machado (named after Alice's fa-ther, João Baptista Machado) that served as Liga headquarters after 1929 and the state Children's Department after 1935.[133]

A colonial institution and favored charity of elite families, the brother-hood of the Santa Casa de Misericórdia modernized according to scientific theories of hygiene and child rearing in the 1930s thanks to its relationship with the Liga and access to public funding. But the brotherhood's position as intermediary for those seeking to bestow Christian alms and patronage to the poor remained intact. José and Sinhazinha Baptista Marques, whose family owned the Passagem sugar refinery in Santo Amaro, sponsored the creation of the Misericórdia's children's polyclinic in 1930. The clinic was named "Arnaldo Baptista Marques" in honor of the couple's deceased son. In 1934, Carlos Costa Pinto, sugar exporter, businessman, and descendant of another influential oligarchic Recôncavo family, largely funded the Ma-ternal Shelter at the completely updated Foundling Home. These surnames, and those of the Liga's benefactors, would have been instantly recognizable in Bahia in the 1930s and 1940s, and the connection to such power and wealth bolstered the stature of the maternalist movement. It allowed wealthy fami-lies to support poor maternity in the abstract without confronting the hier-archies of gender, race, privilege, and servitude within their own households. Their financial support was critical to the institutions' success and part of a long history of elite philanthropy and religious charity.

Because Bahian social assistance organizations had direct ties to the fed-eral government, these financial contributions tie long-standing customs of patronage and even patriarchalism—the concentration of wealth among landed elites and authority among the strongest family patriarchs—with the modern period of state consolidation. This melding of old and new helps ex-plain how the Vargas government executed its call for social projects despite institutional limitations and wavering commitment from top leadership. Much of the work was left to private organizations whose social legitimacy and financial viability depended on relationships with local power holders, many of whom pertained to oligarchic families who had safeguarded and enjoyed the advantages of that power for generations. In Bahia, modernization and patriarchalism were never fully divorced. The rhetoric of aid to deserving single mothers, attempting to fulfill their patriotic duty to rear Brazil's strong future laborers, well suited that discourse of conservative modernization and transition within acceptable limits. Rather than assume a disjuncture between the old rural agricultural interests and Vargas's push to weaken the influence of this class, it is more accurate to understand state dynamics as integral aspects of federal ones—even if sometimes at odds. A close consideration of Bahian social welfare provides a different lens into the modernization fever of the Estado Novo, rather than an exception to it, and elucidates how *trabalhista* politics functioned outside of the industrial South.

WORK, FATHERHOOD, AND DOMESTICITY GIVE LIFE TO the working man, according to the catchy lyrics of the 1941 samba "É negócio casar." In exchange, President Vargas promised an orderly, prosperous nation guided by an ongoing commitment to its "*homens do trabalho*." These men were asked to give even more during wartime, but a legion of Brazilian women, *madrinhas*, and children at home respected their sacrifice because, in a unified nation, all shared the spirit of love of country. Whether in war or in peace, the state would ensure justice and fairness on the factory floor as well as aid and protection of wives and children. This idealized version of *trabalhista* politics reveals the state's emphasis on paternal effort and maternal defense. Despite the rhetoric of citizenship and nationalism, social welfare programs endorsed by the Vargas government were ultimately paternalist in nature, portraying state actions as the extension of patronage from a benevolent Father of the Poor.[134] State paternalism with Getúlio Vargas as figurehead was the national version of the father-headed family structure that the president and his highest authorities hoped would discipline and stabilize Brazil's working class.

Despite the federal government's pact with Brazil's worker-patriarchs, Bahia's welfare model remained maternity focused. Welfare efforts in that state did not seek to assist working-class patriarchy but to act as secondary providers and to ensure all children benefited from proper mothering in the assumed absence of their negligent fathers. The quintessential Bahian public health and welfare client was a single mother who spent her days working in domestic service. This imaginary motherhood left no room for struggling fathers like Joaquim Amancio Pita and Manoel Simplicio dos Santos, introduced in the opening of this chapter. On the labor side, household service was certainly a reality of life for the majority of Bahian women, drawing an unfortunate continuity for women of color with centuries past. In

Bahia, "protection of women and children" always existed in relation to the authority-and-dependence dynamic between servants and their patrons. The single-mother narrative also served a rhetorical purpose. Bahia's public health and welfare system provided badly needed assistance to impoverished children while conveniently avoiding discussion of better education, higher wages, social mobility, or more opportunities for civic participation for their parents. Maternalism, and the single-mother aid recipient, promoted a conservative version of reform, one that did not fundamentally challenge household, community, or social hierarchies. Therefore, despite the orientation toward fatherhood, marriage, and labor within the Estado Novo, Bahian health and assistance took the symbolic abandoned single mother as its point of departure, offering myriad benefit programs but closing the possibility of conceptualizing poor families in alternative ways.

Bahian maternalism did not directly contradict the Estado Novo's male-centered *trabalhista* politics. Local organizations continued and even amplified the maternalist work they had been engaged in for decades while crediting the Father of the Poor for his leadership. Bahia was one of the first states in the nation to pioneer health and welfare services for women and children; it provided foundational ideas, key figures, and model institutions to Brazil's growing welfare state, though this was rarely acknowledged publicly within the official rhetoric of the Vargas government.[135] Between Assis Chateaubriand, Darcy Vargas, Martagão Gesteira, and Minister Capanema, the Bahian maternalist movement certainly had friends in high places. And these were strategic friendships. Though *trabalhismo* promised to elevate working people and their ambitious industrialist employers over the gentry of old, in reality, wealthy benefactors funded a significant portion of social assistance. Thus, the Father of the Poor had many partners on the local level.

When Brazilian elites donated to public-private institutions as a charitable gesture to the disadvantaged, they participated in a slow process that extended the reach of the state into the daily lives and family dynamics of average people. Financial subsidies to private welfare institutions (however limited and inadequate) also helped expand the patronage of the state, setting up the president as the symbolic father to those in need. Like most privileged citizens, benefactors supported a conservative modernization—a reform in harmony with Brazil's foundational fictions: an emphasis on family as the basis of society and the desire to channel social issues through relationships with powerful interests rather than through conflict. In this way, the maternal and child welfare movement offered near universal appeal as a reform option compatible with Bahian concerns and realities. Even the most ardent Vargas detractors would not argue against strengthening family or the importance of women's roles as mothers to the potential of future generations. This movement also promoted the mobilization of upper-class (newly enfranchised) women into an acceptable public arena that was "civic-minded" and therefore "modern," yet not threatening or politically controversial. In Bahia, the marriage of local commitment to maternity and childhood (filtered through traditional social hierarchies) with the family-centered rhetoric and patronage politics of the Estado Novo created an alternative claim to modernization in a state that lacked the industrialization spurring economic development in the South.

The development of maternal and child welfare sheds light on the tension between social welfare as a state obligation and the continued reliance on private organizations, both civic and religious, as well as altruistic individuals to fund and implement social assistance. Idealistic welfare advocates promoted ambitious programs, but they always seemed to outpace the financial resources available. The reform of the Brazilian family was a favorite topic of the president, and important legislative and institutional precedents were set during the Estado Novo, but transformative investment in health care and social welfare was neither a priority nor a reality in the 1930s and 1940s. Although Brazil's highest leaders worked toward centralization and the subjugation of state interests to federal authority, the realization of this responsibility was slow and uneven. Despite Vargas's commitment to the end of regionalism, for example, the central importance of webs of local and national patronage demonstrates that the actual dynamics of the Estado Novo contributed to regional divergence—at least on issues of social welfare. In Bahia, the apparent commitment of the nation's leader to family issues merged with local concerns, recasting federal politics into practical application. This local resonance made maternal and child welfare the most salient "good business" of the Bahian Estado Novo.

Conclusion

*P*LAYING WITH DUALITIES—BLACK MAMMIES/BLACK mothers, empiricist midwives/women of science, failed mothers/mothers redeemed, father of the nation/fathers of children—provides an intriguing entry point into the multiple and overlapping discourses and realities of Brazil's maternalist movement. I have argued that these dual-sided characters alternatively reinforced and challenged the assumptions undergirding the medicalization of motherhood, but those tropes nonetheless remained profoundly engrained. The case of Salvador da Bahia (the Mulata Velha), a city largely defined by its racialized maternal metaphors, adds a spatial and regional dimension to this complexity. These cultural icons, including the Mulata Velha as place, demonstrate that medical knowledge and cultural knowledge were not mutually exclusive. In Brazil, the intersecting historical dynamics of race, gender, and privilege proved essential in the institutionalization of maternalism and social assistance. Nineteenth-century Brazilian medicine took on maternal and infant health for the first time, identifying women's child-care practices (as mothers, servants, and midwives) as hazardous to children's survival and well-being. Physicians presumed that women manifested collective illnesses and deficiencies in the body of the nation, and medical professionals articulated these concerns about society at large through maternalist discourse.

Social problems, even in medical theory, do not have a simple linear relationship to social realities. Brazilian families undoubtedly suffered greatly from the prevalence and severity of infant morbidity and mortality, and they found no assistance from state public health agencies, as such programs did not exist until the twentieth century. Families struggled during periods of epidemic disease, they suffered the devastating effects of poor sanitation, and they grieved and buried their young children and their friends and relatives who did not survive the experience of childbirth. The weight of poverty exacerbated the challenge of staying healthy, and children living in poverty were most vulnerable to the dangers of their own or their parents' illnesses. For prevention, treatment, and birthing, mothers turned to local midwives, who shared knowledge and introduced families to home remedies and procedures that became generational wisdom. For mothers of color, the "compounded exploitation" of productive and reproductive labor meant that healthy child rearing and the perpetuation or transformation of the wider social hierarchy literally and figuratively occurred through their bodies and their domestic work.[1]

Bahian families experienced these tendencies in general and in particular fashion, making them both typical and distinctive. And the state of Bahia made unique contributions to the history of Brazilian maternalism between 1850 and 1945. Some of the goals of this book have been to prioritize mothers of color and to problematize the question of whose experiences count as representative of the general trends of the era and which regions of Brazil tell the history of the *modern* nation. Thus, I have argued that the exploration of motherhood, race, and family health constitutes not a folkloric, peripheral, or idiosyncratic study but rather a critical analysis of the central currents in Brazilian cultural politics and social policy. Bahian maternalism both helped craft and responded to dynamic local realities and the broader Brazilian quest for "modernity" within a national imaginary that threatened to write Bahia out.

By the mid-nineteenth century, the handwriting was on the wall for slavery, and pro-republic voices increasingly exposed the lie of Brazilian liberalism. For the political and intellectual elite, including the small but aspirant sector of physicians, the nation seemed to be stumbling toward chaos with the impending fall of slavery and empire. They rigorously debated the appropriate means of guiding the transition to the new century in ways that would stabilize and reorder state and society, maximize national potential, and engineer a progressive labor force—all without unleashing radical change. Within medicine, this process began with study and diagnosis. French science and medicine provided the frameworks, but Brazilian medicine's prognosis for their anxious society remained deeply rooted in local realities and prevailing cultural logics of gender, race, and class inequalities. I have argued that, as slavery and monarchy threatened to come to an end, medical attention turned to public health, biological and social reproduction, and progressive mothering and child rearing. Maternalist theories—and eventual public health projects—resulted from complex and contradictory debates about nation.

Progressive mothering turned the medical gaze toward Brazilian households. The household was not only a laboratory for determining the insufficiencies in family health and their relation to society at large; it was also a key site where the larger dynamics of social differentiation and inequality were intensely experienced, generated, and replicated. Within the domestic sphere, mothers of means and their female servants shared mothering duties. For generations, the *famílias baianas* had employed free women and bonded enslaved women to care for children. In Bahia and across Brazil, mothering was a form of wage and slave labor. Nineteenth-century physicians largely identified this household situation as dangerous, deadly in fact, for the health of children entrusted to the care of women they labeled as "ignorant," "primitive," and "careless." My argument is that these labels are racially loaded, marking these women as not only incompetent but also uncivilized and polluting artifacts of a bygone era. Added to these presumed hazards, most Bahian women sought out "roving" midwives for medical care, women who moved in and out of their households to attend them. The public nature of this occupation resonated with poor urban women's work in general, requiring a mobility that often fell beyond patrons' tight control. To mitigate the risk poor women and women of color posed, nineteenth-century physicians prescribed a sanitation of child rearing within the "respectable" home, warning privileged mothers to carefully supervise what Sônia Roncador has called the "grotesque" (read: bodily) aspects of maternity.[2]

What that early generation of maternalist physicians did not investigate with any depth was the relation *between* Bahian households. Even after abolition in 1888, hierarchies within households impacted the practices of mothering and child rearing, but so did hierarchies between households. Families of means experienced the household as a protected space of privacy and intimacy; servants experienced those households as demanding workplaces where their own family responsibilities and attachments often went unrecognized or belittled. Domestic servants who slept in lived in separate households from their own children. Mothering of birth children and charges directly and problematically correlated, since the livelihood of domestics' families depended on successful mothering of their charges, not their children. Mothers who worked in domestic service undoubtedly made sacrifices to ensure the income generated by their mothering of others' children. For their own children, these sacrifices may have led to conditions rife for illness. And such crises too frequently led to the steps of the Foundling Home.

As the twentieth century opened, Brazilian maternalism moved in new directions. Rather than enhancing differentiations, this generation of reformists put their faith in "modernization" premised on national cohesion and working-class incorporation under the new republic's rallying cry of "Order and Progress." Incorporation itself could be a means of solidifying a

so-called race-in-formation, promoting economic growth, and avoiding social conflict. Scientific and social scientific ideologies bolstered new conceptions of national change, such as the international rise of eugenics as well as
Brazilian theories of racial improvement through generational whitening
and later "social democracy." Physicians found an opportunity in these dialogues about national reform, racial improvement, and republicanism to
press for the centrality of their profession in steering a modernizing nation
and implementing the interventions it would require.

Within this national context, Bahian medicine made new interpretations
of family life and its health risks. The result was that servitude was no longer the primary axiom through which early-twentieth-century physicians
thought about poor women's mothering and child rearing. They maintained
a concern about midwifery and continued to denigrate their midwife competitors as part of the professionalization of biomedicine. But biomedicine
was increasingly practiced and championed by men *and* women, diversifying
the gender of scientific expertise. Within the spirit of racial democracy and
laying the groundwork for progress, medical experts increasingly considered
the popular classes and the health of mothers and children of everyday families. In Bahia, maternalist advocates sought to medicalize the standard dynamics of average families—to make preventative and restorative biomedical care a routine aspect of family life. This would be the starting point for
reducing infant mortality and helping poor mothers and their children live
longer, healthier, and more productive lives. It would also keep mothers and
children together if possible, and where impossible, place children under
medical supervision at the Foundling Home. Though "populist" oriented,
twentieth-century medicine certainly did not break free of racial and gender
biases and assumptions about the lives and lifestyles of women and men of
color. With regard to women of color, maternalist advocates assumed poor
mothers were ignorant of the proper care of their children and abandoned to
their own misery by the fathers of their children. Thus, reformists continued
to see Bahians of the popular classes as impediments to progress; but by using the tools of medical intervention, they could also be the cure.

The federal government had not yet consolidated a true welfare state with
national scope and reach, supported by a legal apparatus and a comprehensive network of local service agencies. That process would only begin in the
1930s and 1940s under the presidency of Getúlio Vargas. In Bahia, local organizations stepped in to assist mothers and children in the absence of state institutions. They made an enormous impact by serving thousands of families
between those two decades, but their range was largely limited to the capital
city of Salvador and its immediate vicinity. Infrastructural and financial constraints meant that these organizations never adequately addressed all the
health and welfare needs of Bahian families. Yet organizations like the Ba-

hian League against Infant Mortality assembled an impressive roster of free services.

By the 1940s, the Liga and their partners at the Santa Casa de Misericórdia and in state government could consider themselves successful in helping reduce the catastrophic infant mortality rates in Bahia. For the years between 1939 and 1941, the Brazilian Geographic and Statistical Institute (IBGE) recorded the mortality of *soteropolitano* babies under one year of age as 206.3 per 1,000.[3] Between 1948 and 1950, the mortality rate for this age group had fallen to 162.57, still surpassing the national average of 146.4 per 1,000.[4] Improvements in sanitation, hygiene, vaccination, and medical technology undoubtedly contributed to this falling child mortality. Yet the preventative, nutritional, and treatment options that private and public organizations sponsored must have played a significant role as well, since no such services existed in the nineteenth century.

The state of Bahia worked cooperatively with private organizations because both sides needed the other for structural reasons, for legitimacy, and for resources. Private financial support came from wealthy Bahian families, allowing even traditional patronage to modernize along with social medicine. This meant a blending of networks of influential patrons with the growing state bureaucracy, reinforcing my argument that social reform through maternalism did not fundamentally challenge the privilege of Brazilians of means. Their sponsorship of "poor, single mothers" and "redeemed Brazilian children," fundamental to the creation and survival of aid programs, was in itself an act of privilege. Family advocates and politicians constructed the problem in ways that fit their expectations of race, gender, and class. They framed health and welfare assistance as an extension of charity and benevolence rather than an explicit recognition of state responsibility to those structurally kept from any realistic expectation of social mobility. In Bahia, these continuities proved plainly visible into the 1940s, where the cultural language of slavery—its gendered and racialized "order of things"—persisted alongside the invariability in occupation for women of color.

The maternalist movement and the nascent welfare state institutionalized and increasingly amplified its radius of action in new ways, thereby linking families to the state, the state to private organizations and practitioners, and ultimately Bahian organizations to national ones. By the third decade of the new century, in the context of growing nationalism, a push for economic growth, and mobilization for warfare, Bahian maternalism found its paternal champion in President Getúlio Vargas. And President Vargas was the ultimate patron/*pai* of the Brazilian poor. The Vargas administration codified family and labor policy while organizing a new health and social welfare bureaucracy. Though Bahians and their reformers may not have seen a self-reflection in Vargas's Estado Novo and its promotion of industry and working-class patriarchy, they did hold on to the president's rhetorical commitment to poor families. Bahian organizations practiced maternalism in the face of masculine *trabalhista* politics and a paternalist national project. In Bahia, maternalism institutionalized to a greater extent than in the previous thirty years while maintaining a local character in the many spaces left for regional autonomy and traditional patronage. I have argued that a gendered reading of the Vargas era elucidates those spaces of interdependence between old politics, old ideologies, and New State.

The everyday child-rearing activities of poor black and brown women remained central to these public projects, and medical intervention, while often built on problematic assumptions, was only possible through connecting to women's occupational and familial experiences. Maternalist advocates read reform through women's bodies, through mothering as a service to the nation, and through the relationship and ranking of female and male expertise. Yet scientific texts and maternalist publications were certainly not the only significant sites of the production of knowledge about mothering. Bahian women connected to reformists when and where health and aid projects served them and intersected with their own understandings, capacities, and challenges of motherhood. These mothers knew that "woman" as a category and mothering, domesticity, and service were racialized and hierarchal experiences. They knew that cultural icons like the *mãe preta*, the *curiosa*, and the *mãe desamparada* were just that, but they also knew that these were stereotypes, distortions, and abstractions obscuring real lived experiences of motherhood. Bahian women elected to participate in the maternalist movement, within constrained situations of health/illness, welfare/need, and generational poverty. And through their actions, Bahia's mothers of color helped jointly construct the maternal form of social assistance (however partial and insufficient).

The maternal and child health and welfare movement opened new opportunities for poor women of color and their children in Bahia, but within "acceptable" limits. The birth of the Brazilian public health system and its emphasis on family welfare redefined the relationship between the popular classes and their state. It set a precedent for the expectation that the state would provide for Brazilians of all economic and social stations, and this marked a type of differentiated, incomplete, and contingent citizenship. For Bahian women of color, accessing those services entailed navigating a health and welfare system that presumed their incompetence and saw their children as future national commodities. But the rather functional meanings behind maternalism and public health could be reappropriated and repurposed. Bahian mothers utilized those services where needed and useful, and responded to their reformists' own lack of practical knowledge about motherhood. The health, well-being, and survival of their families were literally at stake.

A Suggestive Epilogue

MATERNITY CONTINUES TO BE A HIGHLY POLITI-cal issue in Brazil. Just as in the period examined in this book, contemporary experiences of motherhood and public health reflect broader social dynamics of racial and class inequality. In the early twenty-first century, however, social activism around mothering and childbirth has taken new directions, particularly for black women. This suggestive epilogue explores recent black activism around childbirth. I use the term "black" as a translation of the commonly employed "*negra*," an inclusive term for Brazilians of African descent that is a deliberate rejection of the separation of black from brown. The political resonance of the inclusive "*população negra*" or "*comunidade negra*" reveals the growing national strength of black activism during the past thirty years, taking the fall of the military dictatorship in 1985 as a marker. And we must understand political activism around healthy and safe maternity as one element of that larger project, though one where the particular intersection of race and gender for black women pushes to the fore. Black Brazilian women, either historical or present-day, remain grossly understudied, while their political organization and family experiences continue to be absolutely essential to any consideration of public health and social welfare. As in the preceding chapters, this epilogue responds to what Isabel Cristina Fonseca da Cruz identifies as the failure to see black Brazilian women as "researchable" or to consider their experiences as "real" and "relevant" to the world of public health.[1] I would add as a source of that failure a reticence or refusal to consider black Brazilian women as representative of the general patient experience. Their activist politics respond to a specific set of historical and contemporary structures of inequality, but their conceptualizations of the black female experience in public health and their involvement within it is the only means of understanding the system as a whole.

Therefore, my aim with this epilogue is both synthetic (providing inroads into a crucial study) and argumentative, and I hope to encourage further research on black women's activism around maternity and public health.

I select a specific framework for opening the question of black women's activism and maternal health politics: a critical reading of the "*humanização do parto*" movement that seeks reform in childbirthing practices. Today, as in decades past, racialized cultural politics intersect with the lived experiences of privilege versus poverty. The compounded weight of cultural narratives of black womanhood and the realities of mothering with scarce resources bear upon childbirth in Brazil and help us understand the complexities of the *humanização do parto* movement. "*A humanização*" of childbirth does not translate smoothly into English. The connotation in Portuguese is the action or process of adding a human dimension to childbirth. The ambiguity within this translation echoes the various meanings attached to the concept in Brazilian usage. The phrase "*humanizar o parto*" is employed in many ways and embodies several different elements even within the civil society mobilizations in favor of it. Though diverse and diffuse, two strains can be disaggregated while keeping in mind that both have had an important impact on health policy.

The first and perhaps most familiar expression of the *humanização do parto* movement calls for a valorization of women's bodies and a recasting of birthing as a natural event rather than a medical crisis. These advocates encourage vaginal birth with as little intervention as possible for mothers and babies at "low risk." It is a movement for women's empowerment and a critique of "technocratic" or physician-centered birthing. Its origins trace back to 1960s international dialogues on natural birthing, painless birth, and the Lamaze method. Furthermore, from within Brazil, a small group of obstetricians in the 1970s published on the potential benefits of incorporating elements of folk midwifery and Amazonian women's birthing culture into clinical practice. A politics of indigenist traditionalism was at play there, along with an uncritical vision of the female body as closer to nature than the male body and an equating of womanhood with reproduction. But all these currents served as inspiration for the *humanização do parto* movement.[2] By the 1980s, Brazil had an identifiable campaign in favor of "humanizing" childbirth, particularly after 1985 when the World Health Organization (WHO) published a series of recommendations for clinical birthing. Among many recommendations, the WHO endorsed vaginal birth for routine deliveries, the elimination of unnecessary procedures (such as episiotomy, amniotomy, and enema), the presence of the father or other companion in the birthing room, wider use of obstetric nurses to deliver in routine conditions, as well as greater incorporation of folk midwives in areas with limited access to biomedical clinics.[3] These guidelines became the point of departure for civil society organizations that were urging Brazilian clinics to reform their practices. As in many contexts, the majority of Brazilian natural childbirth advocates came from (and come from) middle-class backgrounds.

The second strain of the *humanização do parto* movement, however, is the focus of this epilogue. Concurrent with the more middle-class campaign in favor of vaginal birth and reduced medical intervention, Brazilian activists have also called for an overhaul in the childbirth practices employed in the unified public health system, the Sistema Único de Saúde (SUS), which falls under the auspices of the Ministry of Health (Ministério da Saúde). Black women's voices are more audible in this branch of the *humanização do parto* movement, as users of SUS maternity clinics; as advocates, activists, and academics; and as health-care providers. The websites of various NGOs as well as the community of black feminist bloggers provide a means of tracing popular conversations and of visualizing how knowledge is produced and shared between black women experts and activists as well as between black women generally. These blogs and sites do vital political work and provide educational information for all women about health resources and their rights as Brazilian citizens.

That SUS maternity wards serve primarily young, underresourced women of color; "low-income black women with little or no education"[4] is a type of popular truth, though racial data on birthing in the clinics are difficult to pin down. Statistical patterns help substantiate the assumption that most women who deliver in SUS clinics are Afro-Brazilian. Most Brazilian women give birth in SUS hospitals, around 77 percent, but there are significant differences between regions, and this has racial implications. In the poorer regions of the North and Northeast, between 85 percent and 90 percent of women use the public clinics to deliver their children, whereas in the most economically vibrant regions of the South, Southeast, and Center-West, this statistic falls significantly (70%–75%).[5] Income disparities are racial disparities in Brazil. In Bahia, the Brazilian Institute of Geography and Statistics (IBGE) household survey of 2008 found that black women use the in-patient services of the SUS system at about a 20 percent greater frequency than do white women, who are more likely to utilize private facilities.[6] Taken with the anecdotal experiences of Brazilians who actually use and work in public maternity clinics, we must take seriously the popular wisdom that the majority of maternity ward patients are black women.

Returning to the *humanização do parto*, many of the concerns with SUS birthing are the same as those expressed by women who use private clinics: safe options for natural childbirth, eliminating the culture of shaming women who elect vaginal delivery, and increased incorporation of laboring women and their loved ones in decision making. Yet some of the recurrent grievances against SUS are particular to Afro-Brazilian women, who receive less of SUS clinicians' time on average than white women do.[7] Particular points of mobilization for black women include the low incidence of prenatal care, the outrageous maternal mortality rate of black women (Afro-Brazilian women's maternal mortality rate was six times that of white women in 2005 but appears to be on the decline),[8] and the specific conditions of childbirth in SUS clinics elaborated below. Because there are divergent health indicators and racialized experiences in the public maternity wards, contemporary calls for SUS reform must also be historicized within Brazil's process of redemocratization post-1985 that opened space for women's, feminist, and Afro-Brazilian civil society organizations, among many other movements. This era saw the foundation of the first three black women's NGOs with national scope: Geledés (1988), Criola (1992), and Fala Preta! (1997). All three had the health of black communities among their political action areas from their inception; they drew attention to the structural racism undergirding health disparities as well as the institutional failures that limit access to adequate health care.[9]

I place black women's activism around reproductive health, safety, and equity in SUS childbirth within the larger call for black women's citizenship and human rights. The politics in this branch of the *humanização do parto* movement are distinct, and black women encounter specific scenarios of institutional violence, access, and objectification in SUS clinics. Because of this, and because Brazilians recognize health care as a universal right, the mobilization of black women on these issues is an element of a larger struggle for self-definition, social justice, and full citizenship.[10] The "humanity" under discussion here is unique to the black female experience, and we can easily observe the salience of these arguments in activists' and academics' writing. They make a clear association between a long history of symbolic violence and the material alienation from the right to one's own body, which has an obvious and unconscionable relevance to childbirth. Sueli Carneiro explains it thus, "There is a specific form of violence that constrains one's right to a positive image or representation, that limits one's options in the affective marketplace, that inhibits or compromises the free expression of one's sexuality, that restricts access to work, and that lowers one's aspirations and self-esteem."[11] In calling for a humanized birthing experience, activists, academics, and practitioners insist upon dignity and respect for black female bodies alongside respect for women's intimacy, sexuality, and relationships. They insist that these parameters guide the conditions in which they bring their children into the world.

Both strains of the *humanização do parto* movement have impacted Brazil's public health system. To understand this influence as well as black activism around public health in general, we must consider the circumstances of birthing that have engendered such vehement calls for reform. Activists across the spectrum denounce the "technocratic model" of birthing assistance so prevalent in Brazil and embodied in the extremely high rates of delivery by cesarean section. Proponents of humanization, within and without the Ministry of Health, refer to the hierarchical, mechanized model of birthing where the surgeon exerts full authority over a disenfranchised patient as "technocratic."[12] I use the high rates of cesarean births as an entry point into this critique but also into the important contrasts of privilege and marginalization that cause divergent experiences in the public system versus in private facilities.

Brazil has one of the highest incidences of cesarean birth in the world, hovering around 50 percent of all annual births. Brazil's statistics far exceed the recommended proportion of fifteen cesareans to eighty-five vaginal births established by the WHO. And, astonishingly, Brazil's numbers are on the rise; a recent study by the Oswaldo Cruz Institute found that cesarean births quadrupled between 1970 and 2010.[13] How do we account for this? And what is the resonance for black women's experiences in SUS and their activism around "humanizing" the childbirth process? I argue that two overlapping and overarching realities explain these extraordinarily elevated numbers. Yes, it is true that Brazilian obstetricians prefer scheduled birth and consider birth inherently dangerous. Yes, women in private hospitals, who presumably enjoy greater decision making than women in SUS facilities, overwhelmingly elect cesarean birth—and are encouraged to do so. These truths are commonly invoked, but their explanatory power goes only so far and cannot account for Brazil's elevated numbers vis-à-vis other nations. Closer attention to birthing experiences and the cultural articulations of race and gender indicates larger mechanisms that are specific to Brazil. I argue that socioeconomic inequalities and general disrespect for the rights of the multiracial poor—expressed politically as an attenuated citizenship or a "poverty of rights"[14] and institutionally as the appalling conditions of SUS birthing—produce and reflect a cultural narrative of vaginal birth as only appropriate for the impoverished: a dangerous, inferior, and painful birth without any mitigating relief. These interlocking factors inform one another.

Explicating further, expectant families associate cesarean birth with safety and comfort for both mother and baby. Private hospitals serve families of means and overwhelmingly deliver babies via cesarean surgeries. According to the Oswaldo Cruz study, cesareans account for nearly 90 percent of births in private hospitals.[15] Vaginal birth in private hospitals is unusual even for "low-risk" pregnancies. Public hospitals do perform cesareans, approximately 40 percent of births, which still far exceeds the recommended 15 percent.[16] However, vaginal delivery is much more common in SUS hospitals than in private facilities. There are class and racial implications in the election of cesarean birth. Privileged mothers pay to give birth with privacy, convenience, and superior technology—read as cesarean—whereas poor mothers enjoy none of these and are left to the uncertainties and discomfort created by their laboring bodies. These distinctions recall the same old racialized tropes that associate cultural whiteness with cleanliness and protection and cultural blackness with disorder and work. But the distinction between privileged and impoverished birthing goes far beyond the symbolic.

Activists, health professionals, and scholars draw our attention to various disturbing realities of SUS childbirth. One recurring denouncement is difficulty of access. Women in labor report having to search from one clinic to the next to locate an open bed. SUS has also been roundly criticized for the conditions and care awaiting women once admitted. Activists cite the frequent employment of "unnecessary" and painful interventions such as pubic shaving before delivery and episiotomy.[17] The usage of episiotomy in Brazilian birthing is alarmingly high, on approximately 90 percent of all women who deliver vaginally.[18] Once again, this falls out of line with the WHO recommendation that this procedure only be utilized when absolutely necessary and under strict indication protocols. In the public clinics, at times there is a lack of any form of anesthesia even for episiotomy; anesthesia is reserved for cesareans.[19] *Humanização do parto* advocates characterize the indiscriminate and routine use of episiotomy as a form of sexual and reproductive violence against women and an infraction against human rights through the total disregard of their "corporal integrity."[20] Finally, women who have delivered in public hospitals report being denied a companion to offer support during the process, particularly male companions/fathers. SUS hospitals have further maintained strict protocols that alienate laboring women and their companions from any decision making, such as failing to provide women with information about their labor process as well as denying them the freedom to move out of the bed should they choose. Activists report forced cesareans and tubal ligations completed without patient consent; some such incidences have garnered national media coverage.[21] In SUS clinics, laboring women are to remain silent, supine, and obedient. Women in public hospitals are more likely to deliver vaginally, "normal" birth in Brazilian parlance, and the experience of delivery between the two systems is stark. In an actual and a comparative sense, vaginal birth is distressing and even humiliating; it is *"parto para pobres"* (birthing for the poor).

Furthermore, activists report acts of obstetric violence as commonplace. I would assert that the frequency of violence in SUS childbirth has become a type of predictable and recognized cultural knowledge. It is a recurrent theme of blogs and popular responses.[22] Violence includes the forced and unnecessary procedures listed above as well as gross neglect and aggression against patients, but it also refers to the Ministry of Health's paradigm for "institutional violence." The ministry defines as "institutional violence" any violence committed with or by agents of public services by omission or commission. There are various scenarios that fall under the official rubric; I highlight a few that relate directly to accusations made against SUS birthing. For the ministry, "institutional violence" includes allowing circumstances in which patients must travel from one clinic to another in search of assistance, poor treatment due to discrimination (by race, age, sexual orientation, gender, physical deficiency, or mental illness), violation of reproductive rights (including accelerating childbirth to free up beds), physical violence, prohibiting the presence of guests or companions, and aggression against patients expressing or crying out in pain.[23] For activists and academics, "institutional violence" in SUS facilities tightly correlates with "institutional racism."[24] They argue that acts of violence against patients are not race-neutral anomalies but rather evidence of the structural racism that exists in Brazil. Adding gender to this, the specific consequences of institutional racism on black women's access to quality health care is a critical quality-of-life and life-expectancy issue. As experts remind us, "To neutralize institutional racism and its impact on the health and well-being of the black woman, it is necessary to promote a political context [within SUS] oriented around equity, citizenship, and emancipation."[25]

What activists uncover in SUS maternity wards is less of a commodification of black reproduction, which would recall a centuries-old practice in the Americas, and more of an abject devaluation. Certainly, the sexual commodification of black women's bodies is alive and well. But the type of devaluation attributed to SUS clinics is an objectification in which the female body is treated as an object through which a surgeon reaches his goal: to extract the child. The surgeon performs his expertise upon the laboring woman's body. Mothers themselves, and often their companions, are treated as hindrances. They report being treated as if their presence were a problem or inconvenience, and Ministry of Health data show that only 27 percent of black women have companions with them during childbirth compared to 46.2 percent of white women, even though companionship is all women's legal right.[26] Mothers report being subjected to various forms of disrespect and negligence, their sexuality ridiculed and their cries of pain and discomfort chastised and even punished.[27] The technocratic model has been and is under fire in Brazil, as are institutional racism and sexism in birthing assistance. But the reality is that too often black women do not have access to the safe health services to which they are entitled as citizens.

A number of high-profile cases of neglect and abuse of black women in

SUS hospitals have been reported, including the cruel death of six-months-pregnant Alyne da Silva Pimentel in 2011. Pimentel died in a Rio de Janeiro maternity ward "after her local health centre misdiagnosed her symptoms and delayed providing her with emergency obstetric care."[28] "Pregnant, poor, and black" Pimentel endured a horror that entailed a tragic succession of utter disregard: being turned away from care in severe pain, induction two days later into what turned out to be a fourteen-hour delivery of a stillborn baby, surgery that came too late, hemorrhage, and an eight-hour wait for an ambulance to transfer her to another facility, where she arrived in a coma.[29] A United Nations human rights investigation of Pimentel's death resulted in censure against Brazil for violating the "Convention on the Elimination of All Forms of Discrimination against Women." The Convention requires that states "guarantee women of all racial and economic backgrounds timely and non-discriminatory access to appropriate maternal health services."[30] For the WHO, Pimentel's death, like far too many others, was preventable. And "preventable maternal deaths seem to be concentrated among marginalized groups of women and they are marked by a lack of accountability."[31]

Pimentel's death illuminates the omnipresent and forceful specters of racial inequality and violence against women. *Humanização do parto* activists explain disenfranchisement, unnecessary procedures, and humiliation in birthing as a form of male-to-female violence, part of a larger contemporary dialogue about the multiple expressions of violence against women in Brazil.[32] And Afro-Brazilian activists remind us that many women's experiences belie the claim of "universality" in the unified health system. All of their work has been pivotal in initiating reform in SUS. In fact, though perhaps slow, uneven, and incomplete, SUS reform has progressed in partnership with social movements rather than in opposition to it. The Ministry of Health has taken steps to respond to the lack of accountability in health care decried by Afro-Brazilian political organizations, women's organizations, and black women's organizations.

Civil-society pressure has led to various concrete gains within the past ten years, and these gains are the accomplishment of social activism work. Perhaps the most impactful achievement has been getting the Ministry of Health to commit to the participation of Afro-Brazilian activists and researchers with expertise in the health of black communities in policy making, and then those activists and academics have had success in directing the conversation to questions of racism and equity. Beyond committees and conventions, such as the significant 2004 accord signed by the Special Secretariat for the Promotion of Racial Equality Policies (SEPPIR) and the Ministry of Health, the tangible fruits of black health activists' work are clearly evident. In 2003, for example, SUS agreed to collect data on race as a result of activists' insistence that accurate and complete statistics are fundamental to addressing health disparities. In 2009, SUS restated and reaffirmed the importance of data collection for properly addressing the health of black communities.[33] Today even the ministry acknowledges that inequalities in health care are a citizenship issue, that health disparities between racial groups are a historically manufactured problem, and that the gains made in combating both of these realities are a result of the ongoing work of civil organizations. Moreover, the ministry confirms that a "silent racism" persists in Brazilian society and *within* the practices of SUS.[34] The most extensive regulation came in the form of the "Política nacional de saúde integral da população negra," or the "National Policy for the Whole Health of the Black Population" (2009), interestingly ratified on May 13, the day Brazil commemorates the 1888 abolition of slavery.[35] Once again, the ministry explicitly cast this regulation as a governmental response to civil society pressure. Its major aims are the improvement of health conditions and "the promotion of equity in health" for Brazil's black population.[36]

We can further see the impact of women's activism in SUS's own initiatives to humanize childbirth. SUS currently maintains several projects to "humanize" various aspects of patient services. The ministry published its first framework for humanizing birth in 2005 in the form of a technical manual. Though rather general by later standards, the criteria outlined therein clearly reflected the World Health Organization's 1985 recommendations as well as the demands of women's organizations. In 2005, the ministry affirmed that humanized childbirth would be ethical and evidence based, avoiding unnecessary procedures and valuing the protagonism of mother and newborn as subjects with rights.[37] That same year the right to a companion of one's choice during and after labor was codified as the "Companion Law," the "Lei do acompanhante." Since 2005, researchers and practitioners have launched several pilot projects and opened many birthing centers that are *humanizados* and funded by SUS. Only very recently, however, has the Ministry of Health crafted a national mandate to introduce humanized processes into all birthing clinics and to widely establish humanized facilities that attend exclusively to vaginal birth, called Centros de Parto Normal. The diligent work of *humanização do parto* activists is stamped all over that 2013 policy, in which the Ministry pledges

> humanized attention to delivery and birth: respecting childbirth as
> a personal, cultural, sexual, and family experience founded on the
> importance of fortifying women's protagonism and autonomy; on
> [women's] participation in decisions; on protection against abuse, vi-
> olence, or negligence; on a recognition of women's and children's fun-

damental rights; on [the use] of appropriate health technology and the adoption of evidence-based practices, including freedom of movement and of position during labor; on the right to a companion of their choice; and on the preservation of their corporal integrity.[38]

Greater Salvador has two SUS natural childbirth centers: the Centro de Parto Normal da Mansão do Caminho, founded in 2011, and the Centro de Parto Normal de Lauro de Freitas, founded in 2012. Both guarantee procedures *humanizados* for vaginal birth, including choice of birthing position; freedom to have a companion bedside; and freedom to eat, drink, and walk during labor. Additionally, they offer water birth and the ability to keep newborns in the birthing room alongside their mothers. One clear pronouncement of the Centros de Parto is the promise of respect, respect for mothers in labor and for their companions. A recent news report confirms that approximately fifty babies are born monthly at Mansão do Caminho, also known as the Centro de Parto Normal Marieta de Souza Pereira. As of November 2014, the center had assisted Bahian mothers in the delivery of more than fifteen hundred infants.[39]

On November 25, 2014, just days after Brazil's annual Black Consciousness Day, the Ministry of Health launched a number of new initiatives to combat racism in SUS, using the slogan "racism is bad for health."[40] The new initiative includes a direct and simple way for Brazilians to denounce experiences of racism in the clinics, reinforcing the right of the public to demand accountability from their universal health system. In January of 2015, the ministry signed an accord with the Agência Nacional de Saúde Suplementar (the regulatory agency for private health insurance companies) to promote vaginal birth and reduce the number of unnecessary cesarean surgeries performed in private hospitals.[41] These and other recent policies are unquestionably steps in the right direction, but the continued critiques of *humanização do parto* advocates and circulating stories of women's experiences demonstrate that practice, certainly in the public maternity clinics, has been slow to change.[42] Institutional failures like that which took the life of Alyne da Silva Pimentel remind us that there is still much work to be done in health equity; in the elimination of racism; and in ensuring safe, respectful, and nonviolent birthing conditions for black women. Given this, the educational and informational work that bloggers, scholars, activists, and patients do is essential. They continue to raise awareness and call the state to task for unacceptable conditions and racialized health disparities. And the policy changes of the past ten years confirm the efficacy of their actions.

Maternity retains the charged political and social power it has wielded since the nineteenth century, now within a new context and an era of national civic activism. In the world of birthing, black activists classify health reform as one element of the larger struggle for full citizenship, equity, and justice, and rightfully so. But I further argue that there is also something more difficult to define in this particular expression of black social activism and feminist activism: an elusive concept appropriately captured with the word "humanity."[43]

Notes

INTRODUCTION

1. Fundação Cultural do Estado da Bahia, *Legislação da Província da Bahia*, 75; and João Henriques, *Falla* . . . , 6–7. This translation and all translations from Portuguese to English in this book are my own unless otherwise noted.

2. Chalhoub, *Machado de Assis, historiador*, 172.

3. Following from Roman legal principles, Portuguese and then Brazilian imperial law held that children inherited the legal status of their mothers, *partus sequitur ventrem*. See Cowling, *Conceiving Freedom*, 53–56.

4. Freire, *Mulheres, mães e médicos*.

5. Gesteira, *Discurso proferido*, 17.

6. Ibid.

7. Leticia Trigueiros, quoted in "Inculcada nas puericultoras o desejo de servir," *Estado da Bahia* (Salvador), November 25, 1941.

8. See Getúlio Vargas, Telegram of December 24, 1932 (Circular aos Interventores dos Estados), Centro de Pesquisa e Documentação de História Contemporânea do Brasil (hereafter CPDOC), GC, rolo 60, 538.

9. Magalhães, *Estado da Bahia*, 9.

10. Departamento de Saúde, Inspetoria de Higiene Pré-Natal e Infantil, "Serviço de auxilio as nutrizes, prêmio de amamentação," Liga Álvaro Bahia contra a Mortalidade Infantil (hereafter Liga), Pasta: "Prêmio de amamentação, 1940–1943."

11. "Campanha de Redenção da Criança," *Pediatria e Puericultura* 13, no. 3-4 (March/June 1944), 154–156.

12. See Richard Graham, *Feeding the City*; Anadelia A. Romo, *Brazil's Living Museum*; and Donald Pierson, *Negros in Brazil*.

13. See Freyre, *Bahia e baianos*, 17.

14. This is verse six of "Bahia de Todos os Santos e de quase todos os pecados." See Freyre, *Bahia e baianos*, 17. The translation of this excerpt was taken from Patricia de Santana Pinho, *Mama Africa*, 190.

15. Freyre, *Bahia e baianos*, 17.
16. Pinho, *Mama Africa*, 190.
17. Romo, *Brazil's Living Museum*, 1.
18. Freyre, *Bahia e baianos*, 13.
19. Landes, *The City of Women*.
20. Graham, *House and Street*.
21. Cunha, "Learning to Serve," 456.
22. Cunha, "Learning to Serve," 460.
23. Cowling, *Conceiving Freedom*.
24. George Reid Andrews, *Blacks and Whites in São Paulo*; Thomas Skidmore, *Black into White*; and Lilia Moritz Schwarcz, *Spectacle of the Races*.
25. See Schwarcz, *Spectacle of the Races*.
26. Blake, *Vigorous Core of our Nationality*.
27. On sanitation, race, and nation building, see Lima and Hochman, "Condenado pela raça, absolvido pela medicina," 23–40.
28. See Guy, *Women Build the Welfare State*.
29. Several recent histories explore medical competition in terms of gender, race, and imperial politics. See Ellen J. Amster, *Medicine and the Saints*; Steven Paul Palmer, *From Popular Medicine to Medical Populism*; Warwick Anderson, *Colonial Pathologies*; and Matthew M. Heaton, *Black Skin, White Coats*.
30. Schwarcz, *Spectacle of the Races*.
31. Dávila, *Diploma of Whiteness*, 9.
32. Ibid., 15.

CHAPTER 1

1. Graham, *Feeding the City*, 23.
2. On the Malé Revolt and Bahian anti-Africanism, see two publications by João José Reis, *Slave Rebellion in Brazil* and *Domingos Sodré, um sacerdote africano*.
3. See chapter 1, "Mãe Africana, Pátria Brasileira: Negotiating the Racial Politics of Identity, Freedom and Motherhood in Nineteenth-Century Bahia, Brazil," of Jane-Marie Collins's forthcoming book *Intimacy and Inequality*, which is available online at http://eprints.nottingham.ac.uk/2192/.
4. Chalhoub, "Precariousness of Freedom," 405–439.
5. Reis, "Presença negra: Conflitos e encontros," 91.
6. Nishida, *Slavery and Identity*.
7. Athayde, *Salvador e a grande epidemia de 1855*; Mattoso and Athayde, "Epidemias e flutuações de preços na Bahia no século XIX," 183–202.
8. Graden, *Disease, Resistance, and Lies*, 66.
9. Graden, *From Slavery to Freedom in Brazil*, 12.
10. Nascimento, *Dez freguesias da cidade do Salvador*.
11. See Borges, *The Family in Bahia Brazil, 1870–1945*.
12. Magalhães, "Falla que recitou o presidente," 32.

13. Vianna, *Memoir of the State of Bahia*, 325–326.

14. Graham, *House and Street*, and Leite, *A condição feminina no Rio de Janeiro*.

15. Reis, *Histórias de vida familiar*; Mattoso, "Slave, Free, and Freed Family Structures," 69–84.

16. Mott, *Os pecados da família*.

17. See Mott, *Os pecados da família*. Also see Kuznesof, "Sexual Politics."

18. Dain Borges reached a similar estimate in *The Family*, 86. Later estimates from the early twentieth century also support this conclusion.

19. Barreto, "Assistência ao nascimento"; Peard, *Race, Place, and Medicine*, 117; Vianna, *As aparadeiras e as sendeironas*.

20. Barreto, "Doenças de mulheres."

21. Peard, *Race, Place, and Medicine*, 16.

22. Ibid., 35.

23. Barreto, "Entre brancos e mestiços."

24. Brenes, "História da parturição no Brasil."

25. Fróes, "Estatística da clinica obstétrica," 324–325.

26. Archives of the Santa Casa de Misericórdia da Bahia (hereafter SCMB), "Livro da Roda ou Registro de Admissão de Expostos, 1889–1945," Livro #29, código 1799. On the colonial history of the Misericórdia, see Russell-Wood, *Fidalgos and Philanthropists*.

27. Reis, *Death Is a Festival*.

28. Rohden, *Uma ciência da diferença*.

29. Lesser, *Negotiating National Identity*.

30. Skidmore, *Black into White*; Schwarcz, *Spectacle of the Races*; and Peard, *Race, Place, and Medicine*.

31. Raeders, *O inimigo cordial do Brasil*.

32. Gobineau, *The Inequality of Human Races*, 25.

33. Raeders, *O conde de Gobineau no Brasil*, 79–80.

34. Louis Agassiz, quoted in Skidmore, *Black into White*, 32.

35. Borges, "'Puffy, Ugly, Slothful and Inert,'" and "Salvador's 1890s."

36. Brazil, *Synopse do recenseamento de 31 de dezembro de 1890*. Also see Levine, "The Singular Brazilian City of Salvador."

37. Andrews, *Blacks and Whites in São Paulo*; Butler, *Freedoms Given, Freedoms Won*.

38. Rodrigues, "Anthropologia pathologica—os mestiços brasileiros," and "Mestiçagem, degenerescência e crime."

39. On the Bahia School of Medicine as a center of race science, see Peard, *Race, Place, and Medicine*, and Schwarcz, *Spectacle of the Races*.

40. I adapt this version of this phrase from Jerry Dávila, who wrote, "Advocates imagined the 'Brazilian Race' to be white, but this whiteness was to be achieved through participation, and Norma participated." Dávila, "Norma Fraga," 179.

41. On Brazilian eugenics, see Boarini, "Higienismo, eugenia e a naturalização do social"; and Mai, "Difusão dos ideários higienista e eugenista no Brasil"; Mota, *Quem é bom já nasce feito*; Stepan, "The Hour of Eugenics."

42. Costa, *The Brazilian Empire*.

43. Comtean positivism, "the religion of humanity," gained adherents across Latin America in the late nineteenth century and would profoundly influence Brazilian politics for decades, predominantly in its emphasis on the application of scientific methods to social phenomena. See Hale, "Political Ideas and Ideologies"; Skidmore, *Black into White*; and Carvalho, "The Unfinished Republic."

44. On the notion of Brazilian "racial perfectability," see Schwarcz, *Spectacle of the Races*.

45. Schneider, "The Eugenics Movement in France," 72.

46. Ibid.

47. Martins, "Políticas públicas."

48. Freire, *Mulheres, mães e médicos*.

49. Lima, "Hygiene pública," 497; and Leite, "Conseqüência para a mulher do casamento de um syphilitico," 14.

50. "Registros da Secretaria de Polícia da Bahia para a inscrição das pessoas que sendo livres ou libertas queiram trabalhar como empregados domésticos," 1887–1893, APEB, Polícia, Série: Correspondência/Registros.

51. Freire, *Mulheres, mães e médicos*.

52. Collins, "Mãe Africana, Pátria Brasileira," 16.

53. Borges, *The Family in Bahia*.

54. Lima, "Hygiene pública," 497–498.

55. Vianna, "Breves considerações sobre o aleitamento," 24.

56. Caldas, "Syphilographia," 55.

57. A. S. Vianna, "Do regimen lacteo," 30.

58. A. S. Vianna, "Do regimen lacteo"; Tanajura, "Letalidade infantil"; and Oliveira, "Aleitamento materno."

59. Moncorvo de Figueiredo, "Projeto de regulamento das amas de leite," 498–504.

60. Moncorvo Filho, "Do exame das amas mercenarias" 236–237, and "Do exame das amas de leite no Brazil."

61. Sandra Lauderdale Graham describes a similar passbook system in Rio de Janeiro; see *House and Street*, 123 and 128–130.

62. Fraga Filho, *Encruzilhadas da liberdade*, 333.

63. "Registros da Secretaria de Polícia da Bahia para a inscrição das pessoas que sendo livres ou libertas queiram trabalhar como empregados domésticos," 1887–1893, APEB, Polícia, Série: Correspondência/Registros.

64. Cowling, *Conceiving Freedom*.

65. Callaway, "Mothers, Orphans, and the Law of the Free Womb," and Collins, "Bearing the Burden of Bastardy."

66. Portella, *Falla*, 46.

67. Homem de Mello, *Falla*, 29.

68. Venâncio, *Famílias abandonadas*, 190.

69. Nazzari, "An Urgent Need to Conceal."

70. Venâncio, *Famílias abandonadas*.

71. Gonçalves, "Expostos, roda e mulheres," and Castro, *A mulher submissa*.
72. Aprígio Amâncio Gonçalves, quoted in Castro, *A mulher submissa*, 155.
73. Landes, *The City of Women*, and Harding, *A Refuge in Thunder*.
74. Peard, *Race, Place, and Medicine*, 117.
75. Mott, "Parto e parteiras no século XIX."
76. Barreto, "Corpo de mulher," and Brenes, "História da parturição."
77. Pontes, "O aborto criminoso," 29. Also Barreto, "Corpo de mulher," and Castro, *A mulher submissa*.
78. Tourinho, "Abortamento criminoso," 32.
79. Mott, "Parteiras: O outro lado da profissão."

CHAPTER 2

1. Alberto, *Terms of Inclusion*. For a comparative history case, see McElya, *Clinging to Mammy*.
2. Roncador, *Domestic Servants in Literature*, 73–86. See also Seigel, *Uneven Encounters*.
3. Freyre, *The Masters and the Slaves*, xxix.
4. Ibid., 380.
5. Rocha, "Nati-Mortalidade na Cidade do Salvador." On the conference itself, see "Noticario—Conferencia Nacional de Protecção á Infância," *Pediatria e Puericultura* 3, no. 2 (1933): 276; "Conferencia Nacional de Protecção á Infância," *Correio da Manhã* (Salvador), September 17, 1933; and "Conferencia Nacional de Protecção á Infância," *Jornal do Commercio* (Rio de Janeiro), September 22, 1933.
6. Secretária de Saúde, Departamento de Saúde, "Registro de matrícula do 3º Centro de Saúde," 1933–1934, APEB, Caixa 4050/ Maço 56. Also see "Sumula do serviço de higiene infantil no ano de 1933," Liga Álvaro Bahia contra a Mortalidade Infantil (hereafter Liga), Pasta: "Expedidos 1933–1935."
7. Souza and Sanglard, "Saúde pública e assistência," and L. A. Santos, "As origens da reforma sanitária."
8. Freire and Leony, "A caridade científica," 219.
9. Wadsworth, "Moncorvo Filho e o problema da infância." Moncorvo Filho also founded another landmark institution in 1919, the Departamento da Creança.
10. Diacon, *Stringing Together a Nation*, and Vital, "Comissão Rondon, doenças e política."
11. Magalhães, "Assistencia e protecção á infancia." Also see Freire, "Os filantropos da nação."
12. Magalhães, "Instituto de Protecção e Assistencia á Infancia."
13. Borges, *The Family in Bahia*, 86. Martagão Gesteira, "Relatório do Chefe dos Serviços de Hygiene Infantil," 1924, APEB, Caixa 3697/Maço 1031 and [Álvaro da Franca] Rocha, "Nati-Mortalidade na cidade." The French statistic is cited in Klaus, *Every Child a Lion*, 13. For US infant mortality statistics, see Meckel, *Save the Babies*.
14. Mott, "Maternal and Child Welfare."

15. Maria Egydia Magalhães, quoted in Márcia Maria da Silva Barreiros Leite, "Educação, cultura, e lazer das mulheres," 125. On the work of the IPAI, see Magalhães, "Instituto de Protecção e Assistencia á Infancia." Also see Gesteira, "As affecções digestivas no Instituto," and Magalhães, "Instituto de Protecção e Assistencia á Infancia da Bahia," 31–32; continues to no. 4 (April 1935): 102.

16. Initially proposed by Magalhães in 1903, the Hospital para Crianças was not operational until 1936. Ferreira and Freire, "Medicina, filantropia e infância na Bahia."

17. Davin, "Imperialism and Motherhood"; Guy, "Pan American Child Congresses," and "Politics of Pan-American Cooperation"; and Birn, "'No More Surprising Than a Broken Pitcher'?"

18. Da Cunha's epic *Os Sertões*, published in 1902, was an interpretive account of the Brazilian government's war against the Bahian rural community of Canudos (1896–1897). The text is a highly detailed account of the racial and climatic conditions of the Brazilian Northeast, a psychological analysis of the unstable yet courageous character of people of mixed race, and a denunciation of the failures of the Brazilian army. See Cunha, *Rebellion in the Backlands*; Johnson, *Sentencing Canudos*; and Levine, *Vale of Tears*.

19. Neiva and Penna, *Viagem científica pelo norte da Bahia*; Hochman, *A era do saneamento* and "Logo ali, no final da avenida"; Lima, "Missões civilizatórias da República"; and Stepan, *Beginnings of Brazilian Science*.

20. Stepan, "The National and the International in Public Health," and Williams, "Nationalism and Public Health."

21. Souza and Barreto, *História da saúde na Bahia*.

22. Souza, *A gripe espanhola na Bahia*, 42–51.

23. Castellucci, "Flutuações econômicas."

24. Williams, "Nationalism and Public Health," 28.

25. See Santos, "As origens," and Blake, *The Vigorous Core*.

26. Gesteira, *Discurso proferido*, 2.

27. The most proximate data come from the year 1925, in which the state recorded 275 deaths under age one for every 1,000 registered births. "Mensagem apresentada pelo Exmo Snr. Dr. Francisco Marques de Goés Calmon, Governador do Estado da Bahia, a Assembléa Geral Legislativa por occasião da abertura da 2ª reunião ordinária da 18ª legislatura em 7 de abril de 1926" (Bahia: Imprensa Official do Estado, 1926), 148.

28. Gesteira, *Discurso proferido*, 2.

29. Ibid., 5.

30. State of Bahia, "Lei N. 1811 de 29 de Julho de 1925: Organiza a Sub-Secretaria de Saúde e Assistência Pública; Decreto-lei no. 4144, de 20 de novembro de 1925: Approva o Código Sanitário do Estado (Salvador: Imprensa Official do Estado, 1926).

31. The Liga's inaugural activities were heavily covered in the press. "A Liga Bahiana contra a Mortalidade Infantil: Já foram approvados os estatutos," *A Tarde* (Salvador), June 18, 1922; "Liga Bahiana contra a Mortalidade Infantil—É para já a primeira creche," *A Tarde* (Salvador), August 22, 1922; "A Liga Bahiana contra a Mor-

talidade Infantil," *Diário da Bahia* (Salvador), July 6, 1923; "A Liga Bahiana contra a Mortalidade Infantil," *Diário da Bahia* (Salvador), July 20, 1923; "Salvemos as Criancinhas de Peito! A cruzada da Liga Bahiana contra a Mortalidade Infantil," *A Tarde* (Salvador) October 11, 1923.

32. Martagão Gesteira, "Relatório Serviço de Higiene Infantil da Bahia," 1924, APEB, Caixa 4084/ Maço 117; "Boletim Estatístico do movimento dos consultórios Regina Helena, Adriano Gordilho, Hospital Santa Izabel," 1926, APEB, Caixa 4032/ Maço 24; "Relatório da Inspetoria de Higiene Infantil," 1926, APEB, Caixa 4082/ Maço 114.

33. Martagão Gesteira, "Relatório dos Trabalhos executados pela Diretoria de Higiene Infantil e Escolar no anno de 1928," APEB, Secretária de Educação e Saúde, Grupo—Gabinete do Secretário, Série, 1928/1929, Caixa 4026/Maço 14.

34. Martins, "Entre a benemerência e as políticas públicas."

35. Alberto, *Terms of Inclusion*, 145.

36. The local papers provided extensive coverage of Salvador's Mãe Preta Day. "Actuou na formação da raça: As homenagens de amanhã á 'Mãe Negra,'" *Diário de Noticias* (Salvador), September 27, 1929; "Uma copia do celebre quadro a 'Mãe preta,'" *A Tarde* (Salvador), September 27, 1929; "Uma data nacional: As homenagens á 'Mãe preta' no dia 28 de setembro," *A Tarde* (Salvador), September 27, 1929; "Homenagem da Bahia á mãe preta," *Diário da Bahia* (Salvador), September 27, 1929; "As festas da mãe preta," *Diário de Noticias* (Salvador), September 29, 1929; "Uma commemoração que institui na cidade," *A Tarde* (Salvador), September 30, 1929; "Estiveram imponentes as festas em homenagem á 'Mãe preta,'" *Diário da Bahia* (Salvador), September 29, 1929.

37. "A mãe preta," *Diário de Noticias* (Salvador), September 28, 1929.

38. "Boletim Estatístico do movimento dos consultórios Regina Helena, Adriano Gordilho, Hospital Santa Izabel," 1926, APEB, Caixa 4032/Maço 24.

39. Secretária de Saúde, Departamento de Saúde, "Registro de matrícula do 3° Centro de Saúde," 1933–1934, APEB, Caixa 4050/ Maço 56.

40. Martagão Gesteira, "Relatório Serviço de Higiene Infantil da Bahia," 1924, APEB, Caixa 4084/ Maço 117; "Boletim Estatístico"; and "Relatório, 1926."

41. Secretária de Saúde, Departamento de Saúde, "Registro de matrícula do 3° Centro de Saúde," 1933–1934, APEB, Caixa 4050/ Maço 56.

42. Landes, *City of Women*, 74.

43. Secretária de Saúde, Departamento de Saúde, "Registro de matrícula do 3° Centro de Saúde," 1933–1934, APEB, Caixa 4050/Maço 56.

44. See Gesteira, "Os serviços de hygiene infantil," and "Relatório do Serviço de Higiene Infantil da Bahia, apresentado ao 4° Congresso Americano da Criança," 1924, APEB, Caixa 4084/Maço 117.

45. Scheper-Hughes, *Death without Weeping*.

46. Gesteira, "Relatório do Serviço, 1924."

47. Meade, *"Civilizing" Rio*.

48. Álvaro Bahia to Luiz Lessa, General Director of the Health Department, June 17, 1943, APEB, Caixa 4039/Maço 36; and Secretária de Educação e Saúde, "Re-

latório apresentado ao Diretor do Dept. de Saúde pela Inspetoria de Higiene Pré-Natal e Infantil," 1939, APEB, Caixa 4062/Maço 81. See also "Caravana da Caridade! O que é o serviço suburbano de hygiene infantil e maternal," *O Imparcial* (Salvador), December 16, 1937; and "Nova mobilisação para o soccorro á infância dos subúrbios," *Estado da Bahia* (Salvador), January 10, 1941.

49. "Movimento do estado civil do município de Santo Amaro, durante o anno de 1929," Departamento de Saúde, APEB, Departamento de Saúde: Serviço de Saneamento Rural, Caixa 4082/Maço 114.

50. "Mapa do movimento de inquérito sobre a mortalidade infantil no Estado da Bahia," 1938, Departamento de Saúde, APEB, Caixa 4038/Maço 34; "Relatório do Departamento de Saúde Pública," 1934, APEB, Caixa 4060/Maço 77; Álvaro Bahia, "Departamento de Saúde, Divisão de Saúde Publica—Inspetoria de Higiene Pré--Natal e Infantil," 1938, APEB, Caixa 4032/Maço 24. Also see "Serviços de Hygiene Infantil no Interior," *A Época de Itabuna* (Itabuna, BA), May 12, 1936; and "Lactario Lavinia Magalhães," *O Castroalvense* (Castro Alves, BA), October 10, 1936.

51. Bahia, "Noticiário," 152–153.

52. "Relatório da Inspetoria de Higiene Infantil," 1926, APEB, Caixa 4082/Maço 114.

53. All examples of the pamphlets were taken from Martagão Gesteira, "Relatório Serviço de Higiene Infantil da Bahia," 1924, APEB, Caixa 4084/ Maço 117; and "Relatório da Inspetoria de Higiene Infantil," 1926, APEB, Caixa 4082/Maço 114.

54. Ibid.

55. Photographic archive, Liga, Folder 11, image 142. Also, Gesteira, "Relatório Serviço de Higiene Infantil da Bahia," 1924, APEB, Caixa 4084/ Maço 117.

56. This idea came from the French legislator and pronatalist Paul Strauss's vision that poor mothers should be the "paid wet nurses of their children." To Strauss, children belonged as much to the state as to their own mothers because of the future utility of their labor for industry, agriculture, and warfare. See Fuchs, "Right to Life," 90.

57. Klaus, *Every Child a Lion*, 145.

58. Sociedade de Medicina da Bahia, "A semana da criança."

59. "A 'Semana da Creança' está despertando grande interesse," *O Imparcial* (Salvador), October 10, 1936; "Para formar uma nação populosa e forte—instituído o culto annual á creanças brasileiras," *A Tarde* (Salvador), October 10, 1938; "Sadias creanças para um Brasil melhor," *Estado da Bahia* (Salvador), October 10, 1938; "Inaugurada, solenemente, ontem, a Semana da Criança," *Diário de Notícias* (Salvador), October 19, 1942; "Iniciada ontem a Semana da Criança," *Estado da Bahia* (Salvador), October 19, 1942; "A criança robusta antecipa o futuro sadio da raça," *A Tarde* (Salvador), October 12, 1943; and "Prosseguem as comemorações da 'Semana da Criança,'" *Diário da Bahia* (Salvador), October 14, 1944.

60. See "A Bahia Hospeda desde ontem o Ministro de Educação e Saúde," *Estado da Bahia* (Salvador), October 18, 1937. Also see "Bases do concurso de robustez entre lactentes, a realizar-se nesta capital, por iniciativa e sob os auspícios do 'Rotary Club' com a colaboração da Liga Bahiana contra a Mortalidade Infantil e da 'Asso-

ciação Bahiana de Imprensa,'" Liga, Pasta: "Expedidos 1933–1935"; and "Concurso de robustez: folha de inscrição, October 10, 1941," Liga, Pasta: "Mov. Financeiro, 1943."

61. Mott, "Maternal and Child Welfare," and Martins, "Políticas públicas."

CHAPTER 3

1. "Livro da Roda ou Registro de Admissão de Expostos, 1889–1945," SCMB.

2. Collins, "Bearing the Burden."

3. Gouveia, "Fisiopsicologia social da maternidade," 291.

4. Ibid., 293.

5. On the institutional history of the Santa Casa de Misericórdia, see Russell-Wood, *Fidalgos and Philanthropists*; Venâncio, *Famílias abandonadas* and "Maternidade negada"; and Costa, *Ações sociais*.

6. Russell-Wood, *Fidalgos and Philanthropists*, 295.

7. Marcílio, *História social da criança abandonada*, 147.

8. Reis, *Death Is a Festival*, 69.

9. Venâncio, *Famílias abandonadas*, 108–119.

10. Between 1892 and 1894, for example, the ratio of girls to boys was almost 4:1. Santa Casa de Misericórdia da Bahia, "Relatório apresentado a Meza e junta da Casa da Santa Misericórdia da capital do Estado da Bahia pelo Provedor Commendador Manoel de Souza Campos no Biennio de 1892 a 1894" (Salvador: Litho-typographia de João Gonçalves Tourinho, 1895).

11. See Russell-Wood, *Fidalgos and Philanthropists*, and Costa, *Ações sociais*. Also see Nascimento, "A pobreza e a honra."

12. "Livro da Roda, 1889–1945," SCMB.

13. "Livro da Roda, 1889–1945," Livro #29, código 1799, SCMB; "Crianças entradas, mensalmente nos cinco anos posteriores á abertura do Escritorio," SCMB; and "Asilo dos Expostos, Ano de 1935–Ano de 1942," Liga, Pasta: "Correspondências com a Sta. Casa de Misericórdia, 1933–1956, Expedidas."

14. "Os serviços federaes de Hygiene Infantil e a Liga Bahiana contra a Mortalidade Infantil," *Diário da Bahia* (Salvador), May 15, 1924.

15. "10.738 litros de leite humano para os bebes!," *Estado da Bahia* (Salvador), January 30, 1941.

16. Rodrigues, *A infância esquecida*.

17. Gesteira, "Assistencia aos menores," 280.

18. Nazzari, "An Urgent Need to Conceal."

19. Gesteira, "Em prol dos nossos enjeitados" and "Assistencia aos menores."

20. "Cifras apavorantes: Das creanças que passam na 'Roda' 90% não vingam!," *A Tarde* (Salvador), November 20, 1924.

21. "Cifras apavorantes"; "O Progresso vence a rotina: Os dias da 'Roda' estão contados," *A Tarde* (Salvador) December 3, 1924; "'A roda sinistra,' Porque morrem as crianças do Asylo dos Expostos?," *A Tarde* (Salvador) November 26, 1925.

22. Venâncio, *Famílias abandonadas*, 108.

23. Gesteira, "Assistencia aos menores," 288.

24. "Crianças entradas, mensalmente," SCMB.

25. Código de Menores, Decreto-lei no. 5.083, de 1º de dezembro de 1926.

26. "Livro da Roda, 1889–1945," Livro #29, código 1799, SCMB.

27. Ibid.

28. Marcílio, *História social*.

29. The proportion of white Bahians in the 1930s cannot be precisely identified because racial data were not collected in the 1920 or 1940 censuses. According to the 1890 census, 26 percent of Bahians were white. Forty-six percent were listed as *mestiço* and 20 percent as black. A small number, 8 percent, were listed as *caboclo*. By the 1950 census, Bahia was 30 percent white, 51 percent "brown" or *pardo*, and 19 percent black.

30. There were actually 453 foundlings in the 1934–1942 sample; however, racial data were only recorded for 400 children. I collapse 6 children labeled as "*moreno*" into the "*pardo*" category. See "Livro da Roda, 1889–1945," Livro #29, código 1799, SCMB; "Crianças entradas, mensalmente," SCMB; and "Asilo dos Expostos," Liga.

31. "Livro da Roda, 1889–1945," SCMB.

32. This number includes children specifically listed as "legitimate," and those whose parents' shared surnames can reliably be assumed to be married names.

33. Of the remaining children, 27 percent were sent to live with tutors or adoptive families, and 4 percent were sent to other institutions. No information was recorded on the destinations of 8 percent of the children.

34. "Acordo com a Sta. Casa de Misericórdia, 1930"; "Dados para organisação do escritorio de admissão"; and "Crianças atualmente internadas no Asilo N. S. da Misericordia," Liga, Pasta: "Correspondências com a Sta. Casa de Misericórdia, 1933–1956, Expedidas."

35. "Relação do Material Adquirido pela Liga, Durante o Anno de 1937 para os Serviços do Asylo de Expostos," Liga, Pasta: "Correspondências com a Sta. Casa de Misericórdia, 1933–1956, Expedidas."

36. "Livro da Roda, 1889–1945," SCMB.

37. "Relatório da Provedoria da Santa Casa de Misericórdia da Bahia, relativo ao biênio de 1939 e 1940, Apresentado á nova administração em sessão de 1º de Janeiro de 1940 pelo Provedor Clovis Moreira Spinola," SCMB, 303.

38. "Livro da Roda, 1889–1945," SCMB.

39. "Plano de profilaxia do engeitamento e assistência aos engeitados organizado para o Asilo de Expostos," Liga, Pasta: "Correspondências com a Sta. Casa de Misericórdia, 1933–1956, Expedidas."

40. Souza and Barreto, *História da saúde na Bahia*.

41. Gesteira to Arthur Newton de Lemos, August 18, 1934, Liga, Pasta: "Correspondências com a Sta. Casa de Misericórdia, 1933 a 1956, Expedidas."

42. "Relatório da Provedoria," SCMB.

43. Guy, *Women Build*, 8.

44. Audíface, "A pupileira e sua organização." On the foundation of the Maternal Shelter and Milk Dispensary, see "A grande obra de assistência á infancia," *A Tarde*

(Salvador), April 14, 1934; "Fundações benemeritas que a philantropia bahiana ampara e protege," *Estado da Bahia* (Salvador), April 14, 1934; "Lactário Julia Carvalho" and "Protecção á Infancia na Bahia," both in *Pediatria e Puericultura* 3, no. 3/4 (March–June 1934); and Departamento de Saúde Pública, "Relatório do Departamento de Saúde Pública," 1934, APEB, Caixa 4060/Maço 77.

45. "Inauguração da Pupileira Juracy Magalhães," *Diário da Bahia* (Salvador), December 20, 1935. Also, "É uma joia e um encanto o pavilhão da Pupilleira," *Diário de Notícias* (Salvador), December 19, 1935; and "As festas tradiccionaes da Bahia," *Estado da Bahia* (Salvador), December 26, 1935.

46. "Inauguração da Pupileira Juracy Magalhães," *Diário da Bahia* (Salvador), December 20, 1935.

47. "Relatório da Provedoria," SCMB, 303.

48. "Notas relativas á assistencia ás crianças de primeira infancia no Asilo N.S. da Misericórdia, coligidas a pedido do Ilmo. Sr. Oscar Magalhães, digno Mordomo do referido Asilo," Liga, Pasta: "Correspondências com a Sta. Casa de Misericórdia, 1933–1956."

49. "Discursos" graduation speech made by Alvaro Bahia to the graduates at the Escola de Puericultura, undated, Liga.

50. "A familia é indispensavel á creança," *O Imparcial* (Salvador), June 7, 1940.

51. "O discurso do Dr. Álvaro Bahia—Ante-Hontem," *O Imparcial* (Salvador), October 11, 1938.

52. Escola de Puericultura, receipts from several boxes on "Prestação de contas, Mov. Financeiro," Liga.

53. See Fuchs, *Poor and Pregnant in Paris*.

54. Martagão Gesteira, "Discursos pronunciados na inauguração dos novos melhoramentos do Asilo de Expostos da Bahia," January 28, 1933, Liga, Pasta: "Expedidos 1933–1935—JA."

55. Ruth Aleixo to Dr. Álvaro Bahia, director of the Liga Bahiana contra a Mortalidade Infantil, February 23, 1943, Liga.

56. "O discurso do Dr. Álvaro Bahia—Ante-Hontem," *O Imparcial* (Salvador), October 11, 1938.

57. Infants labeled as "illegitimate" were not necessarily raised by single mothers. For Fernanda Lopes, consensual union seems probable, given the compound surnames of her children: Cleonice and Carlos Cunha Camacho.

58. "Relatório, Conselho de Assistencia Social," 1941, Liga, Pasta: "Expedidos 1941–1946—AB" and "Prêmio de amamentação, ano de 1940"; "Prêmio de amamentação, 1942–1943," Pasta: "Expedidos 1941–1946—AB"; and "Movimento do ano, 1944," Pasta: "Recebidos 1936–1945—BC."

59. "A familia é indispensavel á creança," *O Imparcial* (Salvador), June 7, 1940.

60. "10.738 litros," *Estado da Bahia* (Salvador), January 30, 1941.

61. "Aquisição de leite humano," Dezembro 14 de 1943, Liga (no folder).

62. "Desde 1937 que há, na Bahia, serviço de fornecimento de leite humano," *Estado da Bahia* (Salvador), (no date legible) 1943.

63. "Folha de Observação de Nutriz, 1950–1951" and "Folha de observação de

Nutriz, 1952–1953," Liga, Caixa: "Mapa de Lactario/ Cantina, Folha de Observação a Nutriz, Mapa de Alimentação (Creche) 1939–1951."

64. Ibid.

65. Departamento de Saúde, Divisão de Saúde Publica—Inspetoria de Higiene Pré-Natal e Infantil, "Boletins do movimento da seção de expediente," 1938/1939, APEB, Caixa 4032/Maço 24.

CHAPTER 4

1. "Boletim de notificações da assistência indouta ao parto do 30 Centro de Saúde," APEB, Caixa 4033/ Maço 27.

2. Freire, "'Ser mãe é uma ciência,'" 166.

3. Mott, "Maternal and Child Welfare."

4. Mott, "Parto e parteiras no século XIX," and Barreto, "Assistência ao nascimento."

5. Mott, "A parteira ignorante."

6. Peard, *Race, Place, and Medicine*.

7. Rocha, "Nati-mortalidade."

8. Adeodato Filho and Machado, "Assistencia social-obstetrica na Bahia."

9. In 1926, of the 2,332 infants enrolled in three clinics, 77 percent had been delivered by traditional midwives. The remaining children were delivered by physicians (13%) and nurse-midwives (10%). The Infant and School-Age Children's Hygiene Directory enrolled 1,986 infants in 1928; 74 percent had been delivered by folk midwives. Of the remaining enrollees, 20 percent were delivered by physicians and 6 percent by nurse-midwives. "Relatório da Inspetoria de Higiene Infantil," 1926, APEB, Caixa 4082/Maço 114; Martagão Gesteira, "Relatório Serviço de Higiene Infantil da Bahia," 1924, APEB, Caixa 4084/Maço 117; and "Relatório dos Trabalhos executados pela Diretoria de Higiene Infantil e Escolar no anno de 1928," APEB, Secretária de Educação e Saúde, Relatório dos Trabalhos executados pela Diretoria de Higiene Infantil e Escolar, 1928/1929, Caixa 4026/Maço 14.

10. Mott cites the data from this journal in "Assistência ao parto," 206.

11. Ibid., 207.

12. Silva and Ferreira, "A higienização das parteiras curiosas."

13. Adeodato Filho and Machado, "Assistencia social-obstetrica na Bahia."

14. Machado, "A proposito do exame pré-natal," 60–61.

15. Ibid., 61.

16. Progianti, "Modelos de assistência," 303–305; and Martins, "Políticas públicas," 112–115.

17. Costa, *Puericultura e maternidade*, 144.

18. Ibid., 145.

19. Ibid.

20. On the larger discourse of the "urban *sertão*," see Hochman, "Logo ali, no final."

21. Mott, "Assistência ao parto," 217.

22. Vinhaes, "Assistencia obstétrica," 92.

23. Pimenta, "Barbeiros-sangradores e curandeiros."

24. Costa, *Puericultura e maternidade*, 143.

25. António Simões, "Medicina e higiene: Casa da mãe pobre," *A Tarde* (Salvador), June 17, 1943.

26. Ferreira, "A puericultura intra-uterina e formação da prole," 45–46.

27. Oscar Oliveira to Ademir de Oliveira, July 9, 1931, APEB, Secretária de Educação e Saúde, Caixa 4034/Maço 28.

28. See Caulfield, *In Defense of Honor*.

29. Governo Provisório da República dos Estados Unidos do Brasil, Decreto-lei no. 20.931, de 11 de janeiro de 1932, "Regula e fiscaliza o exercício da medicina, da odontologia, da medicina veterinária e das profissões de farmacêutico, parteira e enfermeira, no Brasil, e estabelece penas."

30. An older legal tradition had also attempted to govern midwifery. In 1832, imperial law required midwives to become certified thorough the local state physician, the Físico-Mor or Cirurgião-Mor.

31. See Peard, *Race, Place, and Medicine*.

32. The Climério de Oliveira Maternity Center opened its doors on October 30, 1910, in a space donated by the Misericórdia.

33. Estado da Bahia, *Diário Oficial do Estado da Bahia*, 474.

34. Barreto, "Assistência ao nascimento."

35. Amaral, "Da comadre para o doutor," 81.

36. Ibid., 97.

37. "Crianças que entraram pelo escritório aberto, 1934–1945," SCMB.

38. "Maternidade Climério de Oliveira," 134–135; Magalhães, *Estado da Bahia*; and Alves, "Educação e saúde na Bahia."

39. Overmyer-Velazquez, *Visions of the Emerald City*, 35.

40. Amaral, "Mulheres, imprensa e higiene."

41. Instituto Brasileiro de Geografia e Estatística, *Anuário estatístico do Brasil 1936* and *Anuário estatístico do Brasil 1937*.

42. Mott, "Assistência ao parto," 206.

43. Barreto, "Corpo de mulher," 142.

44. See Araujo, "Puericultura intra-uterina," and Magalhães, *Estado da Bahia*.

45. "Amparo á gestante," *O Imparcial* (Salvador), October 26, 1943. Also see "Ata da Sessão da Assembléia Geral do Pro-Matre da Bahia, da Cidade de Salvador," 1941, APEB, Secretária de Educação e Saúde, Conselho de Assistência Social, Caixa 4085/Maço 118; and Adeodato Filho, "Serviço obstétrico domiciliar Pro-Matre."

46. Riesco and Tsunechiro, "Formação profissional de obstetrizes."

47. Secretária de Educação e Saúde, "Relatórios dos trabalhos executados pelo 3º Centro de Saúde," 1933–1947, APEB, Caixa 4060/Maço 76; and Carvalho, "Um ano de atividade pre-natal."

48. See Decreto-lei no. 24.278, of May 22, 1934, creating the Diretoria de Proteção à Maternidade e à Infância.

49. Álvaro Bahia, "Inspetoria de Higiene Pré-Natal e Infantil, Boletins do movimento da seção de expediente," 1938–1939, APEB, Caixa 4032/Maço 24.

50. Secretária de Saúde, Departamento de Saúde, "Decretos de reorganização dos quadros do Departamento de Saúde," 1938, APEB, Caixa 4034/Maço 28.

51. "Amparo á gestante," *O Imparcial* (Salvador), October 26, 1943; Secretária de Educação e Saúde, "Registro de parteiras, 1939–1941," Grupo: Departamento de Saúde. Serie: Relatórios referentes ao Serviço de Fiscalização do Exercicio Profissional e de Hospitais, Asilos e Estabelecimentos Congeneres, 1939, APEB, Caixa 4061/Maço 78.

52. List of graduates, FAMEB (uncataloged).

53. IBGE, *Anuário estatístico do Brasil 1936*.

54. Bahia, "Inspetoria de Higiene," APEB.

55. Carvalho, "Um ano de atividade pre-natal," 142.

56. Silva and Ferreira, "A higienização das parteiras."

57. Mott, "Assistência ao parto," 208–210.

58. Álvaro Bahia, "Departamento de Saúde, Divisão de Saúde Pública, Inspetoria de Higiene Pré-Natal e Infantil," 1938, APEB, Caixa 4032/Maço 24.

59. Bahia, "Estudo do recemnascido," 9.

60. Álvaro Bahia, "Relatório apresentado ao Diretor do Dept. de Saúde pela Inspetoria de Higiene Pré-Natal e Infantil," 1939, APEB, Caixa 4062/Maço 81.

61. Secretária de Educação e Saúde, "Boletim de notificações de assistência indouta ao parto do 3º Centro de Saúde," 1940, APEB, Caixa 4033/Maço 27.

62. Silva and Ferreira, "A higienização das parteiras," 96.

63. Mott, "Maternal and Child Welfare," and Martins, "Políticas públicas."

64. Martins, "'Vamos criar seu filho,'" 137.

65. Carvalho, "Aula inaugural," 64.

66. The Faculdade de Medicina da Bahia has a long history of theses on maternal breast-feeding; for example: Vianna, "Do regimen lacteo," 1881; Tanajura, "Letalidade infantil e suas causas," 1900; Goulart, "Hygiene alimentar na primeira infância," 1900; Freitas, "Ligeiras considerações sobre a hygiene da mulher gravida," 1904; Oliveira, "Aleitamento materno," 1907; Cerqueira, "Prophilaxia alimentar da primeira infancia," 1903; Braga, "Hygiene alimentar na primeira infancia," 1906; and Borba Junior, "O aleitamento materno sob o ponto de vista medico-social," 1913. Also see Almeida, "Noções de higiene infantil."

67. Reis, "Ligeira contribuição," 10.

68. Ibid., 10–11.

69. "Lista das mulheres que obteram grau em medicina, 1887–1968," FAMEB, and "Attestos" (1938–1950), Liga.

70. Gouveia, "Fisiopsicologia social," 295; italics in original.

71. Amaral, "Mulheres, imprensa e higiene," 929.

72. Bahia, "Escola de Puericultura," 39.

73. Adolphe Pinard, quoted in Klaus, *Every Child a Lion*, 79.

74. Estado da Bahia, *Diário Oficial*, 316–317; and Álvaro Bahia, "Relatório dos trabalhos executados pela Diretoria de Higiene Infantil e Escolar no anno de 1929," APEB, Caixa 4026/Maço 14.

75. Neto, "A enfermeira de Puericultura," and Bahia, "Estudo do recemnascido."

76. "A Bahia hospeda desde ontem o Ministro de Educação e Saúde," *Estado da Bahia* (Salvador), October 18, 1937.

77. Bahia, "Escola de Puericultura"; also see "Escola de Puericultura, Linhas gerais da organisação"; "Ata da sessão de diretoria da Liga Bahiana contra a Mortalidade Infantil realizada em 11 de fevereiro de 1938"; and "Ata da sessão de assembléia geral da Liga Bahiana contra a Mortalidade Infantil, do dia 5 de março de 1938," Liga.

78. See Klaus, *Every Child a Lion*, and Meckel, *Save the Babies*.

79. Meckel, *Save the Babies*, 145.

80. Bahia, "Escola de Puericultura."

81. "Escola de Puericultura Raymundo Pereira de Magalhaes, Ano de 1940"; "Ano de 1941"; "Ano de 1942"; "Ano de 1943"; "Ano de 1944"; "Ano de 1945," Liga, Pasta: "Expedidos 1941–1946."

82. Ibid.

83. Álvaro Bahia, graduation speech 1943, Liga, "Discursos."

84. Bahia, "Estudo do recemnascido."

85. "Consultas, ano 1943"; "Consultas, ano 1944"; "Movimento do ano 1945"; "Movimento do ano 1942/1943"; and "Boletim dos Consultorios ano 1944," Liga, Pasta: "Recebidos 1936–1945" and "Expedidos 1941–1946." Also see "Visitando a Escola de Puericultura Raymundo de Magalhães," *Diário da Bahia* (Salvador), June 21, 1942.

86. Álvaro Bahia, "Maternidade desamparada," speech to the Rotary Club, August 13, 1942, Liga.

87. "Relatório do Conselho de Assistencia Social," 1941, and "Consultorio de higiene infantil," 1940 and 1941, Liga, Pasta: "Expedidos 1941–1946."

88. "Exemplo a seguir para todas as moças bahianas," *Estado da Bahia* (Salvador), July 24, 1939.

89. Leticia Trigueiros, quoted in "Inculcada nas puericultoras o desejo de servir," *Estado da Bahia* (Salvador), November 25, 1941. Trigueiros's erudite language and her scholarly, biblical, and scientific references leave no doubt that participants in these courses were among the most educated members of society even prior to their puericulture training.

90. Ibid.

91. "O diploma de puericultora deve ser um ideal de todas as mulheres," *Estado da Bahia* (Salvador), November 22, 1941.

92. "Medicina para todos," *O Imparcial* (Salvador), August 21, 1941.

93. Rocha, "Nati-mortalidade," 230.

94. Maria Esolina Pinheiro, quoted in "Incumbe á mulher o grande papel educador," *Estado da Bahia* (Salvador), November 24, 1941. On Pinheiro's WWII mobilization, see Pinheiro, *Serviço social: Uma interpretação*.

95. "O diploma de puericultora."

96. Gouveia, "Fisiopsicologia social," 295.

97. "O que será o Instituto Nacional de Puericultura," *Estado da Bahia* (Salvador), March 4, 1937; and Ministério de Educação e Saúde, "Sugestão para a criação do 'Instituto de Puericultura Getúlio Vargas' feita ao Professor Olinto de Oliveira,"

CPDOC, GC h 1935.06.22, rolo 60 fot. 416. Before the end of its inaugural year, the National Puericulture Institute became incorporated into the Universidade do Brasil.

98. Freire, "Ser mãe é uma ciência," 168.

CHAPTER 5

1. The lyrics are from "É negócio casar," written by Ataulfo Alves and Felisberto Martins and recorded on Odeon Records in 1941. See Tinhorão, *A musica popular*. I translate the title ambiguously as "Marriage is good business." "É negócio casar" can suggest that "marriage is good" or that "marriage is profitable." See Cunha, "Negócio ou ócio?"

2. Fischer, *A Poverty of Rights*, and Levine, *Father of the Poor?*

3. "Livro da Roda, 1889–1945," SCMB.

4. On the relationship between social policy, philanthropy, and welfare states, see Guy, *Women Build the Welfare State*.

5. Vargas, *A nova política do Brasil*, 158–159.

6. Mott, "Maternal and Child Welfare," and Cynthia Pereira de Sousa, "Saúde, educação e trabalho."

7. Vargas, "Mensagem de Natal" telegram, December 24, 1932, CPDOC.

8. Vargas-era politics have a rich historiography. See Skidmore, *Politics in Brazil*; Hentschke, *Vargas and Brazil*; Gomes, *A invenção do trabalhismo*; and Levine, *The Vargas Regime*.

9. República dos Estados Unidos do Brasil, Constituição de 1934, Título V da Família, da Educação e da Cultura, Capítulo I da Família Art. 144. Brazilian federal legislation is available online on the Senate's website; see http://www.planalto .gov.br.

10. Brasil, Constituição de 1934, Título IV, Art. 121. Some of this was revised in 1943 with the Consolidação das Leis do Trabalho, which guaranteed gender equality but maintained separate sections on women's and children's labor.

11. Governo Provisório da República dos Estados Unidos do Brasil, Decreto-lei no. 21.417 de 17 de maio de 1932.

12. Brasil, Constituição de 1934. Título V, Capítulo I, Art. 138.

13. Williams, *Culture Wars in Brazil*; Hertzman, *Making Samba*; and McCann, *Hello, Hello Brazil*.

14. Vargas, *A nova política*.

15. Ibid., 28.

16. Besse, *Restructuring Patriarchy*.

17. Garfield, *Indigenous Struggle at the Heart of Brazil* and "The Environment of Wartime Migration." Also see Diacon, *Stringing Together a Nation*.

18. Needell, "The Domestic Civilizing Mission."

19. Macedo, *Getúlio Vargas e o culto à nacionalidade*, 50.

20. "Precisamos salvar a vida de milhares de crianças," *Diário de Noticias* (Salvador), January 19, 1944.

21. Minister Capanema to President Vargas, February 12, 1940, CPDOC, GC, rolo 61, 135; and December 1938, GC, rolo 60, 641–643.

22. Stepan, *"The Hour of Eugenics,"* 162–164.

23. Dávila, *Diploma of Whiteness*, and Nava, "Lessons in Patriotism and Good Citizenship."

24. The first Pan American Child Congress was held in Buenos Aires in 1916. Comité Nacional Brasileiro, "Primeiro Congresso Americano da Creança."

25. Pan American Child Congress, *Acta final*, 50.

26. Baker, *Fighting for Life*, and Dwork, *War Is Good for Babies*.

27. Vargas, *A nova política*, 333.

28. Ibid., 91.

29. The Consolidação das Leis do Trabalho had an extensive section on women's and children's protection in the workplace. Also see Decreto-lei no. 21.417, de 17 de maio de 1932.

30. Ministro de Educação e Saúde, "Coleção: Disposições constitucionais, legais, e regulamentares relativos a MENORES," July 8, 1941, CPDOC, GC h, rolo 61/ fot. 437.

31. Sousa Vilhena, "A família na doutrina social."

32. Brasil, Constituição de 1934 and Decreto-lei no. 2.024, de 17 fevereiro de 1940.

33. Fischer, *A Poverty of Rights*.

34. In fact, the Civil Code's lengthy "Patrio Poder" section included seventeen articles, numbers 379–395.

35. Código Civil dos Estados Unidos do Brasil, Article 233.

36. República dos Estados Unidos do Brasil, Decreto no. 17.943-a, de 12 de outubro de 1927.

37. República dos Estados Unidos do Brasil, Decreto-lei no. 2.024, de 17 fevereiro de 1940; Decreto-lei no. 3.200, de 19 de abril de 1941; and amendments Decreto-lei no. 3.284, de 19 de maio de 1941; Decreto-lei no. 5.213, de 21 de março de 1943; and Decreto-lei no. 5.976, de 10 de novembro de 1943.

38. Brasil, Decreto-lei no. 3.200, de 19 de abril de 1941.

39. Caulfield, "Right to a Father's Name," 12. See also Govêrno Provisória da República, Decreto-lei no. 24.273, de 22 de maio de 1934.

40. Weinstein, *For Social Peace in Brazil*.

41. Sousa, "A família na doutrina social."

42. Brazil, Decreto-lei no. 3.200, de 19 de abril de 1941.

43. Wolfe, *Working Women, Working Men*.

44. Instituto Brasileiro de Geografia e Estatística, *Anuário estatístico do Brasil 1946*. Brazil's twentieth-century census data are available online through the IBGE website; see http://seculoxx.ibge.gov.br.

45. On the population of Salvador, see IBGE, Serviço de Estatística Demográfica, Moral e Política, Tabela extraída de: Anuário estatístico do Brasil 1939/1940 and Anuário estatístico do Brasil 1946. On the industrial survey, see Serviço de Inquéritos, da Secretaria Geral do IBGE, Tabela extraída de: Anuário estatístico do Brasil 1941/1945.

46. IBGE, Comissão Censitária Nacional, Sinopse do Censo Industrial e do Censo dos Serviços, 1948, Tabela extraída de: Anuário estatístico do Brasil 1949.

47. Ibid.

48. IBGE, Comissão Censitária Nacional, Sinopse do Censo Demográfico, 1946, Tabela extraída de: Anuário estatístico do Brasil 1949.

49. Ibid.

50. Indústrias de transformação, excluding fishing and forest industry and extractive industry, IBGE, Anuário estatístico do Brasil, vol. 17, 1956.

51. Serviço Nacional de Recenseamento. Tabela extraída de: Anuário estatístico do Brasil 1956. Rio de Janeiro: IBGE, v. 17, 1956.

52. IBGE, "Recenseamento geral do Brasil." See also Ferreira Filho, Quem pariu e bateu; Butler, Freedoms Given, Freedoms Won; and Graham, Feeding the City.

53. Decreto-lei no. 5.452, de 1º de maio de 1943. See also French, Drowning in Laws.

54. Ferreira Filho, Quem pariu e bateu.

55. Bahian physicians had warned of the connection between use of domestic servants, wet nursing, animal milk, and infant mortality since the late nineteenth century. Graduating theses from the School of Medicine are the best source for analyzing this discourse. See Dr. Octaviano de Abreu Goulart, "Hygiene alimentar na primeira infância" (1900); Dr. Joaquim Augusto Tanajura, "Letalidade infantil e suas causas" (1900); and Dr. Mario Cardoso de Cerqueira "Prophilaxia alimentar da primeira infância" (1903), among many others, FAMEB.

56. Ministério da Educação e Saúde, "Proteção à maternidade e à infância," 1940, CPDOC, GC h, rolo 61/fot. 357.

57. Vargas, A nova política, 159.

58. CPDOC, October 13, 1942, GC rolo 07, 690–691 and GC rolo 62, October 1945, 58. Also see Aristides Novis, "Semana da criança," O Imparcial (Salvador), October 10, 1943; and Hosannah de Oliveira, "Mais uma semana da criança," O Imparcial (Salvador), October 16, 1943.

59. CPDOC, October 13, 1942, GC rolo 07, 690–691 and GC rolo 62, October 1945, 58.

60. "Decretos de reorganização dos quadros do Departamento de Saúde," July 29, 1938, APEB, Caixa 4034/Maço 28.

61. "O Presidente Getúlio Vargas governa o Brasil inteiro—Deve ser restaurado a Departamento da Criança na Bahia," A Nota (Salvador), September 10, 1938.

62. Ibid.; emphasis mine.

63. "Em desaccordo com a 'Mensagem do Natal' do Presidente Vargas," Estado da Bahia (Salvador), September 10, 1938.

64. Beyond Bahia, Isaías Alves had his own crucial part to play in the politics of the Estado Novo. See Romo, Brazil's Living Museum.

65. Govêrno Provisório da República, Decreto-lei no. 24.278 de 22 de maio de 1934.

66. "A supressão do Departamento da Criança," A Tarde (Salvador), September 14, 1938; and "O rotula não adeanta—Supresso o Departamento, mas conserva-

dos e até ampliados os serviços de defeza da creança," *A Tarde* (Salvador), September 8, 1938.

67. "Será creado o Departamento Estadual da Criança," *O Imparcial* (Salvador), August 10, 1944.

68. Fonseca, *Saúde no governo Vargas*; Campos, *Políticas internacionais de saúde*; and Hentschke, *Vargas and Brazil*.

69. Ministério da Educação e Saúde, "Departamento Nacional da Criança," CPDOC, GC h, rolo 61/ fot. 135.

70. Minister Capanema to President Vargas, February 12, 1940, CPDOC, GC, rolo 61, 135; emphasis mine.

71. Olinto de Oliveira to Álvaro Bahia, June 30, 1943, Liga, Pasta: "Recebidos 1936-1945"; and Ministério da Educação e Saúde, "Proteção à maternidade e à infância," 1940, CPDOC, GC, rolo 61 fot. 357.

72. These figures are in milreis (meaning 1,000 reis), Brazil's currency until 1942. In amounts of 1,000 reis and above, a dollar sign with double vertical lines was placed just after the thousands digit, as in 1$865 for 1,865 reis. In numbers of one million reis and above, a colon was inserted just after the millions digit, as in 300:000$000 for 300,000,000 reis. Capanema to Appointed Governor Landulfo Alves, July 3, 1940, CPDOC, GC, rolo 61; and Ministério da Educação e Saúde, "Quadro demonstrativo ao auxilio federal aos estados, para o amparo á Maternidade e á Infancia, nos anos de 1939 e 1940," January 6, 1940, CPDOC, GC, rolo 61, fot. 34.

73. Ministério da Educação e Saúde, "Total das subvenções recebidas pelas instituições de proteção à maternidade, à infancia e à adolescencia nos Território do Acre, Estados, e Distrito Federal," October 21, 1944, CPDOC, GC, rolo 62, fot. 26.

74. Levine, *Father of the Poor?*, 118.

75. Ministério da Educação e Saúde, "Total das subvenções," 26.

76. Álvaro Bahia to Minister Capanema, June 3, 1938, CPDOC, GC, rolo 68.

77. Secretária de Educação e Saúde, Serie: Relatório das atividades do Consêlho de Assistência Social, 1940, APEB, Caixa 4092/Maço 181.

78. "A Bahia reinstalada no seu esplendor," *Diário de Noticias* (Salvador), November 20, 1936; "Dias memoráveis para a nossa terra!," *Diário de Noticias* (Salvador), November 21, 1936; "A Bahia cumpriu o seu dever," and "Brasileiros ilustres hospedes da Bahia," *Diário da Bahia* (Salvador), November 20, 1936.

79. "O melhor entre os mais capazes," *Diário da Bahia* (Salvador), November 22, 1936.

80. "A recepção do Ministro Sr. Gustavo Capanema," *Diário de Notícias* (Salvador), October 18, 1937.

81. Ministério da Educação e Saúde, "Atividades da competência dos Deptos. Est. da Criança," CPDOC, GC, rolo 62, 96.

82. Assis Chateaubriand, "A assistencia á infancia," *Estado da Bahia* (Salvador), March 3, 1938.

83. "Recompensando as mães fecundas," *A Tarde* (Salvador), October 11, 1938.

84. Olinto de Oliveira, "Telegramas recebidos pelo Dept. de Saúde, 1939–1949," October 30, 1942, APEB, Secretária de Educação e Saúde.

85. Antonio Simões, "Medicina e higiene—Casa de Mãe Pobre," *A Tarde* (Salvador), June 17, 1943.

86. Borges, *The Family in Bahia.*

87. Gesteira, "Discurso proferido."

88. Gesteira speech at the Asilo dos Expostos on January 28, 1933, Liga, Pasta: "Expedidos 1933–1935."

89. "Precisamos salvar" (see n. 20); Álvaro Bahia, "Refúgios maternais," *O Imparcial* (Salvador), October 14, 1943.

90. "O discurso do Dr. Álvaro Bahia," *O Imparcial* (Salvador), October 11, 1938; "A família e indispensável á creança," *O Imparcial*, June 7, 1940; "Refúgios maternais" (see n. 89); and Álvaro Bahia, "'Maternidade desamparada,'" *Rotary Bahiana*, Separata de no. 38, August 13, 1942.

91. Decreto-lei no. 17.943-a, de 12 de outubro de 1927.

92. Olinto de Oliveira to Capanema, "Exposição de motivos," 1939, CPDOC, GC, rolo 61, fot. 49.

93. "Movimento que emocionam os pobres e os abastados," *Diário de Noticias* (Salvador), January 21, 1944; and "Os direitos da criança brasileira," *O Imparcial* (Salvador), January 6, 1940.

94. "Precisamos salvar" (see n. 20).

95. Fischer, *A Poverty of Rights.*

96. Hahner, *Emancipating the Female Sex*; Butler, *Freedoms Given, Freedoms Won*; Alberto, *Terms of Inclusion.*

97. Caulfield, "Right to a Father's Name," 11.

98. Bahia, "'Maternidade desamparada'" (see n. 89).

99. Conselho Penitenciário do Estado, "Regulamento geral do serviço de assistência á infância e tutelar da juventude do Estado da Bahia," 1939, APEB.

100. Constituição dos Estados Unidos do Brasil, 10 de novembro de 1937.

101. Romo, *Brazil's Living Museum*, and Ickes, *African-Brazilian Culture.*

102. Vargas, *A nova política*, 159.

103. Darcy Vargas, quoted in Silva and Duarte, *As origens da LBA*, 5.

104. "O que é o Serviço de Assistência a Família."

105. *Madrinhas*, or godmothers, were a point of contact for deployed soldiers. They offered moral support and helped facilitate communication between soldiers and their families back home. Many *madrinhas* helped families publish notes to their loved ones in the LBA's journal, *Boletin da LBA*, Arquivo Nacional do Brasil, Recordações da Segunda Guerra Mundial, SM Caixa 16; and Moura e Silva and Duarte, *As origens da LBA*, 8.

106. Legião Brasileira de Assistencia, "Estatutos LBA," Rio de Janeiro, 1942, CPDOC, Arquivo: Alzira Vargas do Amaral Peixoto Classificação: AVAP vpu lba 1942.

107. Decreto-lei no. 4.684.

108. Darcy Vargas, speech before the Executive Board of the LBA, 1953, CPDOC, Alzira Vargas do Amaral Peixoto, AVAP vpu lba, 1942.

109. Brazil, Decreto-lei no. 4.830, de 15 de outubro de 1942. Estados Unidos do Brasil, "Atos do governo," *Diário Oficial da União*, 81, no. 242 (October 17, 1942), 1. The requirement for workers themselves to contribute to the LBA was revoked by Decreto-lei no. 8.252, de 29 novembro de 1945.

110. Decreto-lei no. 5.063, de 10 de dezembro de 1942, and Decreto-lei no. 6.158, de 30 de dezembro de 1943.

111. Carneiro, *Brasil, primeiro*; Ferreira, "Assis Chateaubriand," 1337–1340.

112. "Noticiário: Campanha de Redenção da Criança," 154.

113. "A Campanha de Redenção da Criança instalou, ontem, em São Felix, os trabalhos para a construção do seu primeiro Posto de Puericultura," *Estado da Bahia* (Salvador), March 6, 1944.

114. "Concluidos os trabalhos da caravana da Campanha de Redenção da Criança, na Bahia," *Diário de Noticias* (Salvador), March 8, 1944.

115. "Entra em fase de execução, na Bahia, a Campanha pela Redenção da Criança," *Estado da Bahia* (Salvador), March 2, 1944.

116. "Relatório da Divisão de Proteção Social da Infância," *Anais do Ministério da Educação e Saúde* (June 1945), 162.

117. "Convocadas todas as fortunas para a grande campanha pelo Brasil," *Estado da Bahia* (Salvador), January 13, 1944; "Demos á Criança aquilo que é seu direito exigir," *Diário de Notícias* (Salvador), January 15, 1944; and "Campanha de Redenção da Criança," *Anais do Ministério da Educação e Saúde* (March 1944): 277–278.

118. "Concluidos os trabalhos" (see n. 114).

119. Pang, *Bahia in the First Brazilian Republic*.

120. "Movimento que emocionam" and "Demos á criança aquilo que é seu direito exigir," *Diário de Noticias* (Salvador), January 15, 1944.

121. "Demos á criança" (see n. 120).

122. "A fé no progresso é a fé na criança," *Diário de Notícias* (Salvador), November 29, 1944; and "Convite," *Diário de Notícias* (Salvador), November 23, 1944.

123. Assis Chateaubriand, "O Instituto de Puericultura," *Jornal do Brasil* (Rio de Janeiro), March 24, 1938.

124. Aleixo to Dr. Álvaro Bahia, February 23, 1943, Liga.

125. "Prosseguem as comemorações da 'Semana da Criança,'" *Diário da Bahia* (Salvador), October 12, 1944; and "Inaugurada a creche 'Darcy Vargas,'" *O Imparcial* (Salvador), October 19, 1943.

126. CPDOC, Alzira Vargas do Amaral Peixoto, AVAP vpu lba, 1942.

127. Moura e Silva and Duarte, *As origens da LBA*, 16.

128. Chateaubriand, "O Instituto de Puericultura" (see n. 123).

129. Sousa, "Saúde, educação e trabalho."

130. Guy, *Women Build the Welfare State*.

131. Torres, *As primeiras damas*, 40. Brodwyn Fischer makes a similar argument in chapter 4 of *A Poverty of Rights*.

132. Ministério da Educação e Saúde, Gustavo Capanema to Landulfo Alves, July 3, 1940, CPDOC, GC h/rolo 61.

133. Liga Bahiana contra a Mortalidade Infantil to Vargas, November 20, 1938, Liga, Pasta: "Expedidos 1933–1935"; Silva, "Resenha histórica da Liga Bahiana"; and Souza, *Bahianos ilustres 1564–1925*.

134. Levine, *Father of the Poor?*.

135. "Dr. Isaias Alves—entrevista de S. Ex. ao 'Jornal do Brasil,'" *Diário Oficial* (Salvador), October 3, 1940.

CONCLUSION

1. Collins, "Intimacy, Inequality and Democracia Racial," 28.

2. Roncador, *Domestic Servants*, 41.

3. Instituto Brasileiro de Geografia e Estatística, Laboratório de Estatística, "Pesquisas sobre a mortalidade no Brasil," Tabela extraída de: Anuário estatístico do Brasil 1955, vol. 16 (Rio de Janeiro: IBGE, 1955).

4. Ibid. See also Instituto Brasileiro de Geografia e Estatística, *Estatísticas do século XX*, 240.

EPILOGUE

1. Cruz, "A sexualidade," 450.

2. Tornquist, "Armadilhas da nova era," and Diniz, "Humanização da assistência ao parto."

3. Tornquist, "Armadilhas da nova era," 483–484.

4. Elis Almeida, "Parto humanizado no SUS," Blogueiras Negras (blog), October 13, 2013, http://blogueirasnegras.org/2013/10/04/parto-humanizado-sus/.

5. Ministério da Saúde, *Pesquisa nacional de demografia*, 157.

6. Goes and Nascimento, "Mulheres negras e brancas," 281.

7. Ministério da Saúde, "Campanha mobiliza a população contra o racismo no SUS," Blog da Saúde (blog), November 25, 2014, http://www.blog.saude.gov.br/index.php/34777-campanha-mobiliza-a-populacao-contra-o-racismo-no-sus.

8. Ministério da Saúde, *Perspectiva da eqüidade*, 11.

9. Santos, "Brazilian Black Women's NGOs."

10. Cruz, "Prevenindo a violência."

11. Carneiro, "Mulheres em movimento," 122.

12. Ministério da Saúde, *Cadernos HumanizaSUS*, 26 and 111.

13. Inquérito Nacional sobre Parto e Nascimento, "Nascer no Brasil: Sumário executivo temático da pesquisa" (2012), 4. http://www.ensp.fiocruz.br/portal-ensp/informe/site/arquivos/anexos/nascerweb.pdf.

14. Here I borrow Brodwyn Fischer's very accurate turn of phrase. Fischer, *A Poverty of Rights*.

15. Inquérito Nacional, 3.

16. Agência Nacional de Saúde Suplementar, "Taxa de parto cesáreo," http://

bvsms.saude.gov.br/bvs/publicacoes/qualificacao_saude_sup/pdf/Atenc_saude2 fase.pdf.

17. Senado Federal, Relatório final da "Comissão Parlamentar Mista de Inquérito—com a finalidade de investigar a situação da violência contra a mulher no Brasil e apurar denúncias de omissão por parte do poder público com relação à aplicação de instrumentos instituídos em lei para proteger as mulheres em situação de violência," Brasília, 2013, 62. http://www.senado.gov.br/atividade/materia/getPDF .asp?t=130748&tp=1.

18. Parto do Princípio, "Dossiê da violência obstétrica: Parirás com dor" (2012), 81. http://www.senado.gov.br/comissoes/documentos/SSCEPI/DOC%20 VCM%20367.pdf.

19. "MPF/SP realiza audiência pública para debater episiotomia e humanização do nascimento," População Negra e Saúde (blog), October 21, 2014, http:// populacaonegraesaude.blogspot.com.br/2014/10/mpfsp-realiza-audiencia-publica -para.html.

20. Parto do Princípio, 86.

21. Geledés, "Mulheres criam página na internet para denunciar mortes em hospital do RJ," October 20, 2014, http://www.geledes.org.br/mulheres-criam-pagina -na-internet-para-denunciar-mortes-em-hospital-rj/#ixzz3GhmHC2JR.

22. Geledés, "Vítima de violência obstétrica é retratada como 'comedora de placenta,'" July 15, 2014, http://www.geledes.org.br/vitima-de-violencia-obstetrica-e -retratada-como-comedora-de-placenta/#axzz3Ju76Dzvy.

23. Ministério da Saúde, *Violência intrafamiliar*, 21–22.

24. Silva, "Racismo institucional," 320.

25. Cruz, "A sexualidade," 453.

26. Ministério da Saúde, "Campanha mobiliza," Blog da Saúde (see n. 7).

27. Geledés, "Mulheres negras são 60% das mães mortas durante partos no SUS, diz Ministério," November 26, 2014, http://www.geledes.org.br/mulheres -negras-sao-60-das-maes-mortas-durante-partos-no-sus-diz-ministerio/#axzz3 KHnEYdKg. Also see Aguiar and d'Oliveira, "Violência institucional," 85–87.

28. Bueno de Mesquita and Kismödi, "Maternal Mortality and Human Rights," 79.

29. Juliana Gonçalves, "'Grávida, pobre e negra'—quando a violência e omissão obstétrica matam e parir vira uma questão de coragem," Blogueiras Negras (blog), April 24, 2014; and Senado Federal, "Relatório final," 64.

30. Bueno de Mesquita and Kismödi, "Maternal Mortality and Human Rights," 79.

31. Ibid.

32. Emanuelle Goes, "Mulheres e negras, todas as formas de violência pelo simples fato de existir," População Negra e Saúde (blog), November 25, 2014, http:// populacaonegraesaude.blogspot.com.br/2014/11/mulheres-e-negras-o-todas-as -formas-de.html; and Maria Luciana Botti, "Violência institucional e a assistência às mulheres no parto," *Anais Eletrônicos do I Colóquio Nacional de Estudos de Gênero e História jun. 2013*, ed. Luciana Rosar Fornazari Klanovicz, Laboratório de Histó-

ria Ambiental e Gênero, 649–663, http://sites.unicentro.br/wp/lhag/publicacoes /anais/.

33. Carneiro, "Mulheres em movimento," 123; Ministério da Saúde, *Perspectiva da eqüidade,* 16; and Ministério da Saúde, *Política nacional.*

34. Ministério da Saúde, *Política nacional,* 5.

35. This regulation is Portaria no. 992, de 13 de maio de 2009.

36. Ministério da Saúde, *Política nacional,* 7.

37. Ministério da Saúde, *Pré-Natal e puerpério,* 7.

38. Ministério da Saúde, Portaria no. 904, de 29 de maio de 2013, Art. 2, VI.

39. TV Record, R7 Noticias, "Cresce número de partos humanizados em Salvador," October 18, 2014, http://noticias.r7.com/bahia/fotos/cresce-numero-de -partos-humanizados-em-salvador-centro-de-parto-normal-atende-gratuitamente -18102014#!/foto/1.

40. Geledés, "'Racismo faz mal à Saúde. Denuncie!' Governo lança telefone para denúncia de racismo em hospitais e postos," http://www.geledes.org.br/racismo -faz-mal-saude-denuncie-governo-l...fone-para-denuncia-de-racismo-em-hospitais -e-postos/#axzz3KHnEYdKg; and "Campanha mobiliza população contra racismo na rede pública de saúde," http://www.geledes.org.br/campanha-mobiliza -populacao-contra-racismo-na-rede-publica-de-saude/#axzz3KHnEYdKg, November 27, 2014.

41. Ministério da Saúde, "Ministério da Saúde e ANS publicam regras para estimular parto normal na saúde suplementar," Blog da Saúde (blog), http://www.blog .saude.gov.br/index.php/34963-ministerio-da-saude-e-ans-publicam-regras-para -estimular-parto-normal-na-saude-suplementar, January 6, 2015.

42. Cruz, "Que falta faz uma área técnica!"

43. Paula Vieira, "População Negra e a Luta Diária Pelo Direito à Saúde," População Negra e Saúde (blog), November 27, 2014, http://blogueirasnegras.org/2014 /08/19/populacao-negra-e-a-luta-diaria-pelo-direito-a-saude/.

Bibliography

ARCHIVES CONSULTED

Arquivo da Liga Álvaro Bahia contra a Mortalidade Infantil, Hospital Martagão
Gesteira, Salvador, BA (cited as Liga)
Arquivo da Santa Casa de Misericórdia da Bahia, Salvador, BA (cited as SCMB)
Arquivo Público do Estado da Bahia, Salvador, BA (cited as APEB)
Casa de Oswaldo Cruz, Fundação Oswaldo Cruz, Rio de Janeiro, RJ
Centro de Pesquisa e Documentação de História Contemporânea do Brasil, Funda-
ção Getúlio Vargas, Rio de Janeiro, RJ (cited as CPDOC)
Fundação Instituto Feminino da Bahia, Salvador, BA
Instituto Histórico e Geográfico da Bahia, Salvador, BA
Memorial da Medicina, Arquivo da Faculdade de Medicina da Bahia, Salvador, BA
(cited as FAMEB)

SELECTED THESES, FACULDADE DE
MEDICINA DA BAHIA, SALVADOR

Albernaz, Pedro de Barros. "Primeira infância—hygiene e aleitamento." 1898.
Araujo, Francisco Affonso de. "Puericultura intra-uterina ou feticultura." 1912.
Bahiense, Laura Amalia de Souza. "Da alimentação das crianças na primeira infan-
cia." 1898.
Borba Junior, Antonio de Azevedo. "O aleitamento materno sob o ponto de vista
medico-social." 1913.
Braga, Antonio Fernandes de Carvalho. "Hygiene alimentar na primeira infancia."
1906.
Cerqueira, Mario Cardoso de. "Prophilaxia alimentar da primeira infancia." 1903.
Chavantes, Aprigio José. "O mecanismo do parto natural." 1885.
Ferreira, Alberto Santigo. "Do aleitamento mercenario." 1913.
Ferreira, Arthur Lopes. "Da gravidez e sua hygiene." 1907.

Ferreira, Eduardo Leite Leal. "A puericultura intra-uterina e formação da prole." 1906.

Freitas, Alberto Ferreira. "Ligeiras considerações sobre a hygiene da mulher gravida." 1904.

Gomes, Maria Barbosa. "Contribuição ao estudo jurídico e médico-legal do crime do infanticídio." 1928.

Goulart, Octaviano de Abreu. "Hygiene alimentar na primeira infancia." 1900.

Jatobá, Hildebrando de Freitas. "Contribuição ao estudo da mortalidade infantil na Bahia." 1907.

Leite, Julio Pereira. "Conseqüência para a mulher do casamento de um syphilitico: Transmissão da syphilis pelo casamento." 1893.

Machado, Odilon Ferreira. "Hygiene da gravidez." 1900.

Medeiros, Alfredo Cordeiro Fonseca. "Do infanticidio." 1903.

Moraes, Francisco Wanderley de. "Puericultura prenatal." 1924.

Motta, Amancio de Marsillac. "Considerações geraes sobre o infanticidio." 1891.

Oliveira, Joaquim Gomes Corrêa de. "Aleitamento materno." 1907.

Pontes, Theodoro de Britto. "O aborto criminoso." 1898.

Reis, Cacilda Vieira dos. "Ligeira contribuição ao estudo da sub-alimentação dos lactentes." 1927.

Rocha, Joaquim Gentil Ferreira da. "Hygiene da primeira infancia." 1907.

Rocha, José Cesario da. "Syphilis e casamento." 1906.

Silva, Flaviano Innocencio da. "Aleitamento e syphilis." 1900.

Souza, Ivo Gonçalves de. "Hygiene da procreação." 1919.

Souza, João Prudencio de. "Syphilis e eugenia." 1923.

Tanajura, Joaquim Augusto. "Letalidade infantil e suas causas." 1900.

Telles, Januario Cyrillo da Silva. "Regimen alimentar da primeira infancia." 1909.

Tourinho, Manuel Celso. "Aborto criminoso." 1907.

Vasconcellos, José Soares de. "Profilaxia da syphilis no aleitamento." 1906.

Vianna, Antonio Salustiano. "Do regimen lacteo." 1881.

Vianna, Joaquim Telesphoro Ferreira Lopes. "Breves considerações sobre o aleitamento." 1853.

Vidal, Fulgencio Martins. "Hygiene alimentar na primeira infancia." 1902.

OTHER PRINT SOURCES

Adeodato Filho, José. *O ensino da clínica obstétrica na Universidade da Bahia*. Salvador: Universidade Federal da Bahia, 1967.

———. "Serviço obstétrico domiciliar Pro-Matre da Bahia." *Pediatria e Puericultura* 18, no. 3/4 (March–June, 1949): 225–232.

Adeodato Filho, José, and Domingos Machado. "Assistencia social-obstetrica na Bahia." *Revista Médica da Bahia* 10, no. 5 (May 1942): 111–119.

Agostoni, Claudia. *Monuments of Progress: Modernization and Public Health in Mexico City, 1876–1910*. Calgary: University of Calgary Press, 2003.

Aguiar, Álvaro, and Reinaldo Menezes Martins, eds. *História da pediatria brasileira: Coletânea de textos e depoimentos.* Rio de Janeiro: Sociedade de Pediatria Brasileira, 1996.

Aguiar, Janaína Marques de, and Ana Flávia Pires Lucas d'Oliveira. "Violência institucional em maternidades públicas sob a ótica das usuárias." *Interface: Comunicação Saúde Educação* 15, no. 36 (2011): 85–87.

Alberto, Paulina L. *Terms of Inclusion: Black Intellectuals in Twentieth-Century Brazil.* Chapel Hill: University of North Carolina Press, 2011.

Albuquerque Jr., Durval Muniz de. *The Invention of the Brazilian Northeast.* Durham: Duke University Press, 2014.

Almeida, Dias de. "Noções de higiene infantil." *Gazeta Médica da Bahia* 51, no. 2 (August 1919): 90–101.

Alves, Isaías. *Educação e saúde na Bahia na interventoria Landulpho Alves, abril 1938–junho 1939.* Salvador: Bahia Gráfica e Editora, 1939.

Amador, José. *Medicine and Nation Building in the Americas, 1890–1940.* Nashville: Vanderbilt University Press, 2015.

Amaral, Marivaldo Cruz do. "Da comadre para o doutor: A Maternidade Climério de Oliveira e a nova medicina da mulher na Bahia republicana (1910–1927)." Master's thesis, Universidade Federal da Bahia, 2005.

———. "Mulheres, imprensa e higiene: A medicalização do parto na Bahia (1910–1927)." *História, Ciências, Saúde—Manguinhos* 15, no. 4 (October/December 2008): 927–944.

Amster, Ellen J. *Medicine and the Saints: Science, Islam, and the Colonial Encounter in Morocco, 1877–1956.* Austin: University of Texas Press, 2013.

Anderson, Warwick. *Colonial Pathologies: American Tropical Medicine, Race, and Hygiene in the Philippines.* Durham: Duke University Press, 2006.

Andrews, George Reid. *Blacks and Whites in São Paulo, Brazil 1888–1988.* Madison: University of Wisconsin Press, 1991.

Antunes, José Leopoldo Ferreira. *Medicina, leis e moral: Pensamento médico e comportamento no Brasil (1870–1930).* São Paulo: Fundação Editora da UNESP, 1999.

Apple, Rima D. *Mothers and Medicine: A Social History of Infant Feeding, 1890–1950.* Madison: University of Wisconsin Press, 1987.

———. *Perfect Motherhood: Science and Childrearing in America.* New Brunswick, NJ: Rutgers University Press, 2006.

Athayde, Johildo L. de. "Filhos ilegítimos e crianças expostas." *Revista da Academia de Letras da Bahia* 27 (September 1979): 9–27.

———. *Salvador e a grande epidemia de 1855.* Salvador: Universidade Federal da Bahia, Centro de Estudos Baianos, 1985.

Audíface, Eliezer. "A pupileira e sua organização." *Pediatria e Puericultura* 16, no. 1 (September 1946): 3–14.

Azevedo, Celia Maria Marinho de. *Onda negra, medo branco: O negro no imaginário das elites, século XIX.* Rio de Janeiro: Editora Paz e Terra, 1987.

Bahia, Álvaro. "Escola de Puericultura Raymundo Pereira de Magalhães." *Pediatria e Puericultura* 7, no. 1/2 (1937): 39–48.

————. "Estudo do recemnascido." *Boletim de Educação e Saúde* 1 (October 1940): 1–16.

————. "Noticiário: Centro de Colocação Familiar de Santo Amaro." *Pediatria e Puericultura* 13 (June 1944): 152–153.

Baker, S. Josephine. *Fighting for Life*. New York: Macmillan, 1939.

Barreto, Mary Renilda. "Assistência ao nascimento na Bahia oitocentista." *História, Ciências, Saúde—Manguinhos* 15, no. 4 (October/December 2008): 901–925.

————. "Corpo de mulher: A trajetória do desconhecido na Bahia no século XIX." *História: Questões & Debates, Curitiba* 24 (2001): 127–156.

————. "Doenças de mulheres na Bahia do século XIX." In *Fazendo gênero na historiografia baiana*, ed. Cecilia Maria Bacellar Sardenberg, Iole Macedo Vanin, and Lina Maria Brandão de Aras, 27–34. Salvador: Núcleo de Estudos Interdisciplinares sobre a Mulher, FFCH/UFBA, 2001.

————. "Entre brancos e mestiços: O quotidiano do Hospital São Cristóvão na Bahia oitocentista." In *Historia da saúde: Olhares e veredas*, ed. Yara Nogueira Monteiro, 49–64. São Paulo: Instituto de Saúde, 2010.

Barros Barreto, Antonio Luis C. A. de. "Relatorio da Sub-Secretaria de Saúde e Assistencia Pública, Anno de 1926." Bahia: Imprensa Official do Estado, 1927.

Besse, Susan. *Restructuring Patriarchy: The Modernization of Gender Inequality in Brazil, 1914–1940*. Chapel Hill: University of North Carolina Press, 1996.

Birn, Anne-Emanuelle. "'No More Surprising Than a Broken Pitcher'? Maternal and Child Health in the Early Years of the Pan American Sanitary Bureau." *Canadian Bulletin of Medical History* 19, no. 1 (2002): 17–46.

Blake, Stanley E. *The Vigorous Core of Our Nationality: Race and Regional Identity in Northeastern Brazil*. Pittsburgh: University of Pittsburgh Press, 2011.

Blum, Ann. *Domestic Economies: Family, Work, and Welfare in Mexico City, 1884–1943*. Lincoln: University of Nebraska Press, 2009.

Boarini, Maria Lúcia, ed. *Higiene e raça como projetos: Higienismo e eugenismo no Brasil*. Maringá, Paraná: Eduem, 2003.

————. "Higienismo, eugenia e a naturalização do social." In *Higiene e raça como projetos: Higienismo e eugenismo no Brasil*, ed. Maria Lúcia Boarini, 19–44. Maringá, Paraná: Eduem, 2003.

Borges, Dain. *The Family in Bahia, Brazil, 1870–1945*. Stanford: Stanford University Press, 1992.

————. "'Puffy, Ugly, Slothful and Inert': Degeneration in Brazilian Social Thought, 1880–1940." *Journal of Latin American Studies* 25, no. 2 (May 1993): 235–256.

————. "The Recognition of Afro-Brazilian Symbols and Ideas, 1890–1940." *Luso-Brazilian Review* 32, no. 2 (1995): 59–78.

————. "Salvador's 1890s: Paternalism and Its Discontents." *Luso-Brazilian Review* 30, no. 2 (1993): 47–57.

Brazil, Ministério da Indústria, Viação e Obras Públicas. *Synopse do recenseamento de 31 de dezembro de 1890*. Rio de Janeiro: Directoria Geral de Estatística, 1898.

Brenes, Anayansi Corrêa. "História da parturição no Brasil, século XIX." *Cadernos de Saúde Pública, RJ* 7, no. 2 (April/June 1991): 135–149.

Briggs, Laura. "The Race of Hysteria: 'Overcivilization' and the 'Savage' Woman in Late Nineteenth-Century Obstetrics and Gynecology." *American Quarterly* (2000): 246–273.

Bronfman, Alejandra. *Measures of Equality: Social Science, Citizenship, and Race in Cuba, 1902–1940.* Chapel Hill: University of North Carolina Press, 2004.

Bueno de Mesquita, Judith, and Eszter Kismödi. "Maternal Mortality and Human Rights: Landmark Decision by United Nations Human Rights Body." *Bulletin of the World Health Organization* 90, no. 2 (2012): 79.

Butler, Kim D. *Freedoms Given, Freedoms Won: Afro-Brazilians in Post-Abolition São Paulo and Salvador.* New Brunswick, NJ: Rutgers University Press, 1998.

———. "Slavery in the Age of Emancipation: Victims and Rebels in Brazil's Late 19th-Century Domestic Trade." *Journal of Black Studies* 42, no. 6 (September 2011): 968–992.

Caldas, Claudemiro. "Syphilographia: Ligeiras considerações acerca das principaes theorias syphilographicas." *Gazeta Médica da Bahia* 10, no. 5 (1866): 54–56.

Caldwell, Kia Lilly. *Negras in Brazil: Re-envisioning Black Women, Citizenship, and the Politics of Identity.* New Brunswick, NJ: Rutgers University Press, 2007.

Callaway, Jessica G. "Mothers, Orphans, and the Law of the Free Womb: The Rhetoric of Brazilian Abolition in the Fiction of Aluísio Azevedo, Machado de Assis, and Their Contemporaries." PhD diss., Harvard University, 2008.

"Campanha de Redenção da Criança." *Pediatria e Puericultura* 13, no. 3–4 (March/June 1944), 154–156.

Campos, André Luiz Vieira de. *Políticas internacionais de saúde na era Vargas: O Serviço Especial de Saúde Pública, 1942–1960.* Rio de Janeiro: Editora Fiocruz, 2006.

Campos, Ernesto de Souza. "Santa Casa de Misericórdia da Bahia: Origem e aspectos de seu funcionamento." *Revista do Instituto Geográfico e Histórico da Bahia* 69 (1943): 213–252.

Carneiro, Glauco. *Brasil, primeiro: História dos Diários Associados.* Brasília: Fundação Assis Chateaubriand, 1999.

Carneiro, Sueli. "Mulheres em movimento." *Estudos Avançados* 17, no. 49 (2003): 117–132.

Carrara, Sérgio L. *Tributo a Vênus: A luta contra a sífilis no Brasil, da passagem do século aos anos 40.* Rio de Janeiro: Editora Fiocruz, 1996.

Carvalho, José Murilo de. "The Unfinished Republic." *The Americas* 48, no. 2 (1991): 139–157.

Carvalho, Pinto de. "Aula inaugural da Clinica Pediátrica Medica e Higiene Infantil em 1942." *Revista Médica da Bahia* 10, no. 3 (March 1942): 53–76.

Carvalho, Virgilio de. "Um ano de atividade pre-natal no 3º Centro Sanitario." *Pediatria e Puericultura* 2, no. 4 (1933): 139–143.

Castellucci, Aldrin A. S. "Flutuações econômicas, crise política e greve geral na Bahia da Primeira República." *Revista Brasileira de História* 25, no. 50 (July/December 2005): 131–166.

Castro, Dinorah. *A mulher submissa: Teses da Faculdade de Medicina da Bahia no século XIX.* Salvador, BA, Brazil: Press Color, 1996.

————. *Cartas sobre a educação de Cora do Dr. José Lino Coutinho*. Salvador, BA, Brazil: Beneditina, 1977.

Caulfield, Sueann. *In Defense of Honor: Sexual Morality, Modernity, and Nation in Early-Twentieth-Century Brazil*. Durham: Duke University Press, 2000.

————. "The Right to a Father's Name: A Historical Perspective on State Efforts to Combat the Stigma of Illegitimate Birth in Brazil." *Law and History Review* 30, no. 1 (February 2012): 1–36.

Chalhoub, Sidney. *Cidade febril: Cortiços e epidemias na Corte Imperial*. São Paulo: Companhia das Letras, 1996.

————. *Machado de Assis, historiador*. São Paulo: Companhia das Letras, 2003.

————. "The Precariousness of Freedom in a Slave Society (Brazil in the Nineteenth Century)." *International Review of Social History* 56, no. 3 (December 2011): 405–439.

Collins, Jane-Marie. "Bearing the Burden of Bastardy: Infanticide, Child Murder, Race, and Motherhood in Brazilian Slave Society, Nineteenth-Century Bahia." In *Killing Infants: Studies in the World Practice of Infanticide*, ed. Brigitte Bechtold and Donna Cooper Graves, 199–229. Lewiston, NY: Edwin Mellen Press, 2006.

————. "Intimacy, Inequality and Democracia Racial: Theorizing Race, Gender and Sex in the History of Brazilian Race Relations." *Journal of Romance Studies* 7, no. 2 (2007): 19–34.

————. "Mãe Africana, Pátria Brasileira: Negotiating the Racial Politics of Identity, Freedom and Motherhood in Nineteenth-Century Bahia, Brazil." In *Intimacy and Inequality: Female Histories and Feminist Readings of Manumission and Motherhood in Brazilian Slave Society (Bahia 1830–1888)*. Available at http://eprints.nottingham.ac.uk/2192/.

Collins, Patricia Hill. *Black Feminist Thought*. New York: Routledge, 2009.

Comité Nacional Brazileiro. "Primeiro Congresso Americano da Criança." Rio de Janeiro: Imprensa Nacional, 1917.

Costa, Clovis Corrêa da. *Puericultura e maternidade*. Rio de Janeiro: Imprensa Nacional, 1943.

Costa, Emilia Viotti da. *The Brazilian Empire: Myths and Histories*. Chapel Hill: University of North Carolina Press, 1985.

Costa, Jurandir Freire. *Ordem médica e norma familiar*. Rio de Janeiro: Edições Graal, 1979.

Costa, Paulo Segundo da. *Ações sociais da Santa Casa de Misericórdia da Bahia*. Salvador, BA, Brazil: Contexto e Arte Editorial, 2001.

Couto, Gracília Magalhães de Almeida. *Centenário do Professor Dr. Alfredo Ferreira de Magalhães, Bahia, Brasil, 10 de fevereiro de 1973*. Salvador, BA, Brazil: Gráfica Editora Livro, 1973.

Cova, Anne. "French Feminism and Maternity: Theories and Policies, 1890–1918." In *Women and the Rise of the European Welfare States, 1880s–1950s*, ed. Gisela Bock and Pat Thane, 119–137. London: Routledge, 1991.

Cowling, Camillia. *Conceiving Freedom: Women of Color, Gender, and the Abolition of*

Slavery in Havana and Rio de Janeiro. Chapel Hill: University of North Carolina Press, 2013.

Cruz, Isabel Cristina Fonseca da. "A sexualidade, a saúde reprodutiva e a violência contra a mulher negra: Aspectos de interesse para assistência de enfermagem." *Revista Escola de Enfermagem da USP* 38, no. 4 (2004): 448–457.

———. "Prevenindo a violência (inclusive a simbólica) contra a mulher negra." *Online Brazilian Journal of Nursing* 5, no. 3 (2006), http://www.objnursing.uff.br /index.php/nursing/rt/printerFriendly/721/163.

———. "Que falta faz uma área técnica de saúde da população negra no Ministério da Saúde!" *Revista da ABPN* 5, no. 9 (2013): 163–171.

Cunha, Euclides da. *Rebellion in the Backlands.* Chicago: University of Chicago Press, 1944.

Cunha, Fabiana Lopes da. "Negócio ou ócio? O samba, a malandragem, e a política trabalhista do Vargas." Paper presented at the IV Congreso Latinoamericano de la Asociación Internacional para el Estudio de la Música Popular," Mexico City, April 2–6, 2002.

Cunha, Olívia Maria Gomes da. "Learning to Serve: Intimacy, Morality, and Violence." *Hispanic American Historical Review* 88, no. 3 (2008): 455–491.

Dávila, Jerry. *Diploma of Whiteness: Race and Social Policy in Brazil, 1917–1945.* Durham: Duke University Press, 2003.

———. "Norma Fraga: Race, Class, Education, and the Estado Novo." In *The Human Tradition in Modern Brazil,* ed. Peter M. Beattie, 165–182. Wilmington, DE: Scholarly Resources, 2004.

Davin, Anna. "Imperialism and Motherhood." *History Workshop Journal* 5 (1978): 9–65.

Davis, Darién J. *Avoiding the Dark: Race and the Forging of National Culture in Modern Brazil.* Aldershot, UK: Ashgate, 1999.

De Barros, Juanita. *Reproducing the British Caribbean: Sex, Gender, and Population Politics after Slavery.* Chapel Hill: University of North Carolina Press, 2014.

Diacon, Todd A. *Stringing Together a Nation: Cândido Mariano da Silva Rondon and the Construction of a Modern Brazil, 1906–1930.* Durham: Duke University Press, 2004.

Diniz, Carmen Simone Grilo. "Humanização da assistência ao parto no Brasil: Os muitos sentidos de um movimento." *Ciência & Saúde Coletiva* 10, no. 3 (2005): 627–637.

Doyle, Nora. "'The Highest Pleasure of Which Woman's Nature Is Capable': Breast-Feeding and the Sentimental Maternal Ideal in America, 1750–1860." *Journal of American History* 97, no. 4 (2011): 958–973.

Dwork, Deborah. *War Is Good for Babies and Other Young Children: A History of the Infant and Child Welfare Movement in England, 1898–1918.* London: Tavistock Publications, 1987.

Estado da Bahia. *Diário Oficial do Estado da Bahia: Edição comemorativa ao centenário da independência da Bahia, 1923.* Salvador: Fundação Pedro Calmon, 2004.

Ferreira, Luiz Otávio, and Maria Martha de Luna Freire. "Medicina, filantropia e infância na Bahia: Um hospital para crianças (1920–1930)." *In História da saúde na Bahia: Instituições e patrimônio arquitetônico, 1808–1958*, ed. Christiane Maria Cruz de Souza and Maria Renilda Nery Barreto, 74–100. Rio de Janeiro: Fiocruz, 2011.

Ferreira, Marieta de Morais. "Assis Chateaubriand." In *Dicionário Histórico-Biográfico Brasileiro: Pós-1930*, ed. Alzira Alves de Abreu, Israel Beloch, Fernando Lattman-Weltman, and Sérgio Tadeu de Niemeyer Lamarão, 1337–1340. Rio de Janeiro: Fundação Getúlio Vargas, 2001.

Ferreira Filho, Alberto Heráclito. *Quem pariu e bateu, que balance! Mundos femininos, maternidade e pobreza: Salvador, 1890–1940*. Salvador: Universidade Federal da Bahia, 2003.

Fischer, Brodwyn M. *A Poverty of Rights: Citizenship and Inequality in Twentieth-Century Rio de Janeiro*. Stanford: Stanford University Press, 2008.

Fonseca, Cristina M. Oliveira. *Saúde no governo Vargas (1930–1945): Dualidade institucional de um bem público*. Rio de Janeiro: Editora Fiocruz, 2007.

Foucault, Michel. *The Birth of the Clinic: An Archaeology of Medical Perception*. New York: Pantheon Books, 1973.

———. *The History of Sexuality*. Vintage Books ed. New York: Vintage Books, 1990.

Fraga Filho, Walter. *Encruzilhadas da liberdade: Histórias de escravos e libertos na Bahia, 1870–1910*. São Paulo: Editora UNICAMP, 2006.

Freire, Maria Martha de Luna. *Mulheres, mães e médicos: Discurso maternalista no Brasil*. Rio de Janeiro: Fundação Getúlio Vargas Editora, 2009.

———. "Os filantropos da nação: Alfredo Magalhães e a assistência à infância na Bahia." *Gazeta Médica da Bahia* 80, no. 1 (2010): 117–133.

———. "'Ser mãe é uma ciência': Mulheres, médicos e a construção da maternidade científica na década de 1920." *História, Ciências, Saúde—Manguinhos* 15 (supplement) 2008: 153–171.

Freire, Maria Martha de Luna, and Vinícius da Silva Leony. "A caridade científica: Moncorvo Filho e o Instituto de Proteção e Assistência à Infância do Rio de Janeiro (1899–1930)." *História, Ciências, Saúde—Manguinhos* 18 (December 2011): 199–225.

French, John D. *Drowning in Laws: Labor Law and Brazilian Political Culture*. Chapel Hill: University of North Carolina Press, 2004.

Freyre, Gilberto. *Bahia e baianos*. Ed. Edson Nery da Fonseca. Salvador: Empresa Gráfica da Bahia, 1990.

———. *Casa-grande e senzala: Formação da família brasileira sob o regime economia patriarcal*. 4th ed. Rio de Janeiro: José Olympio Editora, 1943.

———. *The Masters and the Slaves: A Study in the Development of Brazilian Civilization*. Translated by Samuel Putnam. New York: Knopf, 1956.

Fróes, Francisca Prageur. "Estatística da clinica obstétrica da Faculdade de Medicina da Bahia." *Gazeta Médica da Bahia* 34, no. 7 (January 1903): 324–325.

Fuchs, Rachel G. *Abandoned Children: Foundlings and Child Welfare in Nineteenth-Century France*. Albany: State University of New York Press, 1984.

———. *Poor and Pregnant in Paris: Strategies for Survival in the Nineteenth Century.* New Brunswick, NJ: Rutgers University Press, 1992.

———. "The Right to Life: Paul Strauss and the Politics of Motherhood." In *Gender and the Politics of Social Reform in France, 1870–1914,* ed. Elinor A. Accampo, Rachel G. Fuchs, and Mary Lynn Stewart, 82–105. Baltimore: Johns Hopkins University Press, 1995.

Fundação Cultural do Estado da Bahia. *Legislação da Província da Bahia sobre o negro: 1835–1888.* Salvador: Fundação Cultural do Estado da Bahia, 1996.

Garfield, Seth. "The Environment of Wartime Migration: Labor Transfers from the Brazilian Northeast to the Amazon during World War II." *Journal of Social History* 43, no. 4 (July 2010): 989–1019.

———. *Indigenous Struggle at the Heart of Brazil: State Policy, Frontier Expansion, and the Xavante Indians, 1937–1988.* Durham: Duke University Press, 2001.

Gesteira, Joaquim Martagão. "As affecções digestivas no Instituto de P. e A. á Infancia da Bahia." *Gazeta Médica da Bahia* 48, no. 1 (July 1916): 161–177.

———. "Assistencia aos menores: As 'rodas de enjeitados'—necessidade de trabalhar pela sua extinção no Brasil." *Pediatria e Puericultura* 3, no. 3/4 (March–June 1934): 279–289.

———. *Discurso proferido na sessão solenne de inauguração da Liga Bahiana contra a Mortalidade Infantil.* Salvador: Liga Bahiana contra a Mortalidade Infantil, 1923.

———. "Em prol dos nossos enjeitados: A 'roda de expostos.'" *Pediatria e Puericultura* 1, no. 3 (March 1932): 178–205.

———. "Os serviços de hygiene infantil na Bahia em 1924." Salvador: Impresa Official do Estado, 1925.

Giacomini, Sonia Maria. *Mulher e escrava: Uma introdução histórica ao estudo da mulher negra no Brasil.* Petrópolis, RJ: Vozes, 1988.

Giacomini, Sonia Maria, and Elizbeth K. C. Magalhães. "A escrava ama-de-leite: Anjo ou demônio." In *Mulher Mulheres,* ed. Carmen Barroso and Albertina Oliveira Costa, 73–89. São Paulo: Fundação Carlos Chagas, 1983.

Gobineau, Arthur de. *The Inequality of Human Races.* New York: G. P. Putnam's Sons, 1915.

Goes, Emanuelle F., and Enilda R. Nascimento. "Mulheres negras e brancas, as desigualdades no acesso e utilização de serviços de saúde no estado da Bahia, PNAD–2008." In *Saúde da população negra,* ed. Luís Eduardo Batista, Jurema Werneck, and Fernanda Lopes, 274–287. Brasília: Associação Brasileira de Pesquisadores Negros, 2012.

Gomes, Ângela de Castro, ed. *A invenção do trabalhismo.* Rio de Janeiro: Instituto Universitário de Pesquisas do Rio de Janeiro, 1988.

Gonçalves, Margareth de Almeida. "Expostos, roda e mulheres: A lógica da ambiguidade médica-higienista." In *Pensando a família no Brasil: Da colônia à modernidade,* ed. Angela Mendes de Almeida, 37–52. Rio de Janeiro: Espaço e Tempo, 1978.

Gondra, José G. "A sementeira do porvir: Higiene e infância no século XIX." *Educação e pesquisa, São Paulo* 26, no. 1 (January/June 2000): 99–117.

Gormey, Melissa. "Motherhood as National Service: Race, Class, and Public Health Policy in Brazil, 1930–1945." PhD diss., University of California, Davis, 2006.

Gouveia, Almeida. "Fisiopsicologia social da maternidade." *Revista Médica da Bahia* 8, no. 10 (October 1940): 287–295.

Graden, Dale Torston. *Disease, Resistance, and Lies: The Demise of the Transatlantic Slave Trade to Brazil and Cuba.* Baton Rouge: Louisiana State University Press, 2014.

———. *From Slavery to Freedom in Brazil: Bahia, 1835–1900.* Albuquerque: University of New Mexico Press, 2006.

Graham, Richard. *Feeding the City: From Street Market to Liberal Reform in Salvador, Brazil, 1780–1860.* Austin: University of Texas Press, 2010.

Graham, Sandra Lauderdale. *House and Street: The Domestic World of Servants and Masters in Nineteenth-Century Rio de Janeiro.* 1st University of Texas Press ed. Austin: University of Texas Press, 1992.

Guy, Donna J. "The Pan American Child Congresses, 1916 to 1942: Pan Americanism, Child Reform, and the Welfare State in Latin America." *Journal of Family History* 23, no. 3 (1988): 272–291.

———. "The Politics of Pan-American Cooperation: Maternalist Feminism and the Child Rights Movement, 1913–1960." *Gender and History* 10, no. 3 (1998): 449–469.

———. *Women Build the Welfare State: Performing Charity and Creating Rights in Argentina, 1880–1955.* Durham: Duke University Press, 2009.

Hahner, June Edith. *Emancipating the Female Sex: The Struggle for Women's Rights in Brazil, 1850–1940.* Durham: Duke University Press, 1990.

Hale, Charles A. "Political Ideas and Ideologies in Latin America, 1870–1930." In *Ideas and Ideologies in Twentieth-Century Latin America,* ed. Leslie Bethell, 133–206. Cambridge: Cambridge University Press, 1996.

Harding, Rachel E. *A Refuge in Thunder: Candomblé and Alternative Spaces of Blackness.* Bloomington: Indiana University Press, 2000.

Healey, Mark Alan. "'The Sweet Matriarchy of Bahia': Ruth Landes' Ethnography of Race and Gender." *Dispositio/n* 23, no. 50 (1998): 87–116.

Heaton, Matthew M. *Black Skin, White Coats: Nigerian Psychiatrists, Decolonization, and the Globalization of Psychiatry.* Athens: Ohio University Press, 2013.

Henriques, Antonio de Araujo Freitas. *Falla com que o Excellentissimo Senhor Dezembargador João Antonio de Araujo Freitas Henriques abriu a 1ª sessão da 19ª legislatura da Assembléa Provincial da Bahia em 1º de março de 1872.* Salvador: Typ. do Correio da Bahia, 1872.

Hentschke, Jens R. *Vargas and Brazil: New Perspectives.* New York: Palgrave McMillan, 2006.

Hertzman, Marc A. *Making Samba: A New History of Race and Music in Brazil.* Durham: Duke University Press, 2013.

Heywood, Colin. *Growing Up in France: From the Ancien Régime to the Third Republic.* Cambridge: Cambridge University Press, 2007.

Hochman, Gilberto. *A era do saneamento: As bases da política de saúde pública no Brasil.* São Paulo: Editora Hucitec, 1998.

———. "Logo ali, no final da avenida: Os sertões redefinidos pelo movimento sanitarista da Primeira República." *História, Ciências, Saúde—Manguinhos* 5, supplement (1998): 217–235.

———. "Reformas, instituições e políticas de saúde no Brasil (1930–1945)." *Educar* 25 (2005): 127–141.

Homem de Mello, Barão. *Falla com que abriu no dia 1º de maio de 1878 a 57ª legislatura da Assembléa Legislativa Provincial da Bahia o Exm. Sr. Conselheiro Barão Homem de Mello, Presidente da provincia.* Bahia: Typ. do Diário, 1878.

hooks, bell. *Ain't I a Woman: Black Women and Feminism.* Boston: South End Press, 1992.

Hunt, Nancy Rose. "'Le Bebe en Brousse': European Women, African Birth Spacing and Colonial Intervention in Breast Feeding in the Belgian Congo." *The International Journal of African Historical Studies* 21, no. 3 (1998): 401–432.

Hunter, Tera. *To 'Joy My Freedom: Southern Black Women's Lives and Labors after the Civil War.* Cambridge: Harvard University Press, 1997.

Ickes, Scott. *African-Brazilian Culture and Regional Identity in Bahia, Brazil.* Gainesville: University Press of Florida, 2013.

Instituto Brasileiro de Geografia e Estatística (IBGE). *Anuário estatístico do Brasil 1936,* vol. 2. Rio de Janeiro: IBGE, 1936.

———. *Anuário estatístico do Brasil 1937,* vol. 3. Rio de Janeiro: IBGE, 1937.

———. *Anuário estatístico do Brasil 1939/1940,* vol. 5. Rio de Janeiro: IBGE, 1941.

———. *Anuário estatístico do Brasil 1941/1945,* vol. 6. Rio de Janeiro: IBGE, 1946.

———. *Anuário estatístico do Brasil 1946,* vol. 7. Rio de Janeiro: IBGE, 1947.

———. *Anuário estatístico do Brasil 1949,* vol. 10. Rio de Janeiro: IBGE, 1950.

———. *Estatísticas do século XX.* Rio de Janeiro: IBGE, 2007.

———. "Recenseamento geral do Brasil (10 de setembro de 1940): Sinopse do censo demográfico, dados gerais." Rio de Janeiro: Instituto Brasileiro de Geografia e Estatística, 1946.

Johnson, Adriana Michéle Campos. *Sentencing Canudos: Subalternity in the Backlands of Brazil.* Pittsburgh: University of Pittsburgh Press, 2010.

Kehl, Renato. *Eugenía e medicina social: Problemas da vida.* Rio de Janeiro: Livraria Francisco Alves, 1923.

———. *Lições de eugenía.* Rio de Janeiro: Livraria Francisco Alves, 1935.

Klaus, Alisa. *Every Child a Lion: The Origins of Maternal and Infant Health Policy in the United States and France, 1890–1920.* Ithaca, NY: Cornell University Press, 1993.

Klein, Marian van der. *Maternalism Reconsidered: Motherhood, Welfare and Social Policy in the Twentieth Century.* New York: Berghahn Books, 2012.

Koutsoukos, Sandra Sofia Machado. "'Amas mercenárias': O discurso dos doutores em medicina e os retratos de amas–Brasil, segunda metade do século XIX." *História, Ciências, Saúde—Manguinhos* 16, no. 2 (June 2009): 305–324.

Kraay, Hendrik, ed. *Afro-Brazilian Culture and Politics: Bahia, 1790s to 1990s*. Armonk, NY: M. E. Sharpe, 1998.

————. *Race, State, and Armed Forces in Independence-Era Brazil: Bahia, 1790s–1840s*. Stanford: Stanford University Press, 2004.

Kuznesof, Elizabeth Anne. "Sexual Politics, Race and Bastard-Bearing in Nineteenth-Century Brazil: A Question of Culture or Power?" *Journal of Family History* 16, no. 3 (1991) 241–260.

La Berge, Ann. "Mothers and Infants, Nurses and Nursing: Alfred Donné and the Medicalization of Child Care in Nineteenth-Century France." *Journal of the History of Medicine and Allied Sciences* 46, no. 1 (1991): 20–43.

Landes, Ruth. *The City of Women*. New York: Macmillan, 1947.

Legião Brasileira de Assistência. *Súmula histórica da assistência social em São Paulo*. São Paulo: Legião Brasileira de Assistência, 1977.

Leite, Márcia Maria da Silva Barreiros. "Educação, cultura, e lazer das mulheres de elite em Salvador, 1890–1930." M.A. thesis, Universidade Federal da Bahia, 1997.

Leite, Miriam Moreira. *A condição feminina no Rio de Janeiro, século XIX: Antologia de textos de viajantes estrangeiros*. São Paulo: Editora Hucitec, 1984.

Lesser, Jeffrey. *Negotiating National Identity: Immigrants, Minorities, and the Struggle for Ethnicity in Brazil*. Durham: Duke University Press, 1999.

Levine, Robert M. *Father of the Poor? Vargas and His Era*. Cambridge: Cambridge University Press, 1998.

————. "The Singular Brazilian City of Salvador." *Luso-Brazilian Review* 30, no. 2 (December 1, 1993): 59–69.

————. *Vale of Tears: Revisiting the Canudos Massacre in Northeastern Brazil, 1893–1897*. Berkeley: University of California Press, 1992.

————. *The Vargas Regime: The Critical Years, 1934–1938*. New York: Columbia University Press, 1970.

Lima, José Francisco da Silva. "Hygiene pública." *Gazeta Médica da Bahia* 8, no. 11 (1876): 497–498.

Lima, Nísia Trindade. "Missões civilizatórias da Republica e interpretação do Brasil." *História, Ciências, Saúde—Manguinhos* 5, supplement (1998): 163–193.

Lima, Nísia Trindade, and Gilberto Hochman. "Condenado pela raça, absolvido pela medicina: O Brasil descoberto pelo movimento sanitarista da Primeira República." In *Raça, Ciência e Sociedade*, ed. Marcos Chor Maio and Ricardo Ventura Santos, 23–40. Rio de Janeiro: Editora Fiocruz, 1996.

Lowenstein, Karl. *Brazil under Vargas*. New York: Macmillan, 1942.

Luz, Madel Terezinha. *Medicina e ordem política brasileira: Políticas e instituições de saúde (1850–1930)*. Rio de Janeiro: Graal, 1982.

Macedo, Sérgio. *Getúlio Vargas e o culto à nacionalidade*. Rio de Janeiro: Gráfica Olímpica, 1941.

Machado, Domingos F. "A proposito do exame pré-natal." *Pediatria e Puericultura* 11 (1941): 60–61.

Machado, Roberto. *Danação da norma: Medicina social e constituição da psiquiatria no Brasil*. Rio de Janeiro: Graal, 1978.

Magalhães, Alfredo. "Assistencia e protecção á infancia." *Gazeta Médica da Bahia* 35, no. 10 (April 1904): 478–479.

———. "Instituto de Protecção e Assistencia á Infancia." *Gazeta Médica da Bahia* 38, no. 7 (January 1907): 313–331.

Magalhães, João José de Moura. "Falla que recitou o presidente da provincia da Bahia, o dezembargador João José de Moura Magalhães, n'abertura da Assembléa Legislativa da mesma provincia em 25 de março de 1848." Salvador, BA, Brazil: Typ. de João Alves Portella, 1848.

Magalhães, Juracy. *Estado da Bahia: Algumas das realisações do governo, 1931–1937.* Salvador: Estado da Bahia, 1937.

Mai, Lilian Denise. "Difusão dos ideários higienista e eugenista no Brasil." In *Higiene e raça como projetos,* ed. Maria Lúcia Boarini, 45–70. Maringá, Paraná: Eduem, 2003.

Marcílio, Maria Luiza, ed. *Família, mulher, sexualidade e igreja na história do Brasil.* São Paulo: Edições Loyola, 1993.

———. *História social da criança abandonada.* São Paulo: Editora Hucitec, 1998.

Marko, Tamera. "When They Became the Nation's Children: The Foundations of Pediatrics and Its Raced, Classed, and Gendered (Re)Inventions of Childhood in Rio de Janeiro, 1870–1930." PhD diss., University of California, San Diego, 2006.

Marques, Vera Regina Beltrão. *A medicalização da raça: Médicos, educadores e discurso eugênico.* São Paulo: Editora Unicamp, 1994.

Martins, Ana Paula Vosne. "Entre a benemerência e as políticas públicas: A atuação da Liga Bahiana contra a Mortalidade Infantil no começo do século XX." *Gênero, Cadernos do Núcleo Transdiciplinar de Estudos de Gênero* 6, no. 1 (2005): 43–60.

———. "Políticas públicas para a maternidade e a infância no Brasil na primeira metade do século XX." In São Paulo (Brazil: State), *História da Saúde: Olhares e veredas.* São Paulo: Instituto de Saúde, 2010.

———. "'Vamos criar seu filho': Os médicos puericultores e a pedagogia materna no século XX." *História, Ciências, Saúde—Manguinhos* 15, no. 1 (2008): 135–154.

———. *Visões do feminino: A medicina da mulher nos séculos XIX e XX.* Rio de Janeiro: Editora Fiocruz, 2004.

"Maternidade Climério de Oliveira." *Gazeta Médica da Bahia* 69, no. 3 (September 1917): 134–135.

Matos, Lobivar. *A L.B.A. e os soldados do Brasil.* Rio de Janeiro: Departamento Nacional de Informações, 1945.

Mattoso, Kátia de Queirós. *Família e sociedade na Bahia do século XIX.* São Paulo: Corrupio, 1988.

———. "Slave, Free, and Freed Family Structures in Nineteenth-Century Salvador, Bahia." *Luso-Brazilian Review* 25, no. 1 (Summer 1988): 69–84.

Mattoso, Kátia de Queirós, and Johildo de Athayde. "Epidemias e flutuações de preços na Bahia no século XIX." In *L'histoire quantitative du Brésil de 1800 a 1930,* ed. Centre National de La Recherche Scientifique, 183–202. Paris: Éditions du Centre National de La Recherche Scientifique, 1973.

McCann, Bryan. *Hello, Hello Brazil: Popular Music in the Making of Modern Brazil.* Durham: Duke University Press, 2004.

McElya, Micki. *Clinging to Mammy: The Faithful Slave in Twentieth-Century America.* Cambridge: Harvard University Press, 2007.

Meade, Teresa. *"Civilizing" Rio: Reform and Resistance in a Brazilian City, 1889–1930.* University Park: Pennsylvania State University Press, 1997.

Meckel, Richard A. *Save the Babies: American Public Health Reform and the Prevention of Infant Mortality, 1850–1929.* Ann Arbor: University of Michigan Press, 1990.

Medeyros, J. Paulo de. *Getúlio Vargas, o reformador social.* Rio de Janeiro: Gráfica Olímpica, 1941.

Milanich, Nara B. *Children of Fate: Childhood, Class, and the State in Chile, 1850–1930.* Durham: Duke University Press, 2009.

Ministério da Educação e Saúde. *Legislação recente sobre matéria de saúde (1931–1942).* Rio de Janeiro: Imprensa Nacional, 1942.

Ministério da Saúde. *Cadernos HumanizaSUS: Humanização do parto e do nascimento.* Vol. 4. Brasília: Editora Ministério da Saúde, 2014.

———. *Perspectiva da eqüidade no pacto nacional pela redução da mortalidade materna e neonatal: Atenção à saúde das mulheres negras.* Brasília: Editora Ministério da Saúde, 2005.

———. *Pesquisa nacional de demografia e saúde da criança e da mulher—PNDS 2006: Dimensões do processo reprodutivo e da saúde da criança.* Brasília: Editora Ministério da Saúde, 2009.

———. *Política nacional de saúde integral da população negra: Uma política do SUS.* Brasília: Editora Ministério da Saúde, 2013.

———. *Pré-Natal e puerpério: Atenção qualificada e humanizada.* Brasília: Editora Ministério da Saúde, 2005.

———. *Violência intrafamiliar: Orientações para a prática em serviço.* Brasília: Editora Ministério da Saúde, 2001.

Mink, Gwendolyn. *The Wages of Motherhood: Inequality in the Welfare State, 1917–1942.* Ithaca, NY: Cornell University Press, 1995.

Moncorvo de Figueiredo, Carlos Arthur. "Projeto de regulamento das amas de leite." *Gazeta Médica da Bahia* 8 (1876): 498–504.

Moncorvo Filho, Arthur. "Do exame das amas de leite no Brazil." Rio de Janeiro, 1903. Chicago: Center for Research Libraries, Coleção Moncorvo Filho; vol. 12, no. 33.

———. "Do exame das amas mercenarias." *Revista da Sociedade de Medicina e Cirurgia do Rio de Janeiro* (s.d.): 236–237.

———. *Historico da protecção à infancia no Brasil, 1500–1922.* Departamento da Creança no Brasil. Rio de Janeiro: Empresa Gráfica Editora Paulo Pongetti, 1925.

Monteiro, Marcia Rocha. "Homens da cana e hospitais do açúcar: Uma arquitetura da saúde no Estado Novo." *História, Ciências, Saúde—Manguinhos* 18 (December 2011): 67–94.

Monteiro, Yara Nogueira, ed. *Historia da saúde: Olhares e veredas.* São Paulo: Instituto de Saúde, 2010.

Mooney, Jadwiga E. Pieper. *The Politics of Motherhood: Maternity and Women's Rights in Twentieth-Century Chile*. Pittsburgh: University of Pittsburgh Press, 2009.

Morel, Marie-France. "The Care of Children: The Influence of Medical Innovation and Medical Institutions on Infant Mortality 1750–1914." In *The Decline of Mortality in Europe*, ed. Roger Schofield, David Reher, and Alain Bideau, 196–219. Oxford, UK: Clarendon Press, 1991.

Morgan, Jennifer L. *Laboring Women: Reproduction and Gender in New World Slavery*. Philadelphia: University of Pennsylvania Press, 2004.

Mota, André. *Quem é bom já nasce feito: Sanitarismo e eugenia no Brasil*. Rio de Janeiro: Editora DP&A, 2003.

Mott, Luiz. *Os pecados da família na Bahia de Todos os Santos (1831)*. Salvador: Centro de Estudos Baianos, Universidade Federal da Bahia, 1982.

Mott, Maria Lúcia. "A parteira ignorante: Um erro de diagnóstico médico?" *Estudos Feministas* 7, no 1 and 2 (1999): 25–36.

——. "Assistência ao parto: Do domicílio ao hospital (1830–1960)." Revista *Projeto História, São Paulo* 25 (2002): 197–219.

——. "Maternal and Child Welfare, State Policy and Women's Philanthropic Activities in Brazil, 1930–45." In *Maternalism Reconsidered: Motherhood, Welfare and Social Policy in the Twentieth Century*, ed. Marian van der Klein, 168–189. New York: Berghahn Books, 2012.

——. "Parto e parteiras no século XIX: Mme. Durocher e sua época." In *Entre a virtude e o pecado*, ed. Albertina de Oliveira Costa and Cristina Bruschini, 37–56. Rio de Janeiro: Editora Rosa dos Tempos, 1992.

——. "Parteiras: O outro lado da profissão." *Gênero, Cadernos do Núcleo Transdiciplinar de Estudos de Gênero* 6, no. 1 (2005): 117–140.

Moura e Silva, Jayme de, and Paulo Roberto dos Santos Felício Duarte. *As origens da LBA*. Rio de Janeiro: Fundação Legião Brasileira de Assistência, 1977.

Nascimento, Anna Amélia Vieira. "A pobreza e a honra: Recolhidas e dotadas na Santa Casa de Misericórdia da Bahia, 1700–1867." In *Família, mulher, sexualidade e Igreja na história do Brasil*, ed. Maria Luiza Marcílio, 157–170. São Paulo: Edições Loyola, 1993.

——. *Dez freguesias da cidade do Salvador: Aspectos sociais e urbanos do século XIX*. Salvador: Fundação Cultural do Estado da Bahia, 1986.

Nava, Carmen. "Lessons in Patriotism and Good Citizenship: National Identity and Nationalism in Public Schools during the Vargas Administration, 1937–1945." *Luso-Brazilian Review* 35, no. 1 (Summer 1998): 39–63.

Nazzari, Muriel. "An Urgent Need to Conceal." In *The Faces of Honor: Sex, Shame and Violence in Colonial Latin America*, ed. Lyman L. Johnson and Sonya Lipsett-Rivera, 103–126. Albuquerque: University of New Mexico Press, 1998.

Needell, Jeffrey D. "The Domestic Civilizing Mission: The Cultural Role of the State in Brazil, 1808–1930." *Luso-Brazilian Review* 36, no. 1 (July 1, 1999): 1–18.

——. "Identity, Race, Gender, and Modernity in the Origins of Gilberto Freyre's Oeuvre." *The American Historical Review* 100, no. 1 (February 1995): 51–77.

——. *A Tropical Belle Époque: The Elite Culture of Turn-of-the-Century Rio de Janeiro*. New York: Cambridge University Press, 1987.

Neiva, Arthur, and Belisário Penna. *Viagem científica pelo norte da Bahia, sudoeste de Pernambuco, sul do Piauí e de norte a sul de Goiás.* Brasília: Academia Brasiliense de Letras, 1984.

Neto, Hermilo Carneiro. "A enfermeira de Puericultura na proteção à Maternidade e Infância." *Pediatria e Puericultura* 19, no. 2 (1949): 185–193.

Nishida, Mieko. *Slavery and Identity: Ethnicity, Gender, and Race in Salvador, Brazil, 1808–1888.* Bloomington: Indiana University Press, 2003.

"Noticiário: Campanha de Redenção da Criança—O primeiro posto de puericultura." *Pediatria e Puericultura* 13 (June 1944): 154.

Offen, Karen. "Body Politics: Women, Work and the Politics of Motherhood in France, 1920–1950. In *Women and the Rise of the European Welfare States, 1880s–1950s,* ed. Gisela Bock and Pat Thane, 138–159. London: Routledge, 1991.

Oliveira, Hosannah de. "Instituto de Protecção e Assistencia á Infancia da Bahia." *Revista Médica da Bahia* 2, no. 1 (January 1934): 31–32.

Oliveira, Lúcia Lippi, Mônica Pimenta Velloso, and Angela Maria Castro Gomes, ed. *Estado Novo: Ideologia e poder.* Rio de Janeiro: Zahar Editores, 1982.

"O que é o Serviço de Assistência a Família do Convocado da C.B.A." *Cultura Política: Revista Mensal de Estudos Brasileiros* 4, no. 39 (April 1944): 153–162.

Organización de los Estados Americanos; Instituto Interamericano del Niño. *Congresos Panamericanos del Niño: Ordenación sistemática de sus recomendaciones, 1916–1963.* Montevideo: Instituto Interamericano del Niño, 1965.

Otovo, Okezi T. "From *Mãe Preta* to *Mãe Desamparada*: Maternity and Public Health in Post-Abolition Bahia." *Luso-Brazilian Review* 48, no. 2 (2011): 164–191.

Overmyer-Velazquez, Mark. *Visions of the Emerald City: Modernity, Tradition and the Formation of Porfirian Oaxaca, Mexico.* Durham: Duke University Press, 2006.

Owensby, Brian. *Intimate Ironies: Modernity and the Making of Middle-Class Lives in Brazil.* Stanford: Stanford University Press, 1999.

Palmer, Steven Paul. *From Popular Medicine to Medical Populism: Doctors, Healers, and Public Power in Costa Rica, 1800–1940.* Durham: Duke University Press, 2003.

Pan American Child Congress. *Acta final del octavo Congreso Panamericano del Niño.* Washington, DC: US Department of State, 1942.

Pan American Union. *Third American Child Congress, Rio de Janeiro, Brazil, August 27–September 5, 1922.* Washington, DC: Division of Conferences and Organizations, 1954.

Pang, Eul-Soo. *Bahia in the First Brazilian Republic.* Gainesville: University Press of Florida, 1979.

Pappademos, Melina. *Black Political Activism and the Cuban Republic.* Chapel Hill: University of North Carolina Press, 2011.

Peard, Julyan G. *Race, Place, and Medicine: The Idea of the Tropics in Nineteenth-Century Brazilian Medicine.* Durham: Duke University Press, 1999.

Perry, Keisha-Khan. *Black Women against the Land Grab: The Fight for Racial Justice in Brazil.* Minneapolis: University of Minnesota Press, 2013.

Pierson, Donald. *Negros in Brazil: A Study of Race Contact at Bahia.* Carbondale: Southern Illinois University Press, 1967.

Pimenta, Tânia Salgado. "Barbeiros-sangradores e curandeiros no Brasil (1808–1828)." História, Ciências, Saúde—Manguinhos 5, no. 2 (October 1998): 349–372.

Pimpão, Hirosê. Getúlio Vargas e o direito social trabalhista. Rio de Janeiro: Gráfica Guarany, 1942.

Pinheiro, Maria Esolina. Serviço social–documento histórico. São Paulo: Cortez Editora, 1985.

———. Serviço social: Uma interpretação do pioneirismo no Rio de Janeiro. Rio de Janeiro: Edições UERJ, 1985.

Pinho, Patrícia de Santana. Mama Africa: Reinventing Blackness in Bahia. Durham: Duke University Press, 2010.

Portella, Manoel do Nascimento Machado. Falla com que o Illm. e Exm. Sr. Conselheiro Dr. Manoel do Nascimento Machado Portella, Presidente da provincia, abriu a 1ª sessão da 27ª legislatura da Assembléa Legislativa Provincial no dia 3 de abril de 1888. Bahia: Typ. da Gazeta da Bahia, 1888.

Pôrto, Angela, Gisele Sanglard, Maria Rachel Fróes da Fonseca, and Renato da Gama-Rosa Costa, eds. História da saúde no Rio de Janeiro: Instituições e patrimônio arquitetônico (1808–1958). Rio de Janeiro: Editora Fiocruz, 2008.

Primeiro Congresso Brasileiro de Eugenia. "Actas e Trabalhos." Rio de Janeiro: Primeiro Congresso Brasileiro de Eugenia, 1929.

Primeiro Congresso Brasileiro de Protecção á Infancia. Theses oficiaes, memorias e conclusões. Rio de Janeiro: Empresa Gráfica Editora Paulo Pongetti, 1925.

Priore, Mary del. Ao sul do corpo: Condição feminina, maternidades e mentalidades no Brasil colonial. Rio de Janeiro: José Olympio, Editora Universidade de Brasília, 1993.

Progianti, Jane Márcia. "Modelos de assistência ao parto e a participação feminina." Revista Brasileira de Enfermagem 57, no. 3 (2004): 303–305.

Raeders, Georges. O conde de Gobineau no Brasil: Documentação inédita. São Paulo: Secretaria da Cultura, Ciência e Tecnologia, 1976.

———. O inimigo cordial do Brasil: O conde de Gobineau no Brasil. Rio de Janeiro: Paz e Terra, 1998.

Reis, Isabel Cristina Ferreira dos. Histórias de vida familiar e afetiva de escravos na Bahia do século XIX. Salvador: Centro de Estudos Baianos UFBA, 2001.

Reis, João José. Death Is a Festival: Funeral Rites and Rebellion in Nineteenth-Century Brazil. Chapel Hill: University of North Carolina Press, 2003.

———. Domingos Sodré, um sacerdote africano: Escravidão, liberdade e candomblé na Bahia do século XIX. São Paulo: Companhia das Letras, 2008.

———. "Presença negra: Conflitos e encontros." In Brasil: 500 anos de povoamento, ed. Instituto Brasileiro da Geografia e Estatística, 80–99. Rio de Janeiro: Instituto Brasileiro de Geografia e Estatística, 2000.

———. Slave Rebellion in Brazil: The Muslim Uprising of 1835 in Bahia. Baltimore: Johns Hopkins University Press, 1993.

Reis, José Roberto Franco. "'De pequenino é que se torce o pepino': A infância nos programas eugénicos da Liga Brasileira de Hygiene Mental." História, Ciências, Saúde—Manguinhos 7, no. 1 (2000): 135–157.

Riesco, Maria Luiza Gonzalez, and Maria Alica Tsunechiro. "Formação profissional de obstetrizes e enfermeiras obstétricas: Velhos problemas ou novas possibilidades?" *Estudos Feministas* 10, no. 2 (2002): 449–459.

Rizzini, Irene. *A assistência à infância no Brasil: Uma análise de sua construção.* Rio de Janeiro: Editora Universidade Santa Úrsula, 1993.

———. "The Child-Saving Movement in Brazil: Ideology in the Late Nineteenth and Early Twentieth Centuries." In *Minor Omissions: Children in Latin American History and Society,* ed. Tobias Hecht, 165–180. Madison: University of Wisconsin Press, 2002.

Rocha, Álvaro da Franca. "Nati-mortalidade na cidade do Salvador, Bahia, no decennio de 1923–1932." *Pediatria e Puericultura* 3, no. 2 (1933): 229–252.

Rodrigues, Andréa da Rocha. *A infância esquecida: Salvador 1900–1940.* Salvador: Universidade Federal da Bahia, 2003.

Rodrigues, Nina. "Anthropologia pathologica—os mestiços brasileiros." *Gazeta Médica da Bahia* 21, no. 9 and no. 11 (1890): 401–407, 497–502.

———. "Mestiçagem, degenerescência e crime." Originally published 1899; reprinted in *Historia, Ciências, Saúde—Manguinhos* 15, no. 4 (December 2008): 1151–1180.

Rohden, Fabíola. *A arte de enganar a natureza: Contracepção, aborto e infanticídio no início do século XX.* Rio de Janeiro: Editora Fiocruz, 2003.

———. *Uma ciência da diferença: Sexo e gênero na medicina da mulher.* Rio de Janeiro: Editora Fiocruz, 2001.

Romo, Anadelia A. *Brazil's Living Museum: Race, Reform, and Tradition in Bahia.* Chapel Hill: University of North Carolina Press, 2010.

Roncador, Sônia. *Domestic Servants in Literature and Testimony in Brazil, 1889–1999.* New York: Palgrave Macmillan, 2013.

Russell-Wood, A. J. R. *Fidalgos and Philanthropists: The Santa Casa da Misericórdia of Bahia, 1550–1755.* Berkeley: University of California Press, 1968.

Santos, Sonia Beatriz dos. "Brazilian Black Women's NGOs and Their Struggles in the Area of Sexual and Reproductive Health: Experiences, Resistance, and Politics." PhD diss., University of Texas at Austin, 2008.

Santos, Luis A. de Castro. "As origens da reforma sanitária e da modernização conservadora na Bahia durante a Primeira República." *Dados* 41, no. 3 (1998): 593–633.

———. "Power, Ideology and Public Health in Brazil, 1889–1930." PhD diss., Harvard University, 1987.

Santos, Martha S. *Cleansing Honor with Blood: Masculinity, Violence, and Power in the Backlands of Northeast Brazil, 1845–1889.* Stanford: Stanford University Press, 2012.

Santos Filho, Lycurgo de Castro. *História geral da medicina brasileira.* São Paulo: Hucitec, 1991.

Sardenberg, Cecilia Maria Bacellar, Iole Macedo Vanin, and Lina Maria Brandão de Aras, eds. *Fazendo gênero na historiografia baiana.* Salvador: FFCH/Universidade Federal da Bahia, 2001.

Scheper-Hughes, Nancy. *Death without Weeping: The Violence of Everyday Life in Brazil*. Berkeley: University of California Press, 1992.

Schneider, William H. "The Eugenics Movement in France, 1890–1940." In *The Wellborn Science*, ed. Mark B. Adams, 69–109. Oxford: Oxford University Press, 1990.

———. "Puericulture and the Style of French Eugenics." *History and Philosophy of the Life Sciences* 8, no. 2 (1986): 265–278.

Schwarcz, Lilia Moritz. *The Spectacle of the Races: Scientists, Institutions, and the Race Question in Brazil, 1870–1930*. New York: Hill and Wang, 1993.

Schwartzman, Simon. "A Igreja e o Estado Novo: O Estatuto da Família." *Cadernos de Pesquisa da Fundação Carlos Chagas* 37 (May 1981): 71–77.

Schwartzman, Simon, Helena Maria Bousquet Bomeny, and Vanda Maria Ribeiro Costa, eds. *Tempos de Capanema*. São Paulo: EDUSP, 1984.

Seigel, Micol. *Uneven Encounters: Making Race and Nation in Brazil and the United States*. Durham: Duke University Press, 2009.

Semley, Lorelle D. *Mother Is Gold, Father Is Glass: Gender and Colonialism in a Yoruba Town*. Bloomington: Indiana University Press, 2011.

Silva, Augusto da. "Resenha histórica da Liga Bahiana contra a Mortalidade Infantil ao transcurso de seus 40 anos de fundação." *Pediatria e Puericultura* (1963): 71–83.

Silva, Maria Lúcia. "Racismo institucional." In *Nascer com equidade: Humanização do parto e do nascimento, questões raciais/cor e de gênero*, ed. Suzana Kalckmann, Luís Eduardo Batista, Cláudia Medeiros de Castro, Tânia Di Giacomo do Lago, and Sandra Regina de Souza, 317–320. São Paulo: Instituto de Saúde, 2010.

Silva, Tânia Maria de Almeida and Luiz Otávio Ferreira. "A higienização das parteiras curiosas: O Serviço Especial de Saúde Pública e a assistência materno-infantil (1940–1960)." *História, Ciências, Saúde—Manguinhos* 18 (December 2011): 95–112.

Silveira, Éder. *A cura da raça: Eugenia e higienismo no discurso médico sul-rio-grandense nas primeiras décadas do século XX*. Passo Fundo, RS: Editora UPF, 2005.

Skidmore, Thomas. *Black into White: Race and Nationality in Brazilian Thought*. 2nd ed. Durham: Duke University Press, 1993.

Smith, Susan L. *Sick and Tired of Being Sick and Tired: Black Women's Health Activism in America, 1890–1950*. Philadelphia: University of Pennsylvania Press, 1995.

Sociedade de Medicina da Bahia. "A semana da criança realizada na Bahia, de 5 a 11 de Dezembro de 1927." Salvador: Imprensa Official do Estado da Bahia, 1928.

Sousa, Cynthia Pereira de. "A família na doutrina social da Igreja e na política social do Estado Novo." *Psicologia–USP* 3, no. 1/2 (1992): 45–57.

———. "Saúde, educação e trabalho de crianças e jovens: A política social de Getúlio Vargas." In *Capanema: O ministro e seu ministério*, ed. Angela de Castro Gomes, 221–249. Rio de Janeiro: Fundação Getúlio Vargas Editora, 2000.

Souza, Antônio Loureiro de. *Bahianos ilustres 1564–1925*. Salvador: N.p., 1973.

Souza, Christiane Maria Cruz de. *A gripe espanhola na Bahia: saúde, política e medicina em tempos de epidemia*. Rio de Janeiro: Editora Fiocruz, 2009.

Souza, Christiane Maria Cruz de, and Maria Renilda Nery Barreto, eds. *História da saúde na Bahia: Instituições e patrimônio arquitetônico (1808–1958)*. Rio de Janeiro: Fiocruz, 2011.

Souza, Christiane Maria Cruz de, and Gisele Sanglard. "Saúde pública e assistência na Bahia da Primeira República (1889–1929)." In *História da saúde na Bahia: Instituições e patrimônio arquitetônico (1808–1958)*, ed. Christiane Maria Cruz de Souza and Maria Renilda Nery Barreto, 53–55. Rio de Janeiro: Fiocruz, 2011.

Stepan, Nancy Leys. *The Beginnings of Brazilian Science: Oswaldo Cruz, Medical Research and Policy, 1890–1920*. New York: Science History Publications, 1976.

———. *"The Hour of Eugenics": Race, Gender, and Nation in Latin America*. Ithaca, NY: Cornell University Press, 1991.

———. "The National and the International in Public Health: Carlos Chagas and the Rockefeller Foundation in Brazil, 1917–1930s." *Hispanic American Historical Review* 91, no. 3 (2011): 469–502.

Stern, Alexandra. *Eugenic Nation: Faults and Frontiers of Better Breeding in Modern America*. Berkeley: University of California Press, 2005.

Terceiro Congresso Americano da Creança. *Tomo I: Antecedentes. Organização. Programmas. Delegações e adherentes. Sessões plenarias. Votos*. Rio de Janeiro: Imprensa Nacional, 1924.

———. *Tomo II: Trabalhos da 1ª Secção–Medicina*. Rio de Janeiro: Jornal do Commercio, 1924.

Tinhorão, José Ramos. *A música popular no romance brasileiro*. São Paulo: Editora 34, 2002.

Tomes, Nancy. "The Private Side of Public Health: Sanitary Science, Domestic Hygiene, and the Germ Theory, 1870–1900." *Bulletin of the History of Medicine* 64 (1990): 509–539.

Tornquist, Carmen Susana. "Armadilhas da nova era: Natureza e maternidade no ideário da humanização do parto." *Estudos Feministas* 10, no. 2 (2002): 483–492.

Torres, Iraildes Caldas. *As primeiras damas e a assistência social: Relações de gênero e poder*. São Paulo: Cortez Editora, 2002.

Turner, Sasha. "Home-Grown Slaves: Women, Reproduction, and the Abolition of the Slave Trade, Jamaica 1788–1807." *Journal of Women's History* 23, no. 3 (2011): 39–62.

Vargas, Getúlio. *A nova política do Brasil*. Rio de Janeiro: J. Olympio, 1938.

———. *O governo trabalhista do Brasil*. Rio de Janeiro: J. Olympio, 1952.

———. *"Wherever There Be any American Nation, There Should Be all the Nations of our Hemisphere": Excerpts from Manifests, Speeches, and Interviews Made by President Getúlio Vargas*. Rio de Janeiro: Departamento de Imprensa e Propaganda, 1942.

Venâncio, Renato Pinto. *Famílias abandonadas: Assistência à criança de camadas populares no Rio de Janeiro e em Salvador, séculos XVIII e XIX*. Campinas, SP: Papirus, 1999.

———. "Maternidade negada." In *História das mulheres no Brasil*, ed. Mary del Priore, 189–222. São Paulo: Editora UNESP, 1997.

Vianna, Francisco Vicente. *Memoir of the State of Bahia*. Translated by Guilherme Pereira Rebello. Salvador: Diário da Bahia, 1893.

Vianna, Hildegardes. *As aparadeiras e as sendeironas: Seu folklore*. Salvador: Universidade Federal da Bahia, 1988.

Vinhaes, Diogenes. "Assistencia obstétrica." *Annaes da Sociedade de Medicina da Bahia* 11, no. 1 (1935–1936): 76–96.

Viscardi, Cláudia Maria Ribeiro. "Pobreza e assistência no Rio de Janeiro na Primeira República." *História, Ciências, Saúde—Manguinhos* 18 (December 2011): 179–197.

Vital, André Vasques. "Comissão Rondon, doenças e política: 'Região do Madeira: Santo Antônio,' de Joaquim Augusto Tanajura—uma outra visão do Alto Madeira em 1911." *História, Ciências, Saúde—Manguinhos* 18, no. 2 (2011): 545–557.

Von Vacano, Diego A. *The Color of Citizenship: Race, Modernity and Latin American/Hispanic Political Thought.* New York: Oxford University Press, 2012.

Wadsworth, James E. "Moncorvo Filho e o problema da infância: Modelos institucionais e ideológicos da assistência à infância no Brasil." *Revista Brasileira de História* 19, no. 37 (1999): 103–124.

Wadsworth, James E., and Tamera L. Marko. "Children of the Pátria: Representations of Childhood and Welfare State Ideologies at the 1922 Rio de Janeiro International Centennial Exposition." *The Americas* 58, no. 1 (July 2001): 65–90.

Weinstein, Barbara. *For Social Peace in Brazil: Industrialists and the Remaking of the Working Class in São Paulo, 1920–1964.* Chapel Hill: University of North Carolina Press, 1996.

———. "Racializing Regional Difference: São Paulo versus Brazil, 1932." In *Race and Nation in Modern Latin America*, ed. Nancy P. Appelbaum, Anne S. Macpherson, and Karin Alejandra Rosemblatt, 237–262. Chapel Hill: University of North Carolina Press, 2003.

———. "Unskilled Worker, Skilled Housewife: Constructing the Working-Class Woman in São Paulo, Brazil." In *The Gendered Worlds of Latin American Women Workers: From Household and Factory to the Union Hall and Ballot Box*, ed. John D. French and Daniel James, 72–99. Durham: Duke University Press, 1997.

Williams, Daryl. *Culture Wars in Brazil: The First Vargas Regime, 1930–1945.* Durham: Duke University Press, 2001.

Williams, Steven C. "Nationalism and Public Health: The Convergence of Rockefeller Foundation Technique and Brazilian Federal Authority during the Time of Yellow Fever, 1925–1930." In *Missionaries of Science: The Rockefeller Foundation and Latin America*, ed. Marcos Cueto, 23–51. Bloomington: Indiana University Press, 1994.

Windler, Erica M. "City of Children: Boys, Girls, Family and the State in Imperial Rio de Janeiro, Brazil." PhD diss., University of Miami, 2003.

———. "Honor among Orphans: Girlhood, Virtue, and Nation at Rio de Janeiro's Recolhimento." *Journal of Social History* 44, no. 4 (July 2011): 1195–1215.

Wolfe, Joel. *Working Women, Working Men: São Paulo and the Rise of Brazil's Industrial Working Class, 1900–1955.* Durham: Duke University Press, 1993.

Wood, Marcus. *Black Milk: Imagining Slavery in the Visual Cultures of Brazil and America.* Oxford: Oxford University Press, 2013.

Zulawski, Ann. *Unequal Cures: Public Health and Political Change in Bolivia, 1900–1950.* Durham: Duke University Press, 2007.

Index

Page numbers in italics refer to illustrations.